Emerging Materials and Technologies in Drug Delivery

Emerging Materials and Technologies in Drug Delivery

Editor: Michael Mason

AMERICAN
MEDICAL PUBLISHERS
www.americanmedicalpublishers.com

AMERICAN
MEDICAL PUBLISHERS
www.americanmedicalpublishers.com

Cataloging-in-Publication Data

Emerging materials and technologies in drug delivery / edited by Michael Mason.
p. cm.
Includes bibliographical references and index.
ISBN 979-8-88740-070-9
1. Drug delivery systems. 2. Drugs--Administration. 3. Drugs--Dosage forms.
4. Pharmaceutical technology. 5. Biomedical engineering. 6. Pharmaceutical chemistry.
I. Mason, Michael.
RS199.5 .E44 2023
615.6--dc23

American Medical Publishers,
41 Flatbush Avenue,
1st Floor, New York,
NY 11217, USA

ISBN 979-8-88740-070-9 (Hardback)

Contents

Preface

Drug delivery refers to the process or method of providing a pharmaceutical substance to a human or animal for obtaining a therapeutic effect. Nanomaterials are frequently utilized in pharmaceuticals and medicine due to their unique optical, mechanical and electrical properties. They are also used for developing novel therapeutics, detecting biological molecules and imaging of sick tissues. Emerging technologies such as MEMS, 3DP and MF have been studied for the production of diagnostics or drug delivery systems. These technologies have the potential to fight pandemics by offering a preventive, predictive and personalized (3P) medical approach. New technologies allow for the creation of devices that are simpler to use, which can monitor or diagnose a condition quickly, as well as control the release of biologics or drug molecules. The topics covered in this extensive book deal with the emerging materials and technologies in drug delivery. It provides significant information to help develop a good understanding of the recent studies in this field. The readers would gain knowledge that would broaden their perspective in this area of pharmaceutical science.

Various studies have approached the subject by analyzing it with a single perspective, but the present book provides diverse methodologies and techniques to address this field. This book contains theories and applications needed for understanding the subject from different perspectives. The aim is to keep the readers informed about the progresses in the field; therefore, the contributions were carefully examined to compile novel researches by specialists from across the globe.

Indeed, the job of the editor is the most crucial and challenging in compiling all chapters into a single book. In the end, I would extend my sincere thanks to the chapter authors for their profound work. I am also thankful for the support provided by my family and colleagues during the compilation of this book.

Editor

1

Drug Release of Hybrid Materials Containing Fe(II)Citrate Synthesized by Sol-Gel Technique

Michelina Catauro [1,*], Elisabetta Tranquillo [1], Federico Barrino [1], Ignazio Blanco [2], Francesco Dal Poggetto [3] and Daniele Naviglio [4]

[1] Department of Engineering, University of Campania "Luigi Vanvitelli", via Roma 29, I-81031 Aversa, Italy; elisabetta.tranquillo@unicampania.it (E.T.); federicobarrino92@hotmail.it (F.B.)
[2] Department of Civil Engineering and Architecture and UdR-Catania Consorzio INSTM, University of Catania, Viale Andrea Doria 6, 95125 Catania, Italy; iblanco@unict.it
[3] Ecoricerche srl, via Principi Normanni 36, 81043 Capua Caserta, Italy; ecoricerchesrl@virgilio.it
[4] Department of Chemical Sciences, University of Naples Federico II, via Cintia, 80126 Naples, Italy; naviglio@unina.it
* Correspondence: michelina.catauro@unicampania.it

Abstract: The use of oral iron integration is commonly recommended for the treatment of iron deficiency, nevertheless the diagnosis and treatment of this disease could clearly be improved. The aim of this work was the synthesis of therapeutic systems, iron (II) based, by sol-gel method. In an SiO_2 matrix, we embedded different weight percentages of polyethylene glycol ($PEG_{6,\ 12,\ 24\ wt\%}$) and ferrous citrate ($Fe(II)C_{5,\ 10,\ 15\ wt\%}$) for drug delivery applications. Fourier Transform Infrared (FTIR) spectroscopy was used to study the interactions among different components in the hybrid materials. Release kinetics in a simulated body fluid (SBF) were investigated and the amount of Fe^{2+} released was detected by Ultraviolet–Visible spectroscopy (UV-VIS) after reaction with ortho-phenantroline. Furthermore, the biological characterization was carried out. The bioactivity of the synthesized hybrid materials was evaluated by the formation of a layer of hydroxyapatite on the surface of samples soaked in SBF using FTIR spectroscopy. Finally, also, the potential antibacterial properties of the different materials against two different bacteria, *E. coli* and *P. aeruginosa*, were investigated.

Keywords: sol-gel; ferrous citrate; FTIR analysis; drug release; antibacterial properties

1. Introduction

Iron is very important for many biological functions such as respiration, energy production, DNA synthesis, and cell proliferation [1]. Several ways have been observed by the human body to conserve iron; in fact, it is strongly regulated by different molecular mechanisms, avoiding its accumulation to a toxic level or its deficiency [2]. Iron deficiency is considered the main cause of anemia worldwide, [3] and it is a major health problem that is related to maternal and child mortality [4]. The use of oral iron supplementation for the treatment of iron deficiency is usually recommended, such as ferrous sulphate, anhydrous ferrous sulphate ferrous gluconate, and ferrous fumarate [4], nevertheless, the diagnosis and treatment of this disease could clearly be improved. In fact, although oral iron supplementation is the treatment of choice for the majority of patients because of its effectiveness and safety, oral iron supplementation has disadvantages, including poor compliance, high incidence of adverse gastrointestinal effects and high potential for interactions with other treatments [5,6]. In the last decade, the production of new biological systems able to release iron (II) in a controlled manner are an interesting alternative compared to systemic therapy.

Therefore, the aim of this work was the synthesis of iron (II)-based drug delivery systems, by sol-gel method. In an SiO_2 matrix were embedded different weight percentages of polyethylene glycol ($PEG_{6,\,12,\,24\,wt\%}$) and ferrous citrate ($Fe(II)C_{5,\,10,\,15\,wt\%}$) to obtain several hybrid materials. The advantages of the use of these materials as biomedical implants, for example as prosthesis or subcutaneous implants for local delivery in the systemic circulation of Fe^{2+}, are the continuous release of Fe^{2+}, without the need to remember to take the drug daily, also, it is possible always active coverage, because the molecule could dissolve slowly, giving a delayed effect over time. Furthermore, the use of drug delivery system optimizes the biopharmaceutical, pharmacokinetic and pharmacodynamics properties of a drug, reducing side-effects [6]

The sol-gel method is an interesting technique to prepare organic-inorganic hybrid materials which involves the hydrolysis reactions of the precursor leading to the formation of a colloidal suspension and its evolution in a gel by condensation process [7]. The main advantages of the sol-gel techniques for the preparation of hybrid materials are the low temperatures used during the synthesis and versatility [8]. Judenstein and Sanchez have proposed the classification of the hybrid materials which depends of the interactions between the components. In particular, in the Class I the organic and inorganic compounds are bond by hydrogen bonds, van der Waals, or ionic bonds; in the Class II, the two components are linked by strong chemical bonds (covalent or polar covalent bonds) [9].

In the literature, there are many works about the silica-based materials [10–12], that describe the high biological properties, the cell-material interactions and cell invasion due to their reaction products [10]. The biocompatibility of silica materials has been improved with the addition of polyethylene glycol (PEG), because the presence of the polymer improving cell adhesion and growth for the high hydrophilicity of the materials [13–15]. PEG is used in several biomedical applications such as drug delivery thanks to his versatility and biocompatibility [16]. Moreover, the addition of PEG in the hybrids improve the reduction of toxicity and the extension of the circulation time of many drug nanocarriers [17–19].

Furthermore, in silica/PEG materials has been added ferrous citrate (Fe(II)C), prepared by the redox reaction between iron powder and citric acid, to evaluate the Fe^{2+} release from different materials and, thus, the use of hybrids as systems for controlled iron release.

Fourier Transform Infrared (FTIR) spectroscopy was used to study the interactions among different components in the hybrid materials. Release kinetics in a simulated body fluid (SBF) were investigated and the amount of Fe^{2+} released was detected by UV–VIS spectroscopy after reaction with ortho-phenantroline. In addition, the biological characterization was carried out. The bioactivity of the different hybrids was evaluated by observing the typical peaks of hydroxyapatite on the surface of materials, soaked in SBF, using FTIR spectroscopy. Finally, also, the potential antibacterial properties of the different materials against two different bacteria, *E. coli* and *P. aeruginosa*, were investigated.

2. Materials and Methods

2.1. Ferrous Citrate Preparation

A total of 25 g Citric acid monohydrate (>99.5%, Fluka, Munich, Germany) were completely dissolved in 500 mL of ultrapure water to which 6.0 g of iron powder (>99%, Sigma-Aldrich, St. Louis, MO, USA) were added. The solution was boiled and stirred under magnetic stirring (Sigma-Aldrich, St. Louis, MO, USA) until all iron powder disappeared and consequently appeared the ferrous citrate complex (Fe(II)C). Then the mixture was cooled at room temperature and the precipitate grey/pearly complex was filtered under vacuum with a paper filter and washed with water; finally, the obtained solid was freeze dried.

2.2. Sol-Gel Synthesis of the Hybrid Materials

The hybrid materials with different percentages of polyethylene glycol (PEG, MW = 400, Sigma-Aldrich, St. Louis, MO, USA) and Fe(II)C were synthesized by sol-gel method. Tetraethyl orthosilicate (TEOS; $Si(OC_2H_5)_4$; Sigma-Aldrich, St. Louis, MO, USA) was used as precursor of silica matrix and it was added in a solution of 99.8% ethanol (EtOH, Sigma-Aldrich, St. Louis, MO, USA) and distilled water. In this study the molar ratios of solution were equal to H_2O/TEOS = 26.6 and EtOH/TEOS = 6.

Afterwards, different amount of $PEG_{(6,\ 12,\ 24\ wt\%)}$ and $Fe(II)C_{(5,\ 10,\ 15\ wt\%)}$ were solubilized in 99.8% ethanol and distilled water under stirring at 38 °C, respectively. Afterwards to the gelation process, the residual solvent was removed from the wet gels in an oven at 50 °C for 24 h. The Figure 1 shows the flow chart of the hybrid synthesis.

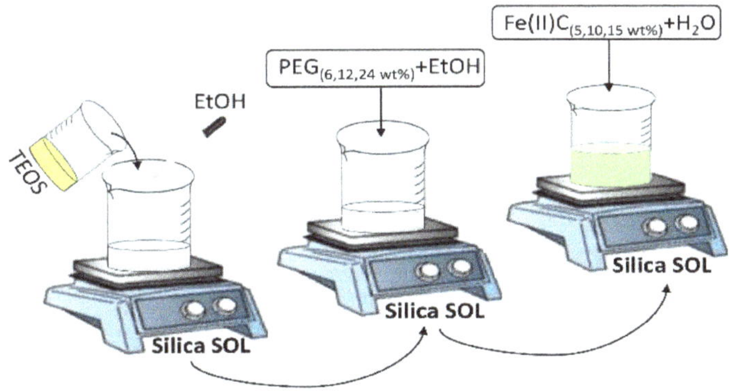

Figure 1. Flow chart of sol-gel synthesis.

2.3. *Fourier Transform Infrared (FTIR) Analysis of the Hybrid Materials*

A Prestige 21 Shimadzu (Kyoto, Japan) FTIR instrument equipped with a DTGS detector was used to study the interactions between the different components. In the 400–4000 cm^{-1} region, with resolution of 4 cm^{-1} (45 scans) were recorded the spectra of the materials by Fourier transform infrared (FTIR) transmittance. KBr pelletized disks containing 2 mg of each sample and 198 mg of KBr were made. The FTIR spectra were processed by Prestige software (IR solution, software version 1.50, Shimadzu, Kyoto, Japan)

2.4. *Study of In Vitro Release*

The hybrid materials were crushed to a powder using an agate mortar (Sigma-Aldrich, St. Louis, MO, USA) and were soaked in 10 mL of simulated body fluid (SBF) solution under continuous magnetic stirring at 150 rpm.

The study of in vitro release is used to evaluated the amount of Fe^{2+} released from the materials in function of the percentages of Fe(II)C in the hybrids.

In particular, the release of Fe^{2+} from different materials was assessed at different exposure time using normative reference APAT IRSA CNR Man. 29/2003 Metodo 3160/A. In this regard, 1mL of SBF solution with the powder was added to a solution of water, hydroxylamine hydrochloride 10%, 1,10-phenanthroline 0.1%, Acetate Sodium 10%.

Release measurements were taken by means of a Shimadzu UV-1700 Double Beam Scanning UV-VIS Spectrophotometer (Kyoto, Japan). Absorbance values were taken at a wavelength λ = 520.0 nm, corresponding to the absorbance of Fe^{2+}. The release experiments were repeated three times on each hybrid. Data are presented as means ± standard deviation for a representative experiment.

The calibration curve was determined by taking absorbance versus concentration between 0 and 4.99 mg/L as parameters. For this interval, the calibration curve fits the Lambert and Beers' law [20]

$$A = \varepsilon\, l\, C = 1.265\ C, \quad (1)$$

where A is absorbance, ε is molar absorptivity coefficient, l is path length and C is concentration (mg/L).

2.5. Bioactivity Test

The simulated body fluid (SBF) solution was used for 7, 14, 21 days at 37 °C to study the hybrids' bioactivity [21]. The materials powders were obtained using a mortar. The FTIR and XRD analysis were used to evaluate the apatite formation. XRD analysis was carried out using a Philips 139 diffractometer (Amsterdam, The Netherlands) equipped with a PW 1830 generator, tungsten lamp and Cu anode, where the source 140 of X-ray is given by a Cu-Kα radiation (λ = 0.15418 nm). The nucleation of biominerals on the samples could allow the depletion of the ionic species in the SBF, to overcome this problem the solution was replaced every 2 days. The ratio between the total exposed surface and the volume solution was chosen in agreement with the literature. After the exposure, the samples powders were dried in a glass desiccator (Sigma-Aldrich, St. Louis, MO, USA), and then subjected to FTIR analysis."

2.6. Antibacterial Activity

In order to study the effect of the samples on the microbial growth, *E. coli* (ATCC 25922) and *P. aeruginosa* (ATCC 10145) were used. *E. coli* was cultured in TBX Medium (Tryptone Bile X-Gluc) (Liofilchem, Roseto degli Abruzzi, Italy), while *P. aeruginosa* in Pseudomonas CN Agar (Liofilchem, Roseto degli Abruzzi, Italy).

Afterwards, the bacterial cultures were diluted in distilled water to produce a bacterial cell suspension of 10×10^5 CFU/mL. Both bacteria were inoculated in absence and in presence of the hybrid materials. *E. coli* was incubated with the materials for 24 h at 44 °C, while the *P. aeruginosa* for 48 h at 36 °C. The microbial growth was evaluated by observing the diameter of the inhibition halo (ID). The obtained values are the mean standard (SD) deviation of measurements carried out on samples analyzed three times.

3. Results

3.1. FTIR Analysis

FTIR analysis is considered as an appropriate method to study the interactions in the hybrid materials. The typical bands of silica matrix and polymer are visible in the hybrids' spectra which are shown in the Figure 2 (curve b–d). The asymmetric and symmetric Si–O–Si stretching, and bending vibrations of the silica are attributed to the band at 1080 cm^{-1} with a shoulder at 1200 cm^{-1} and the peaks at 800 cm^{-1} and 460 cm^{-1}, respectively [22,23]. Furthermore, in the hybrid spectra, it is possible to observe a slight shift toward lower wavenumbers of the Si–OH bond vibrations and O–H stretching compared to pure SiO_2 (curve e) from 960 to 955 cm^{-1} and from 3450 to 3440 cm^{-1} [24,25], suggesting that an interaction between silica matrix, PEG and Fe(II)C occurred.

These interactions can be confirmed, also, by the shift of wavenumbers of some polymer peaks, in the hybrids' spectra, the PEG methylene C–H asymmetric stretching at 2927 cm^{-1} and the band of CH_2 group at 1382 cm^{-1} are observed, while, the same peaks, in the pure PEG spectra (curve a) at 2870 and 1350 cm^{-1} are recorded [26].

The presence of Fe(II)C is confirmed comparing the hybrid spectra with those of the pure Fe(II)C. When the different amounts of Fe(II)C are added in the SiO_2/PEG/Fe(II)C some bands related to citrate are detectable with several intensity. In particular, the peaks at 1734 and 1430 cm^{-1} due to the C=O stretching and COO^- group, respectively, are visible as shoulder in the hybrid spectra (curve b–d) compared to pure Fe(II)C spectra (curve f) [27,28].

Therefore, the formation of hydrogen bonds between the –OH groups of the silica matrix and ethereal oxygen atoms (H-bond donors) or terminal –OH in the polymer chains [25,29], and, also, the interaction with Fe(II)C were suggested by the different shape and position of the silica bands.

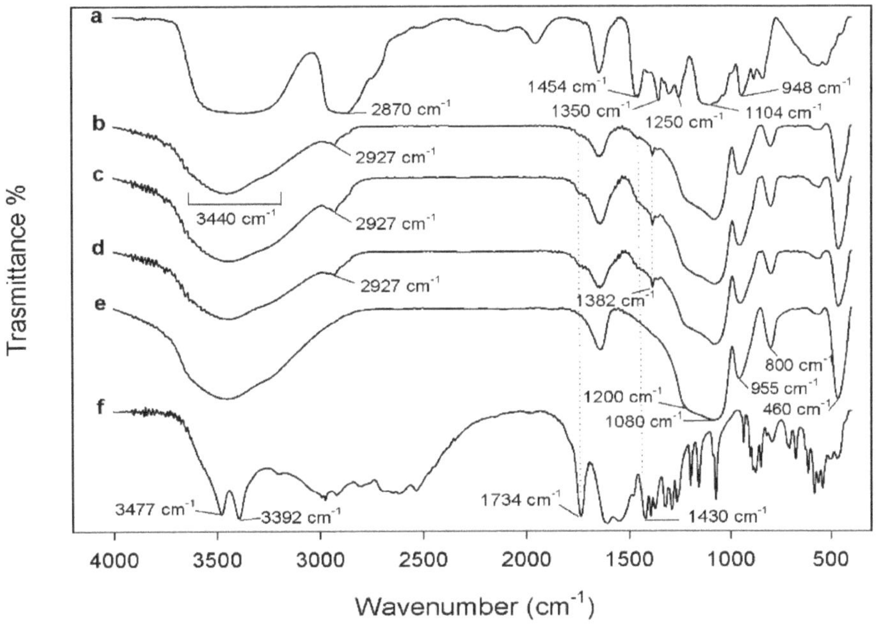

Figure 2. Representative FTIR spectra of (**a**) pure PEG; (**b**) $SiO_2/PEG_{12\ wt\%}/Fe(II)C_{5\ wt\%}$; (**c**)$SiO_2/PEG_{12\ wt\%}/Fe(II)C_{10\ wt\%}$; (**d**) $SiO_2/PEG_{12\ wt\%}/Fe(II)C_{15\ wt\%}$; (**e**) pure SiO_2; (**f**) pure Fe(II)C.

3.2. *Study of In Vitro Release*

Controlled Fe^{2+} release from hybrid materials is an interesting alternative to systemic therapy. The study of drug release is required to understand treatment continuity and its efficacy. The release was assayed by measuring the UV absorbance at λ = 520.0 nm related to the concentration of the solution. The calibration curve was drawn for a standard solution with different concentrations from 0 to 4.99 mg/L (Figure 3).

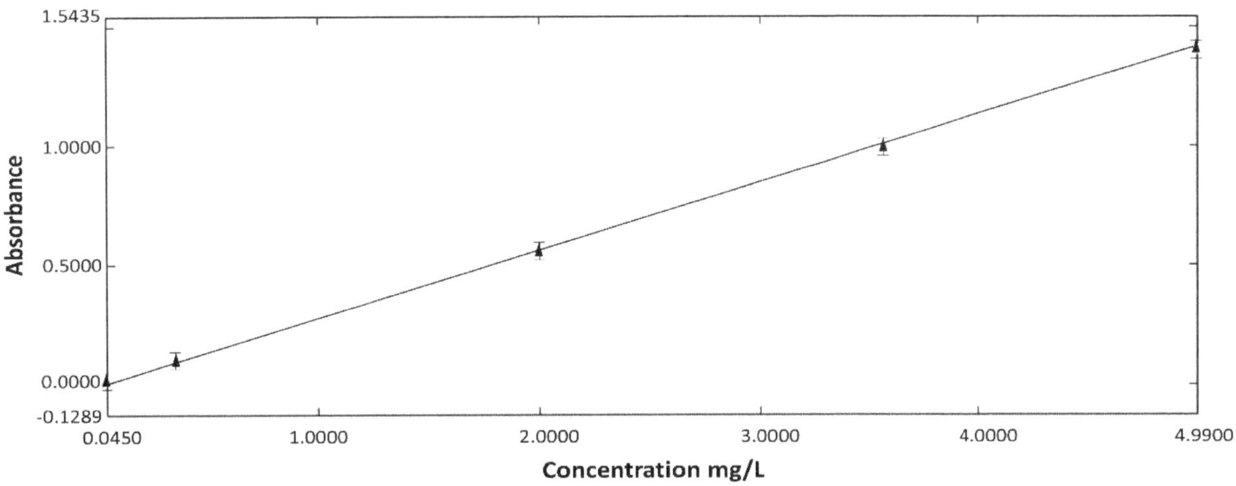

Figure 3. Calibration curve (520.0 nm) based on the concentration of Fe^{2+} (r^2 = 0.9973).

The several amount of the polymer in $SiO_2/Fe(II)C$ hybrids modulates the drug release differently. Comparing the different release plots (Figure 4A–C), it is possible to observed that the release of Fe^{2+} is completed within 8 h without any evident difference in the time of release. Initially, the drug release is due to dissolution and diffusion of the Fe^{2+} incorporated near the surface of the samples, afterwards, the release depends on the different type of interaction between Fe(II)C and PEG and silica.

A similar behavior was observed in the $SiO_2/PEG_{(6,\ 12,\ 24\ wt\%)}/Fe(II)C_{(5\ wt\%)}$ hybrids (Figure 4A–C), despite the different amounts of polymer. Probably, the release of Fe^{2+} do not depend of polymer concentration but it might be due to a low percentage of Fe(II)C in the hybrid that allows many interactions with silica-PEG matrix, reducing the release of Fe^{2+}.

In the release plots (Figure 4A–C) of $SiO_2/PEG_{(6, 12, 24\ wt\%)}/Fe(II)C_{(10\ wt\%)}$ and $SiO_2/PEG_{(6, 12, 24\ wt\%)}/Fe(II)C_{(15\ wt\%)}$ the presence of the different percentages of polymer modified the Fe^{2+} release curves, unlike the hybrids with $Fe(II)C_{(5\ wt\%)}$. The PEG amount equal to 24 wt% (Figure 4C) determines a greater release of the Fe^{2+} compared to another one, probably due to the formation of the silica/PEG network. In particular, when the content of PEG and Fe(II)C is higher in the hybrids, a part of it cannot form H-bonds because all hydroxyl groups of silica are already involved in H-bonds. Probably, the formation of few weak bonds between Fe(II) and silica-PEG matrix allow the greater release of Fe^{2+} [30–32].

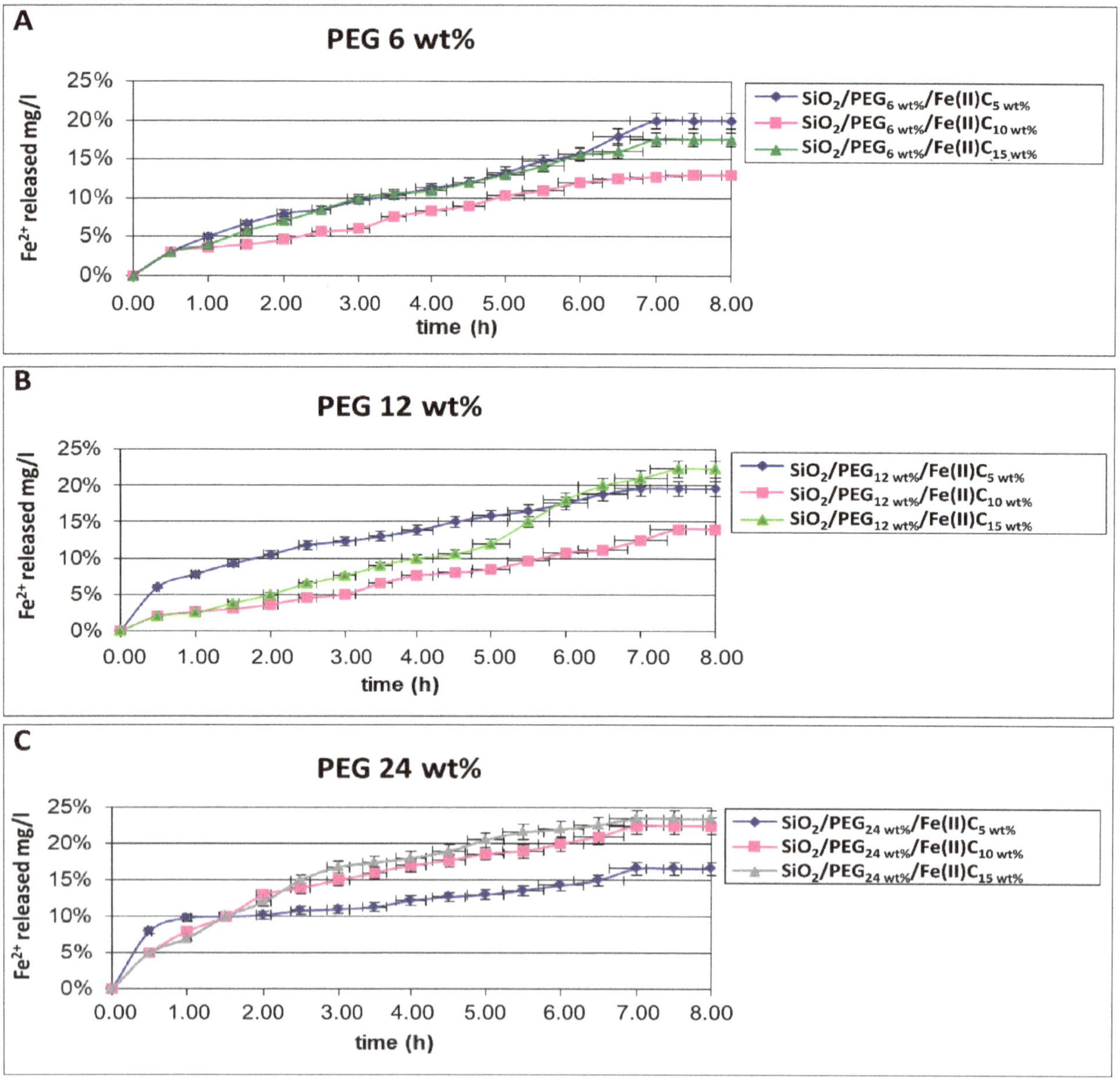

Figure 4. Time-dependent drug release plot for (**A**) $SiO_2/PEG_{6\ wt\%}/Fe(II)C_{5\ wt\%}$; $SiO_2/PEG_{6\ wt\%}/Fe(II)C_{15\ wt\%}$; $SiO_2/PEG_{6\ wt\%}/Fe(II)C_{20\ wt\%}$; (**B**) $SiO_2/PEG_{12\ wt\%}/Fe(II)C_{5\ wt\%}$; $SiO_2/PEG_{12\ wt\%}/Fe(II)C_{10\ wt\%}$; $SiO_2/PEG_{12\ wt\%}/Fe(II)C_{15\ wt\%}$; (**C**) $SiO_2/PEG_{24\ wt\%}/Fe(II)C_{5\ wt\%}$; $SiO_2/PEG_{24\ wt\%}/Fe(II)C_{10\ wt\%}$; $SiO_2/PEG_{24\ wt\%}/Fe(II)C_{15\ wt\%}$. Data are presented as means ± SD for a representative experiment.

3.3. Bioactivity Test

The bioactive materials are able to form an apatite layer on their surfaces in the living body, allowing the bond to living bone. The presence of various functional groups on materials surface induce the hydroxyapatite formation. In this regard, the hybrids were soaked in SBF for 7, 14 and 21 days to evaluate their bioactivity [21]. In particular, the interaction of Si–OH groups on the hybrids' surface with the Ca^{2+} ions present in the fluid allow to the hydroxyapatite nucleation and leading to an increase of positive surface charge. The formation of amorphous phosphate is induced by the combination of the Ca^{2+} ions and negative charges of the phosphate ions, which spontaneously transforms into hydroxyapatite $[Ca_{10}(PO_4)_6(OH)_2]$ [33]. The FTIR was used to identify the typical peaks of hydroxyapatite layer on materials surface (Figure 5). All hybrid materials showed the same results independently of PEG and Fe(II)C content. The displacement of Si–OH band, from 960 to 970 cm^{-1} suggested the interaction of the hydroxyapatite layer with the –OH groups of the silica matrix. Furthermore, comparing the hybrid materials spectra (Figure 5 curve) after 21 days in SBF with those of the same materials not soaked in SBF (Figure 5 curve a), the split of the band at 580 cm^{-1} in two new ones at 575 and 560 cm^{-1}, was visible. The presence of these new bands is caused by the formation of the hydroxyapatite precipitate, in particular, and are due to the stretching of the hydroxyl groups of hydroxyapatite and the vibrations of the PO_4^{3-} groups [34,35]. Moreover, the peak related to citrate at 1430 cm^{-1} attributed to COO^- group, undergoes change in the intensity that might be due to the interaction with the hydroxyapatite layer.

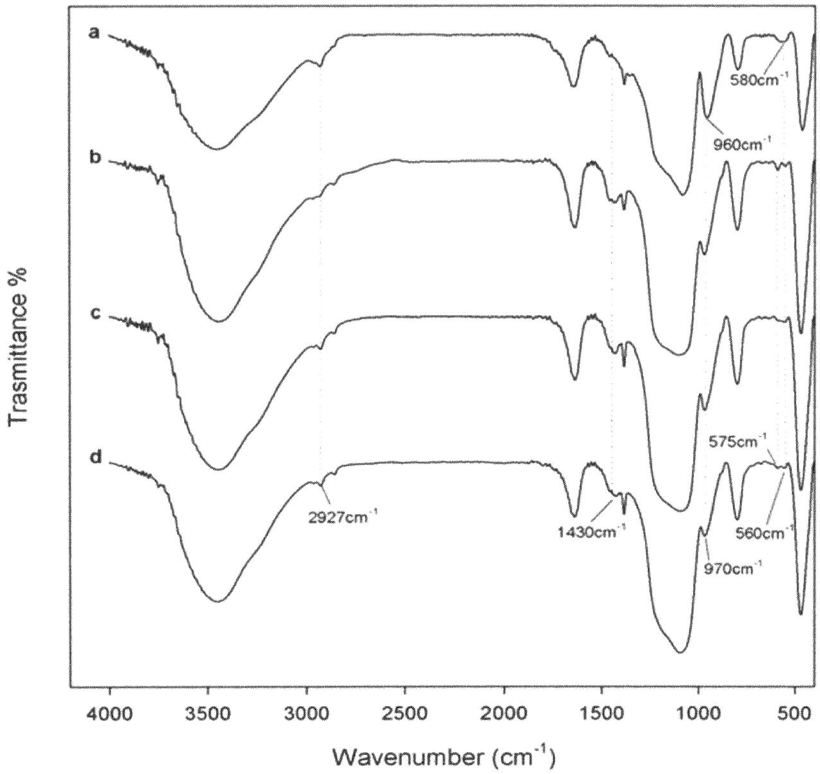

Figure 5. Representative FTIR spectra of (**a**) $SiO_2/PEG_{12\ wt\%}/Fe(II)C_{5\ wt\%}$ not soaked in SBF; (**b**) $SiO_2/PEG_{12\ wt\%}/Fe(II)C_{5\ wt\%}$; (**c**) $SiO_2/PEG_{12\ wt\%}/Fe(II)C_{10\ wt\%}$; (**d**) $SiO_2/PEG_{12\ wt\%}/Fe(II)C_{15\ wt\%}$; after 21 days of exposure to SBF.

Furthermore, XRD measurement was used to identify the presence of hydroxyapatite on the hybrids' surface. The intense peaks of hydroxyapatite crystalline are visible in Figure 6(●), confirming that the materials surface is covered by hydroxyapatite layer after 21 days in SBF. Moreover, this result suggest that the hydroxyapatite layer is very thick to detect XRD signals from hybrids' surface [21,36].

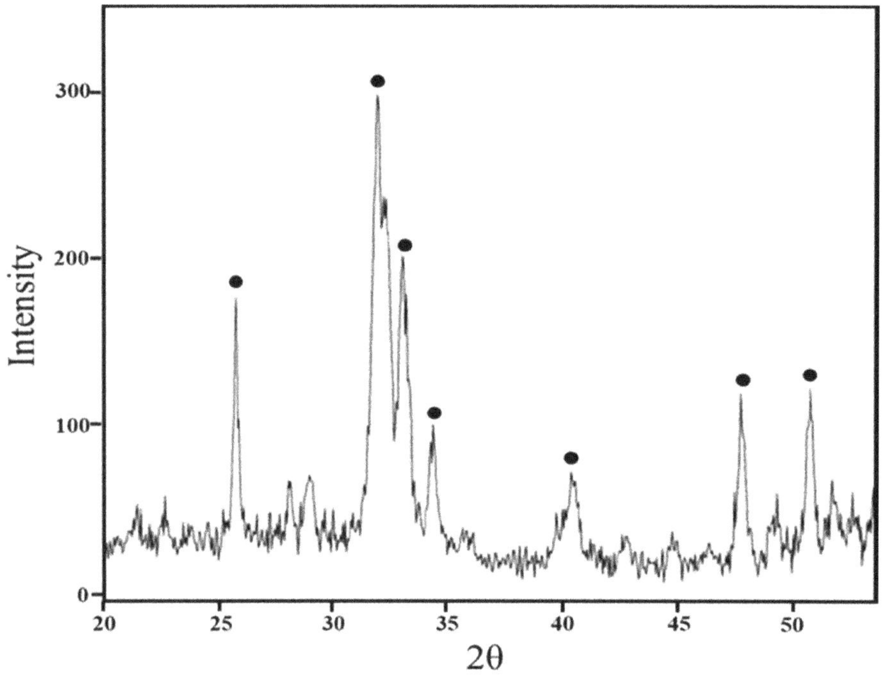

Figure 6. A representative XRD of $SiO_2/PEG_{12\ wt\%}/Fe(II)C_{15\ wt\%}$ soaked in SBF solution for 21 days.

3.4. Antibacterial Activity

In order to evaluate the effect of the hybrids on the microbial growth, *E. coli* and *P. aeruginosa* were used. The different materials were grinded in a mortar to obtain powders. Both bacteria were inoculated in absence and in presence of the 100 mg of hybrids' powders. The zones of inhibition formed by the materials without Fe(II)C and containing different amount of Fe(II)C against *E. coli* are shown in Figure 7A. It is possible to observed that the materials exhibited mild activity against *E. coli*, only the $SiO_2/PEG_{6\ wt\%}/Fe(II)C_{15\ wt\%}$ hybrid induces the inhibition halo around the synthesized hybrid Figure 7C. These results suggest that the microbial growth was inhibited by higher amount of Fe(II)C and by low percentage of PEG. When the *P. aeruginosa* was inoculated in presence of all the hybrids, the inhibition halo was more visible (Figure 7B). In particular, the diameter of zone of inhibition (Figure 7C) increases with 10 and 15 wt% of Fe(II)C, independently of the polymer content. Furthermore, the pigmentation reddish brown of *P. aeruginosa* inoculated with the hybrids containing Fe(II)C is observed (Figure 7B). In literature is reported that *P. aeruginosa* is able to produce a range of pigments under certain growth conditions [37–39]. Probably, the pigmentation reddish brown it is due to the production of pyomelanin which is involved in iron reduction and acquisition [40], resistance to oxidative stress [41] and virulence [38]. The pyomelanin could be produced by the release of Fe^{2+} from hybrids as this phenomenon is not observed with materials without Fe(II)C. Finally, in the Figure 7C are reported the inhibition zones of *E. coli* and *P. aeruginosa*. Comparing the diameter of the inhibition zones of the different hybrids, the better antibacterial activity against *P. aeruginosa* was observed.

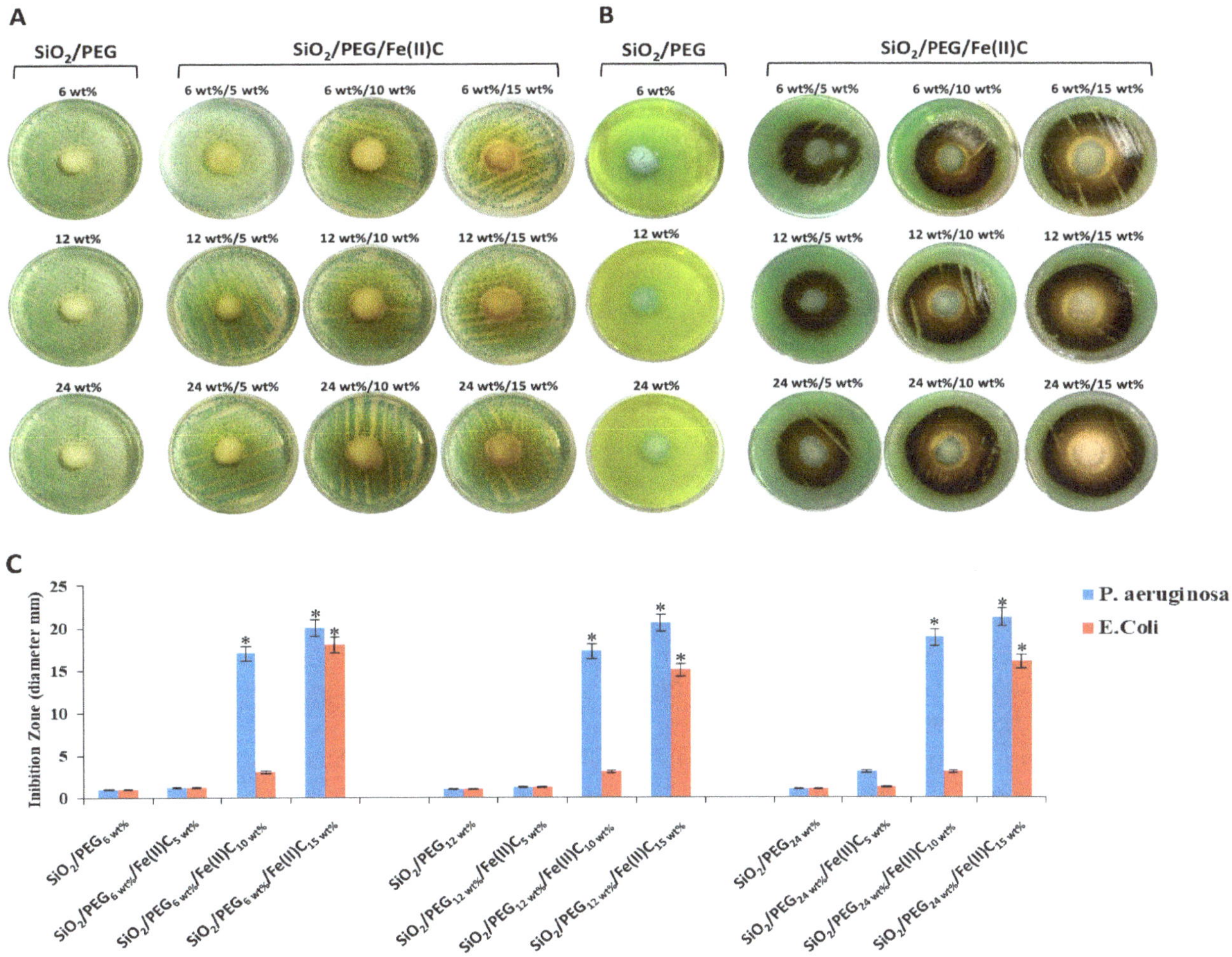

Figure 7. (**A**) Inhibition halo (ID) of *E. coli* with all materials; (**B**) Inhibition halo (ID) of *P. aeruginosa* with all materials; (**C**) Comparison of inhibition zone of *E. coli* and *P. aeruginosa* for all materials. Values are the mean SD of measurements carried out on samples analyzed three times. The means and S.D. are shown. *, $p < 0.05$ vs the bacteria control treated with hybrids without Fe(II)C or vs the bacteria treated with hybrids containing Fe(II)C.

4. Conclusions

In the present study, the different percentage of Fe(II)C and PEG were added in the silica matrix by sol-gel method. FTIR spectra of the obtained hybrids, show all bands of citrate, and also, the typical peaks of polymer and silica. Therefore, the different shape and position of some bands confirm the formation of H-bonds between the inorganic matrix, the PEG chains and, also, the interaction with Fe(II)C. The release of Fe^{2+} from hybrids was studied. Comparing all materials, those containing 24 wt% of PEG determine a greater release of the Fe^{2+}. This result might be due to the high content of PEG and Fe(II)C, that doesn't allow a part of it to form H-bonds because all hydroxyl groups of silica are already involved in weak bonds. Furthermore, the FTIR analysis after 21 days in SBF has suggest that the hybrids are bioactive, and the presence of Fe(II)C or polymer does not affect the bioactivity of silica matrix. Finally, *E. coli* and *P. aeruginosa* were inoculated with the different hybrid materials to evaluate their antibacterial activity. The materials exhibited mild activity against *E. coli* compared to *P. aeruginosa*. In particular the diameter of zone of inhibition of *P. aeruginosa* increases with 10 and 15 wt% of Fe(II)C, independently of polymer content. In conclusion the obtained hybrid materials could be used as biomedical implants to release different controlled amount of Fe^{2+} in the systemic circulation, without going through the gastrointestinal track, in order to allow active coverage. Obviously, these hybrid materials will be investigated further to confirm and extend the obtained results.

Author Contributions: Validation, M.C. and F.D.P.; Formal Analysis, E.T. and F.B.; Data Curation, I.B. and D.N.; Writing-Review & Editing, M.C. and I.B.; Supervision, M.C. and F.D.P. All authors have read and approved.

References

1. Hentze, M.W.; Muckenthaler, M.U.; Galy, B.; Camaschella, C. Two to tango: Regulation of mammalian iron metabolism. *Cell* **2010**, *142*, 24–38. [CrossRef] [PubMed]
2. Camaschella, C. Iron-deficiency anemia. *N. Engl. J. Med.* **2015**, *372*, 1832–1843. [CrossRef] [PubMed]
3. McLean, E.; Cogswell, M.; Egli, I.; Wojdyla, D.; De Benoist, B. Worldwide prevalence of anaemia, WHO vitamin and mineral nutrition information system, 1993–2005. *Public Health Nutr.* **2009**, *12*, 444–454. [CrossRef] [PubMed]
4. Lopez, A.; Cacoub, P.; Macdougall, I.C.; Peyrin-Biroulet, L. Iron deficiency anaemia. *Lancet* **2016**, *387*, 907–916. [CrossRef]
5. Pundir, S.; Badola, A.; Sharma, D. Sustained release matrix technology and recent advance in matrix drug delivery system: A review. *Int. J. Drug Deliv. Res. Technol.* **2017**, *3*, 8.
6. Fragoulakis, V.; Kourlaba, G.; Goumenos, D.; Konstantoulakis, M.; Maniadakis, N. Economic evaluation of intravenous iron treatments in the management of anemia patients in Greece. *ClinicoEconomics Outcomes Res.* **2012**, *4*, 127–134. [CrossRef]
7. Brinker, C.; Scherer, G. *Sol-Gel Science: The Physics and Chemistry of Sol-Gel Processing*; Academic Press: San Diego, CA, USA, 1989.
8. Amiri, S.; Rahimi, A. Hybrid nanocomposite coating by sol–gel method: A review. *Iran. Polym. J.* **2016**, *25*, 559–577. [CrossRef]
9. Judeinstein, P.; Sanchez, C. Hybrid organic–inorganic materials: A land of multidisciplinarity. *J. Mater. Chem.* **1996**, *6*, 511–525. [CrossRef]
10. Owens, G.J.; Singh, R.K.; Foroutan, F.; Alqaysi, M.; Han, C.-M.; Mahapatra, C.; Kim, H.-W.; Knowles, J.C. Sol–gel based materials for biomedical applications. *Prog. Mater. Sci.* **2016**, *77*, 1–79. [CrossRef]
11. Catauro, M.; Bollino, F.; Renella, R.A.; Papale, F. Sol-gel synthesis of SiO_2-CaO-P_2O_5 glasses: Influence of the heat treatment on their bioactivity and biocompatibility. *Ceram. Int.* **2015**, *41*, 12578–12588. [CrossRef]
12. Blanco, I. Polysiloxanes in theranostics and drug delivery: A review. *Polymers* **2018**, *10*, 755. [CrossRef]
13. Kim, G.; Hong, L.Y.; Jung, J.; Kim, D.-P.; Kim, H.; Kim, I.J.; Kim, J.R.; Ree, M. The biocompatability of mesoporous inorganic–organic hybrid resin films with ionic and hydrophilic characteristics. *Biomaterials* **2010**, *31*, 2517–2525. [CrossRef] [PubMed]
14. Nguyen, K.; Garcia, A.; Sani, M.A.; Diaz, D.; Dubey, V.; Clayton, D.; Dal Poggetto, G.; Cornelius, F.; Payne, R.J.; Separovic, F.; et al. Interaction of N-terminal peptide analogues of the Na+,K+-ATPase with membranes. *Biochim. Biophys. Acta* **2018**, *1860*, 1282–1291. [CrossRef] [PubMed]
15. Catauro, M.; Tranquillo, E.; Salzillo, A.; Capasso, L.; Illiano, M.; Sapio, L.; Naviglio, S. Silica/Polyethylene Glycol Hybrid Materials Prepared by a Sol-Gel Method and Containing Chlorogenic Acid. *Molecules* **2018**, *23*, 2447. [CrossRef] [PubMed]
16. Moghimi, S.M.; Szebeni, J. Stealth liposomes and long circulating nanoparticles: Critical issues in pharmacokinetics, opsonization and protein-binding properties. *Prog. Lipid Res.* **2003**, *42*, 463–478. [CrossRef]
17. Salama, A.; El-Sakhawy, M. Preparation of polyelectrolyte/calcium phosphate hybrids for drug delivery application. *Carbohydr. Polym.* **2014**, *113*, 500–506. [CrossRef] [PubMed]
18. Son, K.D.; Kim, Y.-J. Anticancer activity of drug-loaded calcium phosphate nanocomposites against human osteosarcoma. *Biomater. Res.* **2017**, *21*, 13. [CrossRef] [PubMed]
19. Zhou, Z.-F.; Sun, T.-W.; Chen, F.; Zuo, D.-Q.; Wang, H.-S.; Hua, Y.-Q.; Cai, Z.-D.; Tan, J. Calcium phosphate-phosphorylated adenosine hybrid microspheres for anti-osteosarcoma drug delivery and osteogenic differentiation. *Biomaterials* **2017**, *121*, 1–14. [CrossRef] [PubMed]
20. Thomas, M. *The Lambert-Beer Law*; Wiley: New York, NY, USA, 1996.
21. Kokubo, T.; Takadama, H. How useful is SBF in predicting in vivo bone bioactivity? *Biomaterials* **2006**, *27*, 2907–2915. [CrossRef] [PubMed]

22. Catauro, M.; Tranquillo, E.; Risoluti, R.; Ciprioti, S.V. Sol-Gel synthesis, spectroscopic and thermal behavior study of SiO_2/PEG composites containing different amount of chlorogenic acid. *Polymers* **2018**, *10*, 682. [CrossRef]
23. Innocenzi, P. Infrared spectroscopy of sol–gel derived silica-based films: A spectra-microstructure overview. *J. Non-Cryst. Solids* **2003**, *316*, 309–319. [CrossRef]
24. Catauro, M.; Pacifico, S. Synthesis of bioactive chlorogenic acid-silica hybrid materials via the sol-gel route and evaluation of their biocompatibility. *Materials* **2017**, *10*, 840. [CrossRef] [PubMed]
25. Coates, J. Interpretation of infrared spectra, a practical approach. *Encycl. Anal. Chem.* **2000**, *12*, 10815–10837.
26. Catauro, M.; Renella, R.; Papale, F.; Ciprioti, S.V. Investigation of bioactivity, biocompatibility and thermal behavior of sol–gel silica glass containing a high PEG percentage. *Mater. Sci. Eng. C* **2016**, *61*, 51–55. [CrossRef] [PubMed]
27. Bichara, L.C.; Lanús, H.E.; Ferrer, E.G.; Gramajo, M.B.; Brandán, S.A. Vibrational study and force field of the citric acid dimer based on the SQM methodology. *Adv. Phys. Chem.* **2011**, *2011*, 347072. [CrossRef]
28. Tsimbler, S.; Shevchenko, L.; Grigor'eva, V. The IR absorption spectra of the tartrate and citrate complexes of nickel, cobalt, and iron. *J. Appl. Spectrosc.* **1969**, *11*, 1096–1101. [CrossRef]
29. Catauro, M.; Naviglio, D.; Risoluti, R.; Vecchio Ciprioti, S. Sol–gel synthesis and thermal behavior of bioactive ferrous citrate–silica hybrid materials. *J. Therm. Anal. Calorim.* **2018**, *133*, 1085–1092. [CrossRef]
30. Catauro, M.; Bollino, F.; Papale, F.; Gallicchio, M.; Pacifico, S. Synthesis and chemical characterization of new silica polyethylene glycol hybrid nanocomposite materials for controlled drug delivery. *J. Drug Deliv. Sci. Technol.* **2014**, *24*, 320–325. [CrossRef]
31. Catauro, M.; Melisi, D.; Curcio, A.; Rimoli, M.G. Sol-gel processing of anti-inflammatory entrapment in silica, release kinetics, and bioactivity. *J. Biomed. Mater. Res. A* **2008**, *87*, 843–849. [CrossRef] [PubMed]
32. Kruppke, B.; Hose, D.; Schnettler, R.; Seckinger, A.; Rößler, S.; Hanke, T.; Heinemann, S. Drug Release as a function of bioactivity, incubation regime, liquid, and initial load: Release of bortezomib from calcium phosphate-containing silica/collagen xerogels. *J. Biomed. Mater. Res. B* **2018**, *106*, 1165–1173. [CrossRef] [PubMed]
33. Ohtsuki, C.; Kokubo, T.; Yamamuro, T. Mechanism of apatite formation on $CaOSiO_2P_2O_5$ glasses in a simulated body fluid. *J. Non-Cryst. Solids* **1992**, *143*, 84–92. [CrossRef]
34. Kokubo, T.; Ito, S.; Huang, Z.; Hayashi, T.; Sakka, S.; Kitsugi, T.; Yamamuro, T. Ca, P-rich layer formed on high-strength bioactive glass-ceramic A-W. *J. Biomed. Mater. Res.* **1990**, *24*, 331–343. [CrossRef] [PubMed]
35. Kokubo, T.; Kushitani, H.; Sakka, S.; Kitsugi, T.; Yamamuro, T. Solutions able to reproduce in vivo surface-structure changes in bioactive glass-ceramic A-W3. *J. Biomed. Mater. Res.* **1990**, *24*, 721–734. [CrossRef] [PubMed]
36. Xu, J.; Wang, Y.; Huang, Y.; Cheng, H.; Seo, H.J. Surface reactivity and hydroxyapatite formation on $Ca_5MgSi_3O_{12}$ ceramics in simulated body fluid. *Appl. Surf. Sci.* **2017**, *423*, 900–908. [CrossRef]
37. Ben-David, Y.; Zlotnik, E.; Zander, I.; Yerushalmi, G.; Shoshani, S.; Banin, E. SawR a new regulator controlling pyomelanin synthesis in *Pseudomonas aeruginosa*. *Microbiol. Res.* **2018**, *206*, 91–98. [CrossRef] [PubMed]
38. Hunter, R.C.; Newman, D.K. A putative ABC transporter, hatABCDE, is among molecular determinants of pyomelanin production in *Pseudomonas aeruginosa*. *J. Bacteriol.* **2010**, *192*, 5962–5971. [CrossRef] [PubMed]
39. Ketelboeter, L.M.; Potharla, V.Y.; Bardy, S.L. NTBC treatment of the pyomelanogenic *Pseudomonas aeruginosa* clinical isolate PA1111 inhibits pigment production and increases sensitivity to oxidative stress. *Curr. Microbiol.* **2014**, *69*, 343–348. [CrossRef] [PubMed]
40. Chatfield, C.H.; Cianciotto, N.P. The secreted pyomelanin pigment of *Legionella pneumophila* confers ferric reductase activity. *Infect. Immun.* **2007**, *75*, 4062–4070. [CrossRef] [PubMed]
41. Ahmad, S.; Lee, S.Y.; Kong, H.G.; Jo, E.J.; Choi, H.K.; Khan, R.; Lee, S.-W. Genetic determinants for pyomelanin production and its protective effect against oxidative stress in ralstonia solanacearum. *PLoS ONE* **2016**, *11*, e0160845. [CrossRef] [PubMed]

2

Protein-Based Drug-Delivery Materials

Dave Jao [1,2], Ye Xue [1,2], Jethro Medina [1] and Xiao Hu [1,2,3,*]

1. Department of Physics and Astronomy, Rowan University, Glassboro, NJ 08028, USA; jaod07@students.rowan.edu (D.J.); xuey5@rowan.edu (Y.X.); medina99@students.rowan.edu (J.M.)
2. Department of Biomedical Engineering, Rowan University, Glassboro, NJ 08028, USA
3. Department of Biomedical and Translational Sciences, Rowan University, Glassboro, NJ 08028, USA

* Correspondence: hu@rowan.edu

Academic Editors: James Z. Tang and Charley Chuan-yu Wu

Abstract: There is a pressing need for long-term, controlled drug release for sustained treatment of chronic or persistent medical conditions and diseases. Guided drug delivery is difficult because therapeutic compounds need to survive numerous transport barriers and binding targets throughout the body. Nanoscale protein-based polymers are increasingly used for drug and vaccine delivery to cross these biological barriers and through blood circulation to their molecular site of action. Protein-based polymers compared to synthetic polymers have the advantages of good biocompatibility, biodegradability, environmental sustainability, cost effectiveness and availability. This review addresses the sources of protein-based polymers, compares the similarity and differences, and highlights characteristic properties and functionality of these protein materials for sustained and controlled drug release. Targeted drug delivery using highly functional multicomponent protein composites to guide active drugs to the site of interest will also be discussed. A systematical elucidation of drug-delivery efficiency in the case of molecular weight, particle size, shape, morphology, and porosity of materials will then be demonstrated to achieve increased drug absorption. Finally, several important biomedical applications of protein-based materials with drug-delivery function—including bone healing, antibiotic release, wound healing, and corneal regeneration, as well as diabetes, neuroinflammation and cancer treatments—are summarized at the end of this review.

Keywords: protein biopolymer; drug delivery; controlled release; silk; collagen; elastin; keratin

---

1. Introduction

New discoveries in medicine and the way different ailments should be treated create a need for more sophisticated methods of drug delivery. Traditionally, the therapeutic efficacy of biomolecular drugs, such as proteins and oligonucleotides, is often limited by their short half-lives due to proteolysis and renal clearance [1,2]. Drugs in blood circulation could be rapidly filtered in the kidney and cleared via the reticuloendothelial system (RES) before reaching the target site. For drugs administered through injection, the vasculature can provide a direct path to the site of disease or take detours where the drug can be eliminated. However, these drugs have to be administered at a high dosage and frequency to perfuse and circulate through the vasculature, finally diffusing into the tissue interstitium, to achieve the desired therapeutic effect [3]. While the oral route for administering drugs is the most convenient, safe and widely accepted method, these bioactive compounds must be insoluble in the

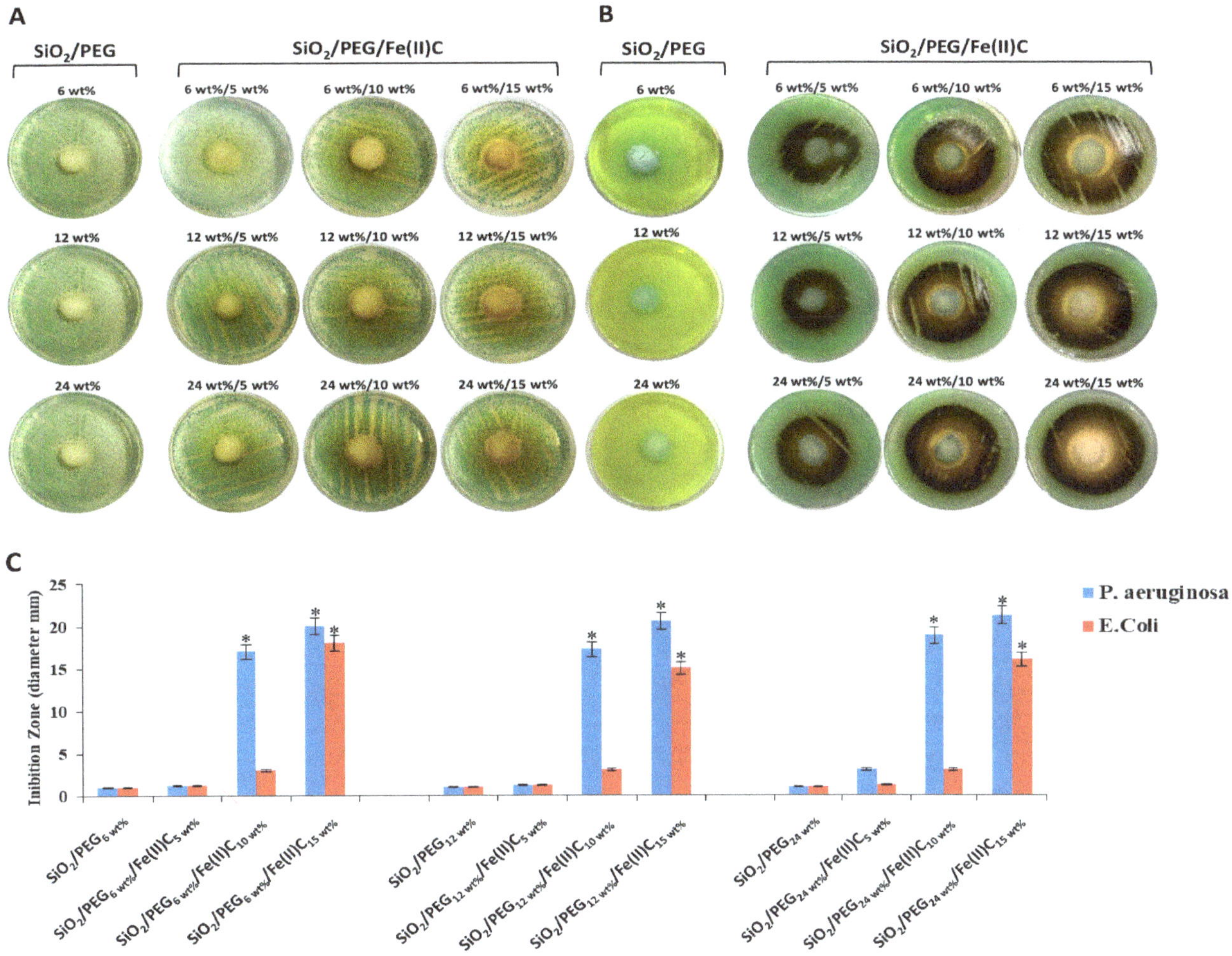

Figure 7. (**A**) Inhibition halo (ID) of *E. coli* with all materials; (**B**) Inhibition halo (ID) of *P. aeruginosa* with all materials; (**C**) Comparison of inhibition zone of *E. coli* and *P. aeruginosa* for all materials. Values are the mean SD of measurements carried out on samples analyzed three times. The means and S.D. are shown. *, $p < 0.05$ vs the bacteria control treated with hybrids without Fe(II)C or vs the bacteria treated with hybrids containing Fe(II)C.

4. Conclusions

In the present study, the different percentage of Fe(II)C and PEG were added in the silica matrix by sol-gel method. FTIR spectra of the obtained hybrids, show all bands of citrate, and also, the typical peaks of polymer and silica. Therefore, the different shape and position of some bands confirm the formation of H-bonds between the inorganic matrix, the PEG chains and, also, the interaction with Fe(II)C. The release of Fe^{2+} from hybrids was studied. Comparing all materials, those containing 24 wt% of PEG determine a greater release of the Fe^{2+}. This result might be due to the high content of PEG and Fe(II)C, that doesn't allow a part of it to form H-bonds because all hydroxyl groups of silica are already involved in weak bonds. Furthermore, the FTIR analysis after 21 days in SBF has suggest that the hybrids are bioactive, and the presence of Fe(II)C or polymer does not affect the bioactivity of silica matrix. Finally, *E. coli* and *P. aeruginosa* were inoculated with the different hybrid materials to evaluate their antibacterial activity. The materials exhibited mild activity against *E. coli* compared to *P. aeruginosa*. In particular the diameter of zone of inhibition of *P. aeruginosa* increases with 10 and 15 wt% of Fe(II)C, independently of polymer content. In conclusion the obtained hybrid materials could be used as biomedical implants to release different controlled amount of Fe^{2+} in the systemic circulation, without going through the gastrointestinal track, in order to allow active coverage. Obviously, these hybrid materials will be investigated further to confirm and extend the obtained results.

Author Contributions: Validation, M.C. and F.D.P.; Formal Analysis, E.T. and F.B.; Data Curation, I.B. and D.N.; Writing-Review & Editing, M.C. and I.B.; Supervision, M.C. and F.D.P. All authors have read and approved.

References

1. Hentze, M.W.; Muckenthaler, M.U.; Galy, B.; Camaschella, C. Two to tango: Regulation of mammalian iron metabolism. *Cell* **2010**, *142*, 24–38. [CrossRef] [PubMed]
2. Camaschella, C. Iron-deficiency anemia. *N. Engl. J. Med.* **2015**, *372*, 1832–1843. [CrossRef] [PubMed]
3. McLean, E.; Cogswell, M.; Egli, I.; Wojdyla, D.; De Benoist, B. Worldwide prevalence of anaemia, WHO vitamin and mineral nutrition information system, 1993–2005. *Public Health Nutr.* **2009**, *12*, 444–454. [CrossRef] [PubMed]
4. Lopez, A.; Cacoub, P.; Macdougall, I.C.; Peyrin-Biroulet, L. Iron deficiency anaemia. *Lancet* **2016**, *387*, 907–916. [CrossRef]
5. Pundir, S.; Badola, A.; Sharma, D. Sustained release matrix technology and recent advance in matrix drug delivery system: A review. *Int. J. Drug Deliv. Res. Technol.* **2017**, *3*, 8.
6. Fragoulakis, V.; Kourlaba, G.; Goumenos, D.; Konstantoulakis, M.; Maniadakis, N. Economic evaluation of intravenous iron treatments in the management of anemia patients in Greece. *ClinicoEconomics Outcomes Res.* **2012**, *4*, 127–134. [CrossRef]
7. Brinker, C.; Scherer, G. *Sol-Gel Science: The Physics and Chemistry of Sol-Gel Processing*; Academic Press: San Diego, CA, USA, 1989.
8. Amiri, S.; Rahimi, A. Hybrid nanocomposite coating by sol–gel method: A review. *Iran. Polym. J.* **2016**, *25*, 559–577. [CrossRef]
9. Judeinstein, P.; Sanchez, C. Hybrid organic–inorganic materials: A land of multidisciplinarity. *J. Mater. Chem.* **1996**, *6*, 511–525. [CrossRef]
10. Owens, G.J.; Singh, R.K.; Foroutan, F.; Alqaysi, M.; Han, C.-M.; Mahapatra, C.; Kim, H.-W.; Knowles, J.C. Sol–gel based materials for biomedical applications. *Prog. Mater. Sci.* **2016**, *77*, 1–79. [CrossRef]
11. Catauro, M.; Bollino, F.; Renella, R.A.; Papale, F. Sol-gel synthesis of SiO_2-CaO-P_2O_5 glasses: Influence of the heat treatment on their bioactivity and biocompatibility. *Ceram. Int.* **2015**, *41*, 12578–12588. [CrossRef]
12. Blanco, I. Polysiloxanes in theranostics and drug delivery: A review. *Polymers* **2018**, *10*, 755. [CrossRef]
13. Kim, G.; Hong, L.Y.; Jung, J.; Kim, D.-P.; Kim, H.; Kim, I.J.; Kim, J.R.; Ree, M. The biocompatability of mesoporous inorganic–organic hybrid resin films with ionic and hydrophilic characteristics. *Biomaterials* **2010**, *31*, 2517–2525. [CrossRef] [PubMed]
14. Nguyen, K.; Garcia, A.; Sani, M.A.; Diaz, D.; Dubey, V.; Clayton, D.; Dal Poggetto, G.; Cornelius, F.; Payne, R.J.; Separovic, F.; et al. Interaction of N-terminal peptide analogues of the Na+,K+-ATPase with membranes. *Biochim. Biophys. Acta* **2018**, *1860*, 1282–1291. [CrossRef] [PubMed]
15. Catauro, M.; Tranquillo, E.; Salzillo, A.; Capasso, L.; Illiano, M.; Sapio, L.; Naviglio, S. Silica/Polyethylene Glycol Hybrid Materials Prepared by a Sol-Gel Method and Containing Chlorogenic Acid. *Molecules* **2018**, *23*, 2447. [CrossRef] [PubMed]
16. Moghimi, S.M.; Szebeni, J. Stealth liposomes and long circulating nanoparticles: Critical issues in pharmacokinetics, opsonization and protein-binding properties. *Prog. Lipid Res.* **2003**, *42*, 463–478. [CrossRef]
17. Salama, A.; El-Sakhawy, M. Preparation of polyelectrolyte/calcium phosphate hybrids for drug delivery application. *Carbohydr. Polym.* **2014**, *113*, 500–506. [CrossRef] [PubMed]
18. Son, K.D.; Kim, Y.-J. Anticancer activity of drug-loaded calcium phosphate nanocomposites against human osteosarcoma. *Biomater. Res.* **2017**, *21*, 13. [CrossRef] [PubMed]
19. Zhou, Z.-F.; Sun, T.-W.; Chen, F.; Zuo, D.-Q.; Wang, H.-S.; Hua, Y.-Q.; Cai, Z.-D.; Tan, J. Calcium phosphate-phosphorylated adenosine hybrid microspheres for anti-osteosarcoma drug delivery and osteogenic differentiation. *Biomaterials* **2017**, *121*, 1–14. [CrossRef] [PubMed]
20. Thomas, M. *The Lambert-Beer Law*; Wiley: New York, NY, USA, 1996.
21. Kokubo, T.; Takadama, H. How useful is SBF in predicting in vivo bone bioactivity? *Biomaterials* **2006**, *27*, 2907–2915. [CrossRef] [PubMed]

stomach to avoid substantial losses due to acid and pepsin in the stomach and pancreatic enzymes in the small intestine [4]. Once it reaches the intestine, drugs must be dissolvable and absorbed through the intestinal mucosa [3]. These above traditional methods are not suitable for chronic and persistent medical conditions requiring drug-delivery systems that are non-toxic, long-term, and controlled to deliver the correct dosage at the correct time. Therefore, there is an overwhelming need for mechanically stable polymer materials as drug-delivery carriers to encapsulate therapeutics from degradation and clearance, while sparing the rest of the body from excess toxicity. Polymer materials can be easily processed into different shapes and structures including films, microcapsules, microspheres, nanoparticles, micelles, gels, and fibers. With the application of polymer carrier systems, therapeutics and biomolecular proteins can protect itself against the harsh environment of the gastrointestinal tract and provide efficient site-specific delivery avoiding the risk of significant side effects and immunological responses.

Interests in protein-based biopolymers for drug delivery have increased in recent years. Compared to synthetic polymers, they have advantages of being water-soluble, biocompatible, biodegradable and non-toxic [4]. Many natural animal proteins such as keratin, collagen, elastin, and silk are relatively inexpensive and sustainable. They are easily derived from their natural sources and simple to process under mild conditions. These proteins have been studied extensively, having high biocompatibility and favorable structural properties for various biomedical applications. Drug-delivery methods using these protein polymers form an essential part of the pharmaceutical applications with release behavior, degradation profile, and mucoadhesive nature. Plant-based proteins, such as zein derived from maize (corn), have also proven to be a very attractive drug-delivery carrier that has enhanced interaction with the biological environment, absorption, and retention time. Zein proteins have been modified and tested in formats of different polarities based on pH via electrostatic interactions or hydrophobic bonds with anti-microbial agents and anticancer drugs for controlled release [5]. Other plant proteins (such as soy protein and wheat gliadin) are also frequently explored for various drug-delivery applications, which can be used to deliver proteins, peptides, DNA, and vaccines [2]. With animal and plant proteins, their respective hydrolysates and small peptides can be recycled from agricultural, aquatic (fisheries) and animal (poultry and meat) sectors and be directly employed in high-priority fields such as biomedical engineering and pharmaceutics [6].

In this review, we will first discuss the structure and potential applications of these natural protein-based polymers. Next, we will discuss the fabrication of various materials from these proteins and their drug-release efficacy. Using these natural protein polymers as an excipient for transdermal, nasal, ocular and oral drug delivery, we will also discuss in detail the effects of drug particle size and density and their binding capacity.

2. Protein Materials

Many fibrous protein materials such as keratin, collagen, elastin and silk have been widely used in drug-delivery research (Figure 1). Since protein materials share similar properties, they can be processed in similar manners [7–9].

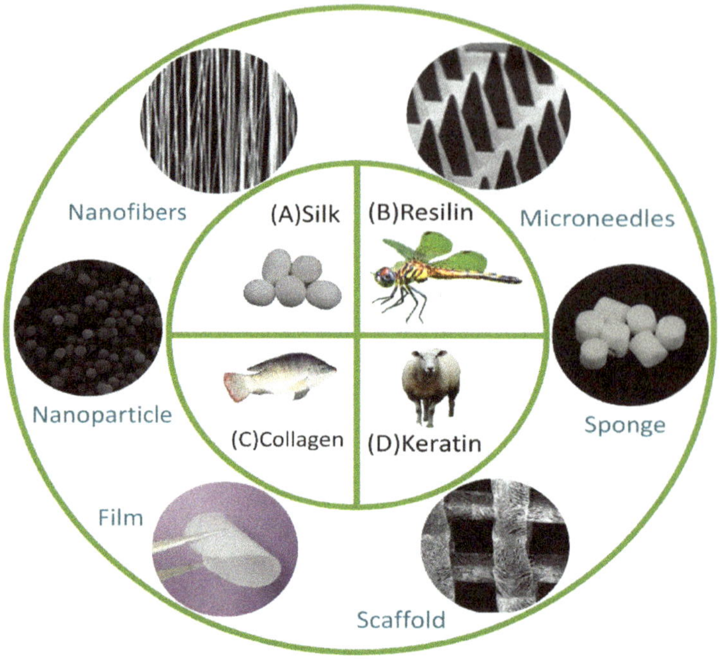

Figure 1. Various proteins and their possible sources under research for drug-delivery applications: (**A**) silk from *Bombyx mori* cocoons; (**B**) resilin from dragonfly; (**C**) collagen from fish scales; (**D**) keratin from goat hairs. These proteins can be fabricated into various drug-delivery vehicles such as films, sponges, gels, fibers, nanoparticles and microneedles. (Reproduced with permission from Reference [7,8,10,11], ACS Publications and Elsevier.)

2.1. Keratin

Keratin is a fibrous protein found in the integumentary system of humans and animals. It can be derived from the outer layer of human skin and the epidermal appendages of animals such as feathers, hair, hooves, horns, nails, scales, and wool [6]. Compared to petroleum-based polymers, keratin is very viable and cost-effective option for biomedical applications. About 95% of pure keratins can be derived from recycled wool with the rest being other components such as hydrocarbons [12]. At the molecular level, keratin can have three different configurations: α-, β- and γ-keratin. The α-keratin is an intermediate filament protein that has an α-helix structure consisting of four right-handed α-helices intertwined to form a protofibril. It has a molecular weight ranging from 40 to 70 kDa and a low sulfur amino acid content of 1.5–2% w/w which can form disulfide bridges from adjacent chains. The β-keratin is also an intermediate filament protein but has a β-sheet structure with amino acids rich in glycine, alanine, serine, lysine, histidine and tryptophan with a molecular weight ranging from 11 to 22 kDa. The structure is stabilized by hydrogen since no cysteine thiol groups are present [6]. The γ-keratin is a matrix protein that has an amorphous structure containing a large amount of cysteine, glycine and tyrosine. It has a molecular weight ranging from 11 to 28 kDa and a high sulfur amino acid content of 4–8% w/w which can form the high degree of intermolecular and intramolecular disulfide bonds. Based on the crosslinking cysteine residues, hard and soft keratins can be generated for mechanical, thermal, and chemical stability [12]. Unlike collagen and elastin, wool is a cheap source of keratin, which is the by-product of the textile industry. Keratin biomaterials extracted from wool and human hairs are biocompatible, biodegradable, nontoxic and very tunable. Further, keratin can contain cell adhesion motifs, RGD (Arg-Gly-Asp) and LDV (Leu-Asp-Val), which mimic the sites of cellular attachment for the development of drug-delivery vehicles [13]. It can be prepared into various forms such as gels, films, fiber, and sponge for various drug-delivery applications, wound dressings and neural tissue-repairing applications.

2.2. Collagen

Collagen is a protein imperative to the structural integrity of tissues and cell growth in vertebrates and other organisms [14]. It is an animal-based protein with three polypeptide chains found in various connective tissues. Accounting for 30% of all proteins in mammals, collagen has various types in most of the extracellular matrix. Type I collagen, in particular, is a major component of different extracellular matrices present in skin, arteries, bone, and corneas [14]. Collagen can be used as a highly biocompatible and versatile protein material. It can be processed into various forms suitable for drug delivery (such as hydrogels, microparticles and films) [15]. One challenge in treating collagen proteins is the heat. To make collagen water soluble, a relatively high amount of heat is necessary to process. Such heat is not suitable for withholding drugs and other substances in collagen films, microparticles, and other materials. As a result, using other solvents such as organic acids can be employed. Areas of applicability for collagen-based materials include bone healing and cancer treatment [15].

Collagen is also a dominant candidate material for corneal regeneration due to its high biocompatibility. Since the cornea is mainly made up of type I collagen, it is a promising drug-delivery biomaterial for corneal repair. Even though collagen fulfills a variety of physiological functions and is very durable in vivo, extracted collagen is easily degradable in vitro, due to the dissociation of natural crosslinks during isolation and purification process [16]. To reduce the rate of enzymatic and hydrothermal degradation, collagen can be chemically crosslinked to provide improved mechanical stability. There are several ways to chemically crosslink collagen molecules, but they are divided into two categories: bi-functional and amide-type. Bifunctional reagents, such as glutaraldehyde, genipin, polyethylene glycol diacrylate (PEG-DBA), and hexamethylene diisocyanate, are used to bridge amine groups of lysine or hydroxylysine residues of collagen polypeptide chains and other natural protein-based polymers [16,17]. However, a major handicap of these chemical crosslinking reagents is the potential cytotoxicity or chromogenic effect of residual molecules or compounds. While genipin and carbodiimide (amide-type) do not have cytotoxicity, most crosslinking agents have the potential to be released into the natural environment during degradation [18]. By selecting and employing safe crosslinking modification methods to collagen, drug stability and retention times can be increased.

2.3. Elastin

Similar to collagen, elastin is a protein within the extracellular matrices of different flexible tissues [19]. It is one of the most stable proteins in the body that can be stretched and relaxed more than a billion times and remain extremely insoluble. Elastin is a heavily crosslinked structure with beta-spiral secondary structure, making up a major component in elastic fibers [19]. While natural elastin is insoluble, there is also research into soluble elastin derivatives, such as human tropoelastin [19,20]. Elastin-like polypeptides (ELP) can also be synthesized. They are biopolymers composed of repetitious chains of the valine, proline, glycine, and unknown (Xaa) amino acids (e.g., VPGXG) from natural elastin protein sequence [21]. With low critical solution temperature and phase transition behavior, elastin composites are feasible materials for stimulus-responsive controlled drug release and vascular stents [22]. Functionalized elastin nanoparticles, microparticles, and macromolecular carriers can also be controlled genetically, resulting in control over size and sequence. The potential diseases/conditions of interest using elastin materials include osteoarthritis, cancer, and type II diabetes [22].

Elastin is also a thermoresponsive protein that provides structure and maintains elasticity of many types of tissues and organs in the human body such as skin, blood vessels, lung, and connective tissues. Various forms of thermoresponsive elastin, such as animal-derived soluble elastin, recombinant human tropoelastin (rhTE), and elastin-like polypeptides (ELPs), have been synthesized and utilized to engineer promising synthetic tissue scaffolds [23]. ELPs are polypeptides derived from the hydrophobic domains of elastin. They are widely used as thermoresponsive units in biomaterials due to the presence of a sharp soluble-to-insoluble phase change at a specific transition temperature. These elastin-derived molecules can be assembled linearly or become star-shaped using lysine amino acids as branching and terminal units with 1–3 pentameric repeats between each branch [24]. The ELP transition temperatures can also be tuned using different forms of the sequence, Xaa-Pro-Gly-Xaa-Gly (XPGXG), where *X* represents different amino acids, to adjust the lower critical solution temperature (LCST) behavior [23]. With the ability to change from random coil to β-turn conformation upon heating through the transition temperatures, ELPs can demonstrate temperature-dependent flow and retention with the opening and closing of pores when processed into various forms of three-dimensional porous hydrogels, elastomeric films, and electrospun scaffolds. Being able to adjust pore size and stress-stiffness, ELPs can enhance cell growth and mediate mesenchymal stem cell fate.

2.4. Silk

Silk is a protein of long historical use in biomedical applications, such as tissue and ligament repair, nerve regenerators, and artificial blood vessels [25]. Silk fibroin protein is mainly derived from silkworm cocoons and spider threads with insoluble beta-sheet crystal structures. Different silkworm silks have been used for drug-delivery applications including *Bombyx mori, Tussah,* and *Eri* silks [26]. Silk proteins can be prepared in various ways, such as films [27], 3D porous scaffolds [28], and micro and nanoparticles [29], with controlled degradation rates. Silk is an excellent material for drug-delivery applications due to its mild processing conditions and aids in reducing cost. With desirable biocompatibility and controllable biodegradability, silk-based materials make ideal long-term drug-eluting depots. Silk-controlled release properties are defined by two primary methodologies: diffusion of substance payload and solubilization/degradation of the silk material [28]. A thin silk film with programmable solubility rate, for example, can release the desired substance as the film degrades within the designated area [28].

Compared to naturally spun silkworm fibers, spider dragline silks have many attractive physical properties that include significantly higher tensile strength and elasticity. The development of silk fibers having the properties of spider silks is of keen interest. However, the generation of a spider silk-manufacturing process faces serious problems through spider farming, since spiders are quite territorial by nature. Therefore, standard recombinant silk protein production platforms were employed. Thus far, only small quantities of artificial spider silk can be produced due to the inability to successfully assemble spider silk proteins into fibers with native-sized recombinant silk protein (250–320 kDa) [30]. While native-sized spider silk protein can be favorably expressed in metabolically engineered *Escherichia coli*, the recombinant proteins can also yield lower molecular weight versions, which leads to inferior fiber properties [31]. To overcome these limitations, Teulè et al. using recombinant DNA introduced a unique genetic engineering vector called 'PiggyBac' [30]. These vectors are pieces of DNA known as a transposon taken from spiders that can insert itself into the genetic machinery of silkworms. The silk fibers produced by these transgenic silkworms were a combination of chimeric silkworm and spider silk proteins. The genetically engineered silk proteins produced are an extremely stable composite material with improved elasticity and strength as native dragline spider silk fibers. By using recombinant DNA, gene manipulations into current commercial silkworm production can be a potentially viable solution for large-scale production of engineered protein fibers with customizable properties of strength and elasticity that can exceed properties of native silkworm silk. This biotechnological approach can lead to a broad range of mechanical properties, optimized for specific biomedical and drug-delivery applications, such as fine suture materials, bandages, or scaffolds for tendon and ligament repair in addition to strong and lightweight structural fabrics.

2.5. Resilin

Resilin is an elastomeric protein first found existing in jumping insects' cuticles of many species [32]. It contains coiled amino acid chains that form a flexible and elastic network structure when the di- and tri-tyrosine links are crosslinked [32]. Under high-frequency deformation, contraction and extension, the dityrosine crosslinked protein structures possess extraordinary resilience and long-range reversible elasticity. Resilin also exhibits high extensibility, low stiffness, efficient energy storage and extraordinary resilience, which enables some jumping insects to jump many times' their body length. The resilin's rubber-like elasticity also possess excellent biocompatibility and mechanical properties, which can be used for a broad range of biomedical applications such as drug delivery and tissue scaffolds [32–34].

2.6. Corn Zein

Many types of plant-based proteins have been used for drug-delivery applications. Zein is a major plant-based storage protein rich in prolamine found in the endosperm of the corn kernel [35]. It is a by-product from the processing of maize corn present in corn gluten meal and from the manufacturing of ethanol during the wet and dry milling processes [36]. Zein has a molecular weight of about 40 kDa and is rich in glutamine, proline, alanine, and leucine residues [5]. It is grouped into four classes, α-, β-, γ- and δ-zein, with varying molecular weights and modes of extraction [36]. The α-zein consists of 70–85% of the total zein with molecular weights ranging from 22 to 24 kDa with a predominant triple super-helix protein structure; followed by 10–20% of γ-zein consists with molecular weights ranging from 18 to 27 kDa. The remaining minor fractions consist of 1−5% of β-zein with a molecular weight of 17 kDa high in methionine and 1−5% of δ-zein with molecular weight of 10 kDa [37]. All zein fractions have hydrophobic and hydrophilic domains but zein is frequently considered to be a hydrophobic protein due to its insolubility in water and solubility in ethanol, acetone, and acetylacetone. The non-polar helical interiors of the zein protein have glutamine-rich turns and loops that allow it to self-assemble into particles and layers [35]. With successive helical segment folding in an antiparallel arrangement, zein can exhibit chemical and thermoplastic properties that are heat and pH stable [37]. Other excellent material properties of zein include biodegradability, mechanical resistance and water barrier ability, making it attractive in applications such as drug delivery and coatings in food and pharmaceuticals [35]. Also, zein has shown to form aggregates and entrap solutes like drugs or amino acids which make it an excellent matrix material for sustained release.

3. Fabrication Methods of Devices Based on Biopolymers

Once the raw protein materials are prepared, there are different ways to process them, and the method ultimately used is determined by their delivery applications (some key examples have been summarized in Table 1). Drug stability, release kinetics, and method of administration are all factors that affect the final form of the material.

Table 1. Biomedical applications of protein biomaterial and their structural design.

Material	Applications	Structural Design
Collagen	Engineering of cartilage, corneal, nerve, ocular, skin, and tendon/ligament tissues, surgical conduits, wound repair, integrated in a variety of composite materials to enhance favorable drug-delivery properties	Hydrogels [15,38–40], Films [17], Fibers [41]
Elastin	Controlled drug delivery, engineering of cartilage, liver, ocular, and vascular graft tissue, highly tunable thermoresponsive intracellular functionalized peptide drugs, wound healing applications	Hydrogels [42–44], Films [45,46], Fibers [47,48]
Keratin	Antibacterial, drug delivery, tissue engineering, trauma and medical devices, wound healing	Hydrogels [49–52], Films, [53], Fibers [54]
Resilin	Engineering of native vocal fold, cardiovascular, human cartilage tissues, protein-engineered bioactive materials to promote cell adhesion, degradation, growth factor delivery, and cell differentiation	Hydrogels [34,55–57], Nanoparticles [58]
Silk	Adhesive fillers, engineering of cartilage or load bearing tissues, wound dressing, enzyme immobilization, drug delivery	Hydrogels [59], Films [60], Microcapsules [61], Microparticles [62]
Zein	Biomineralization, controlled drug release, enhanced mechanical strength, microbial resistance, positive cell attachment and osteoblast growth	Films [63], Microspheres [64], Nanofibers [65], Nanoparticles [66]

3.1. Films and Coatings

Films are thin layers of a particular substance. They are flexible and can cover vast areas. These two properties open avenues for drug delivery on various surfaces using films. Wound dressing, for example, requires a material that can match the flexibility of the skin and the pressure forced onto it. Using protein-based films infused with drug treatment can be continuous while reducing the risk of infection from multiple treatments and drug admissions.

Silk films can be prepared by several steps. First silk cocoons or raw fibers are degummed to separate the sericin from the silk fibroin fibers [67]. The degummed fiber is then dried, followed by dissolution in lithium bromide or other organic solvents. The resulting silk solution is dialyzed for further purification to obtain a silk aqueous solution. This new solution can be then cast into various molds or areas to form silk films [67]. Microparticles and nanoparticles containing a desired drug or substance can be incorporated into silk films in the solution stage for controlled drug-release applications.

Collagen films are fabricated in a similar manner to silk films. The process begins with obtaining dried collagen [68]. The dried collagen is dissolved in an acidic solution and then neutralized. Crosslinkers, such as acrylamide, are added to facilitate crosslinking of collagen protein chains [69]. The resulting solution can be cast into films for drug-delivery applications. The addition of other substances can increase the range of use of the films, such as providing collagen films antimicrobial properties [69].

Elastin protein and ELPs can be fabricated into films as well. HFIP (hexafluoro-2-propanol), ddH_2O, or acetic acid are appropriate solvents for making elastin and ELP solutions [68]. The elastin solutions are cast and set at room temperature for the period aforementioned. As the solvent evaporated, films will be produced within 48 h [68]. Incorporating ELP-drug composites into the films will allow for additional controlled drug release from the fabricated films [68].

3.2. Particles and Spheres

Particles for drug-delivery applications are typically on the micro- and nano-scale. Microparticles are particles with diameters between 0.1 and 100 μm, while nanoparticles measure between 1 and 100 nm in diameter. Encapsulating drugs and other substances into particles of such size will increase release capabilities in a targeted tissue or organ. Using protein-based particles will add the biocompatibility necessary to utilize microparticles and nanoparticles in controlled drug release [70].

Silk nanoparticles can be generated from different solvents such as acetone desolvation [28]. Acetone desolvation involves rapidly introducing aqueous silk fibroin solution to acetone. After drying, water-insoluble nanoparticles can be separated from the solution [71]. Applying an electric field to nanoparticles can also physically produce silk microspheres of 2–3 μm in diameter. Silk nanoparticles, when exposed to a weak electric field, were found to be able to aggregate into microspheres around the positive electrodes [71].

Elastin-based magnetic ELP microparticles can be prepared through a water-in-oil emulsion. Introducing magnetic nanoparticles to the system, Cifani et.al found their magnetic properties can be transferred into the ELP microparticles [72]. Human elastin-like polypeptide (HELP) microparticles can also be prepared using the emulsion mentioned prior and a subsequent enzymatic crosslinking procedure [72]. A typical process for producing magnetic HELPs can be seen in Figure 2. Drug molecules are introduced into the aqueous phase in Figure 2, yielding magnetic, drug-loaded ELP microparticles.

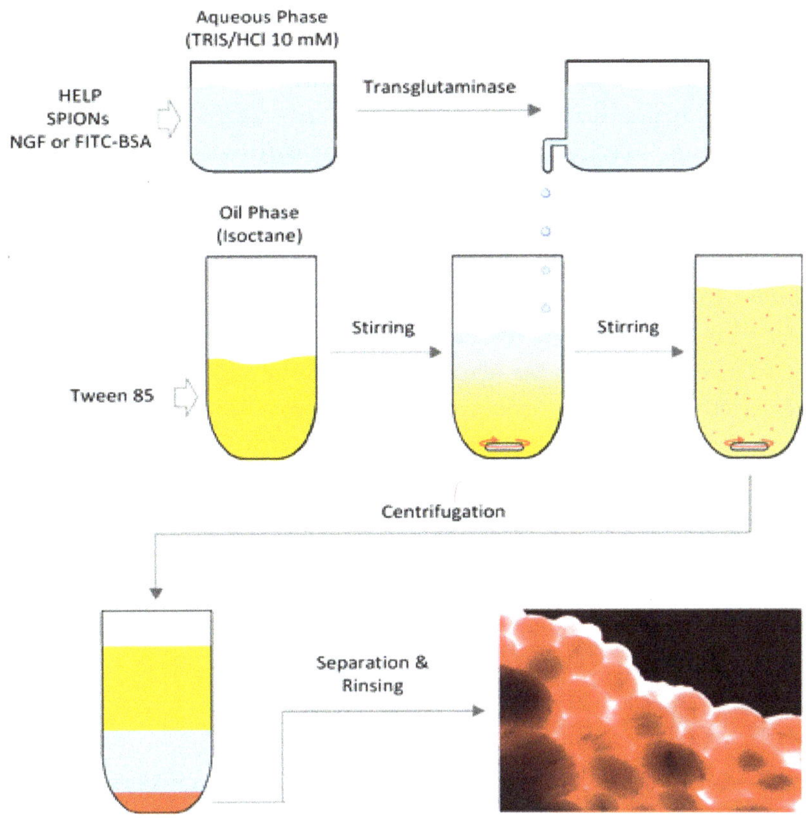

Figure 2. Preparation for the magnetic human elastin-like polypeptide (HELP) microparticles with various controlled drug-delivery applications. (Reproduced with permission from Reference [72], John Wiley and Sons).

Collagen microparticles can be fabricated by two methods: membrane emulsification and the use of microfluidic devices [73]. The membrane emulsion method uses a membrane of uniform pore size and low pressure to produce particles of uniform size [74]. A collagen solution mixed with acetic acid is pumped through a membrane, into a continuous methyl acetate phase [73]. The solution pushed through the membrane was added dropwise to the methyl acetate. Centrifugation was then employed to separate the microparticles from the methyl acetate solution. Microfluidic devices were also used to produce microparticles. Figure 3 depicts the process for the fabrication of collagen microparticles using microfluidics. A diluted collagen solution is first fed through the opening of the device [73] and then introduced into a polar organic solvent (acetic acid). The mixture is finally mixed continuously with the crosslinking reagent (a glutaraldehyde solution) to form the particles [73]. The resulting microparticles are collected at the exit of the device, with a diameter of about 20–50 μm.

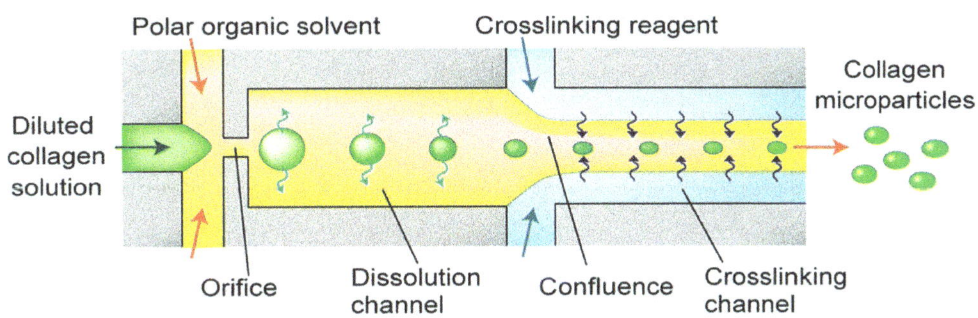

Figure 3. Microfluidic schematic for producing collagen microparticles. (Reproduced with permission from Reference [73], The Royal Society of Chemistry).

3.3. Hydrogels

Hydrogels are networks used in facilitating the controlled release of cells and other bioactive molecules [75]. Their three-dimensional design aids in the controlled release of molecules such as proteins, antibodies, and drugs. Hydrogels are sometimes infused with nanoparticles to further their uses in drug-release applications.

To form collagen hydrogels, a collagen solution is first prepared by dissolving dried collagens in an acidic solution [69]. The solution is then mixed with monomers (HEMA) and crosslinking agent (MBA) and neutralized before producing the hydrogels. Ammonium persulfate can be then be added to initiate crosslinking of the collagen within 12 h [69]. Additional collagen techniques such as plastic compression and vitrification can also be applied to collagen gels to form films. Placing the gels solution in Petri dishes and allowing the reaction to occur gives collagen fibrils the necessary time to reorganize and crosslink during solvent evaporation.

Unlike collagen, silk hydrogels can be prepared using physical methods without additional crosslinkers. This is due to the formation of beta-sheet crystals, which can act as crosslinkers in the hydrogel. To begin silk aqueous solution is prepared [75], then the silk solution is mixed and vortexed gently in an ethanol solution or directly sonicated in ultrasound, resulting in a physically crosslinked hydrogel system. By using an ethanol solution with drug-containing silk particles, the resulting hydrogel can contain the particular drug or substance of interest [75].

3.4. Microneedles

Microneedles can be employed as a method of transdermal drug delivery [10,76]. They can be utilized as a painless alternative to traditional hypodermic needles. Microneedles penetrate skin across the stratum corneum, giving patients a feeling of slight pressure with no pain [77]. Furthermore, sites of microneedle injection showed faster rates to reaching maximum blood flow when compared to topical applications.

Silk-based microneedles have been designed for controlled substance release with relatively mild processing conditions [28]. Controlling drug-release rates is dependent on the secondary structure and beta-sheet crystallinity of the silk materials [28], which can be adjusted by various post-processing procedures. One method of producing silk microneedles is provided in Figure 4. PDMS is first cast over an aluminum mold to create PDMS molds in the proper microneedle shape. The silk-drug solutions are then cast over the PDMS mold and dried. The silk layer is finally separated from the PDMS, resulting in silk-drug microneedles [78].

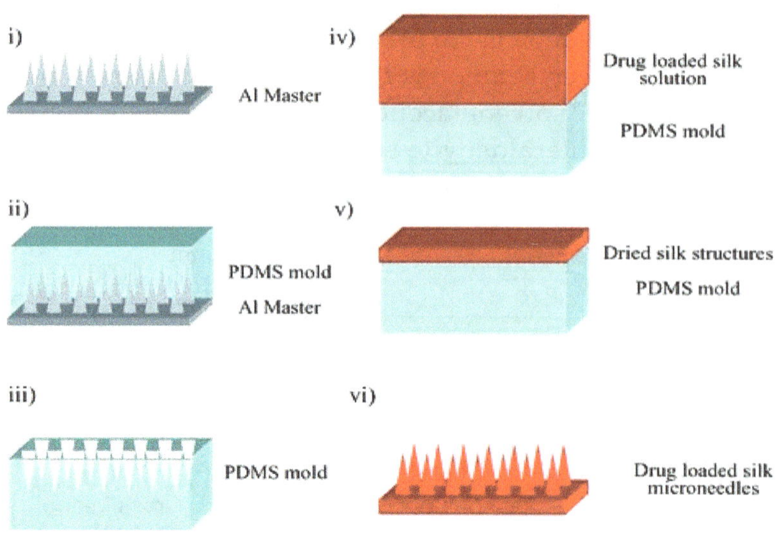

Figure 4. Schematic of silk microneedle fabrication for drug delivery. (Reproduced with permission from Reference [78], John Wiley and Sons).

3.5. Composite Materials

3.5.1. Keratin Composites

Medicated wound dressing-composite scaffolds have been developed using freeze-drying techniques. These solid sponge scaffolds based on keratin (K), fibrin (F) and gelatin (G) obtained show highly interconnected pores with macroporous morphology through SEM analysis. Mimicking extracellular matrix with cell-binding motifs in the keratin and fibrin can enhance NIH 3T3 fibroblast and keratinocyte growth, and adhesion can be seen in vitro fluorescence images. The efficiency of KFG-composite scaffolds have been studied and tested using mupirocin as the model drug. The drug-loaded scaffold showed a gradual, sustained drug release, which suggested that the scaffold could be used as an active antibacterial wound-dressing biomaterial in skin tissue regeneration [79].

Also in tissue regeneration, De Guzman et al. have studied the intermolecular surface and bulk interaction properties of reduced keratin proteins (kerateines) with gold and bone morphogenetic protein 2 (BMP-2) as potential drug carriers [79]. To investigate the gold to kerateines interactions, the group chemisorbed thiol-rich kerateines onto gold substrates to form a 2 nm rigid layer for surface plasmon resonance analysis. The gold substrate showed irreversibly link to the free thiols of kerateines forming strong intermolecular covalent disulfide bonds, which can lead to longer-lasting gels. To study the electrostatic forces between negatively charged keratins and positively charged growth factors, the binding and release kinetics of BMP-2 from the kerateines' network are examined by electrostatic or coulombic interactions in various pH and salt concentrations. These findings contribute to the understanding of the release kinetics of BMP-2-conjugated kerateines systems, which can potentially be employed in bone repair and regeneration as drug-delivery vehicles [79].

Through thiol–ene click chemistry, keratin graft poly(ethylene glycol) (keratin-g-PEG) copolymer nanoparticles can be synthesized [80]. Due to the amphiphilicity and the thiol groups of the graft copolymers, the nanoparticles can self-assemble with PEG chains and keratin as the core in aqueous solutions. The disulfide bonds can crosslink the core of the nanoparticles on the keratin backbones. With cleavable glutathione (GSH) crosslinks, the efficiency of the drug-delivery system has been evaluated using doxorubicin hydrochloride salt (DOX·HCl) as the model drug. The work concluded that the release of the loaded DOX is dependent on the concentration of GSH at the cellular level. The nanoparticles also showed excellent DOX-loading capacity of 18.1% (w/w) and accelerating release into the nucleus of the cells with the dual triggerable release properties of GSH and trypsin. With the controllable and responsive release of the loaded DOX, cells can efficiently internalize the DOX making it a promising carrier for intracellular drug delivery for cancer therapy and other drug-delivery applications [80].

Like other natural polymers, keratin promotes favorable cell interactions and degradable porous non-toxic scaffold for regenerative medicine. Han et al. developed alkylated kerateine hydrogels impregnated with rhBMP-2, rhIGF-1, and ciprofloxacin, for the differentiation of stem cells toward osteogenic lineage [81]. The scaffold was synthesized with an iodoacetamide alkylation (or "capping") of cysteine residues on reductively extracted keratin (kerateines). Unlike the oxidatively derived keratin (keratose) that cannot form disulfide crosslinks, kerateines can provide a more stable crosslinked hydrogel network. Employing alkylation, the levels of disulfide crosslinking in keratin hydrogels can be modulated providing controllable rates of gel erosion and therapeutic agent release. The modification process of kerateines did not lead to increased cytotoxicity in MC3T3-E1 pre-osteoblasts and maintained the ability of cells to attach to the material at levels greater than collagen. The release of therapeutic agents appears to follow the rate of keratin hydrogel erosion with loss of disulfide crosslinking. The alkylated kerateine hydrogels provided good cell attachment and proliferation as while as controlled delivery, leading to drug concentrations appropriate for bone and tissue-engineering applications [81].

3.5.2. Elastin Composites

For thermo-targeted chemotherapy of hyperthermic tumor margins, thermosensitive ELP-based diblock biopolymers have been developed containing functional poly-glutamic/aspartic acid blocks for drug conjugation [82]. The efficiency of ELP-based polymers was tested using geldanamycin (GA) as the model drug. Even though clinical trials of GA have not shown promise due to off-target toxicity and poor formulation design, this study stated that conjugation of geldanamycin (GA) with ELP-based polymer could be used for the thermo-targeted drug-delivery agents of the tumor margins and inhibition of heat shock protein 90 (HSP90), an essential molecular chaperone of several potent pro-oncogenic pathways. The ELP-based polymer-GA conjugates demonstrated high drug loadings and tunable thermo-responsiveness. Thermal precipitation of the biopolymer-GA conjugates at hyperthermic isotherms $T > 40$ °C provide active targeting at the tumor site while the pH-sensitive drug, GA, is released within the acidic tumor microenvironment. This avoids systemic toxicity and off-target effects, which presents a novel platform for anti-cancer treatment [82].

For gene delivery, tunable hollow ELP spheres (~100–1000 nm) were developed by Dash et al. Using the self-assembly property and slight positive charge of ELP, the group fabricated the hollow spheres using polystyrene (PS) beads as a template. Permeation studies of the polyplex (~70 µg pDNA/mg of hollow sphere) were carried out using plasmid DNA (pDNA) as the model drug [83]. To provide stability, the ELP spheres were crosslinked with microbial transglutaminase (mTGase) following the removal of the PS beads. The addition of pDNA into polyplex resulted in higher loading efficiency than that of self-assembled solid particles and controlled release triggered by protease and elastase. Moreover, polyplex-loaded hollow spheres also yielded higher luciferase expression by providing protection against endosomal degradation. Throughout this process, surface functional groups were well maintained. The technique is straightforward and efficient allowing ELP hollow spheres to be produced in large quantities. Designing advanced ELP hollow spheres with the ability to couple targeting ligands can provide exciting new opportunities in gene delivery applications [83].

For tumor-specific delivery and controlled drug release, thermosensitive ELP-grafted dipalmitoylphosphatidylcholine (DPPC)-based liposomes were developed by Kim et al. using a lipid film hydration method [84]. The group designed an ELP with a mild hyperthermia-mediated trigger using an $\alpha v\beta 3$ integrin targeting moiety that induces target-specific endocytosis. Doxorubicin (DOX), an anticancer drug, was used as the model drug. Upon mild hyperthermia, 75% to 83% DOX was able to be released from the thermosensitive ELP at 42 °C and 45 °C. Using an ammonium sulfate-gradient method, the efficiency of cRGD-targeted and ELP-modified DOX-encapsulated liposomes (RELs) were studied. Since cyclic arginine-glycine-aspartic acid (cRGD) is overexpressed in the angiogenic vasculature and tumor cells, RELs showed an 8- to 10-fold overexpression in U87MG and HUVEC cells, which were higher than that of non-targeting liposomes. These highly specific RELs can be guided and activated using currently available external heat-generating devices such as ultrasound or radiofrequency [84].

3.5.3. Collagen Composites

To be applied as drug-eluting implants or a drug-release system, McMaster et al. developed a highly biocompatible and porous collagen-based (CAC) scaffold coated with an alginate polymer [9]. The layer-by-layer collagen scaffold was assembled using a cryogenic plotting system. The efficiency of the drug-delivery system was evaluated using rhodamine B as the model drug. The system exhibited an initial burst release regulated by the porosity of the CAC scaffolds, followed by a constant drug release controlled by the volume percentage of alginate coated on the collagen scaffold. The CAC scaffolds have a Young's modulus of 30 MPa, which is nine times higher than pure collagen scaffolds. With a porosity of 88%, biological function can be maintained. Osteoblast-like cells (MG63) seeded on CAC scaffolds have shown to proliferated and migrated into the interior of the scaffolds. The CAC scaffolds can be tuned for long-term therapeutic applications in tissue engineering [9].

For dentistry applications, glutaraldehyde crosslinked type-I collagen gels were developed by Barbaresso et al. [85] using a freeze-dried technique. Drug permeation studies were carried out on the 3D collagen matrices using niflumic acid as the model drug. Niflumic acid, an anti-inflammatory drug, was embedded into the collagen sponges using glutaraldehyde as the crosslinking agent. The addition of crosslinking agents resulted in the formation of collagen matrices with constant niflumic acid release rate. The crosslinked collagen gels showed reduced swelling and enzymatic degradation. Since the presence of niflumic acid did enhance water absorption, a non-Fickian kinetic mechanism was proposed for drug release. The released niflumic acid percent can be tuned by adjusting the amount of crosslinking agent, thus allowing the optimum release of the desired amount of drug in relation to the application site and therapeutic recommendations [85].

For topical drug delivery applications, antibiotic-loaded collagen (coll)-containing hydrogel films have been fabricated by mixing degraded collagen with synthetic monomers, such as acrylamide (AAm) and 2-hydroxy ethyl methacrylate (HEMA) [69]. Antibiotics, such as gallic acid (GA) and naproxen (NP), were then loaded into the crosslinked composites of p(coll-co-AAm) and p(coll-co-HEMA) hydrogel films to test its efficacy. The drug kinetics studies were carried out in vitro. Linear drug releases were observed in both GA-loaded p(coll-co-AAm) and NP-loaded p(coll-co-HEMA) composite films obtaining up to 32 h and 36 h release, respectively. As other studies have concluded, higher amounts of active agents could be increased by crosslinking collagen. This also provides additional advantages, such as better mechanical strength and absorption. Moreover, metal nanoparticles such as Ag and Cu can be added within these hydrogel films to further enhance the antimicrobial characteristic against known common bacteria such as *Escherichia coli*, *Bacillus subtilis*, and *Staphylococcus aureus*. The investigation showed that antibiotic-loaded collagen hydrogel films could be readily prepared and used as potential wound- and/or burn-dressing materials for drug-delivery and healing purposes [69].

Nanoparticles based on biopolymers or peptides can also be fabricated to have targeted and controlled release. Anandhakumar et al. developed collagen peptide (CP) for the preparation of chitosan (CN) nanoparticles via ionic gelation method by co-precipitation of CN and CP [86]. The CPCN nanoparticles are formed through hydrogen bonding and electrostatic interactions. They are pH-responsive and stable under physiological conditions. The efficiency of the drug-delivery system was evaluated using doxorubicin (DOX) hydrochloride as the model drug. The unique CPCN nanoparticles showed biphasic release with a burst release in the first 20 h, followed by sustained release over 7 days. In response to the extracellular pH of the tumor environment, enhanced delivery of anti-tumor drugs was also seen with 68% controlled release at pH 7.4 and 89% release at pH 1.5. With cell viability studies, DOX-loaded NPs showed excellent anti-proliferative characteristics against HeLa cells with favorable biocompatibility with NIH 3T3 fibroblast cells. Therefore, protein-based NPs have a high potential for encapsulation and release of anti-tumor drugs in the area of cancer drug delivery [86].

4. Factors to Control Drug-Delivery Efficiency

Delivery efficiency is one of the important factors in drug delivery. Protein materials with drug-delivery function need to guarantee that the drug can maintain a continuous release over a period of time at a certain therapeutic level. For poorly soluble drugs in particular, maintaining controllable drug-delivery efficiency is vital. Proper delivery efficiency can optimize the drug absorption and the cure effectiveness. It has been studied that the controllable drug delivery can be achieved through altering the molecular weight or monomer of the protein-polymer system or changing the size, porosity and morphology of the protein-material matrix. The drug-release efficiency may also vary due to the shape of the material, such as ellipsoid, disc or rods, as well as the delivery molecules. In this section, we will discuss the drug-delivery efficiency in the case of molecular weight, particle size, particle shape, morphology, and porosity of protein polymers.

4.1. Molecular Weight

Natural silk fibroin materials, featuring good biocompatibility and biodegradability, have been sufficiently studied as a promising drug-delivery material. Pritchard et al. [87,88] reported that the drug-release rate could be controlled by changing the molecular weight of silk (Figure 5). To process raw silk fibers into desired drug-delivery materials, it is necessary to remove the hydrophilic sericin proteins, which functions as the glue coated on hydrophobic fibroin fibers, through degumming. When subjected to thermal and alkaline conditions during the degumming procedure, the molecular weight of silk fibroin fibers can be controlled by the degumming time. Thereby, the drug-release rate can be controlled by adjusting the duration of degumming, as shown in Figure 5 [27]. With the degumming time increasing, the molecular weight of silk fibroin materials will decrease, which may decrease the crystallinity and molecular chain length, and reduce physical crosslinks of silk materials. Besides the molecular weight, the chain length also has an impact on the drug diffusion through the silk matrix. A correlation between degumming time and silk molecular weight has been thoroughly studied by Pandit et al. [89] and Yamada et al. [90]. The drug-release behavior can be affected by both the diffusion of the drug through the silk-polymer matrix and the degradation of the matrix. Thereby, both factors can be manipulated through controlling the molecular weight of the silk-polymer matrix. Indigo carmine, rifampicin, reactive red 120 and azoalbumin particles have been used to study the relation between drug-release profile and the molecular weight of silk polymer [27]. It was found that the drug release increased while the molecular weight decreased (with longer degumming time). A similar study was also conducted by Fang et al. [91], which confirmed that reducing the molecular weight of silk in silk hydrogels can increase the drug-release rate qualitatively.

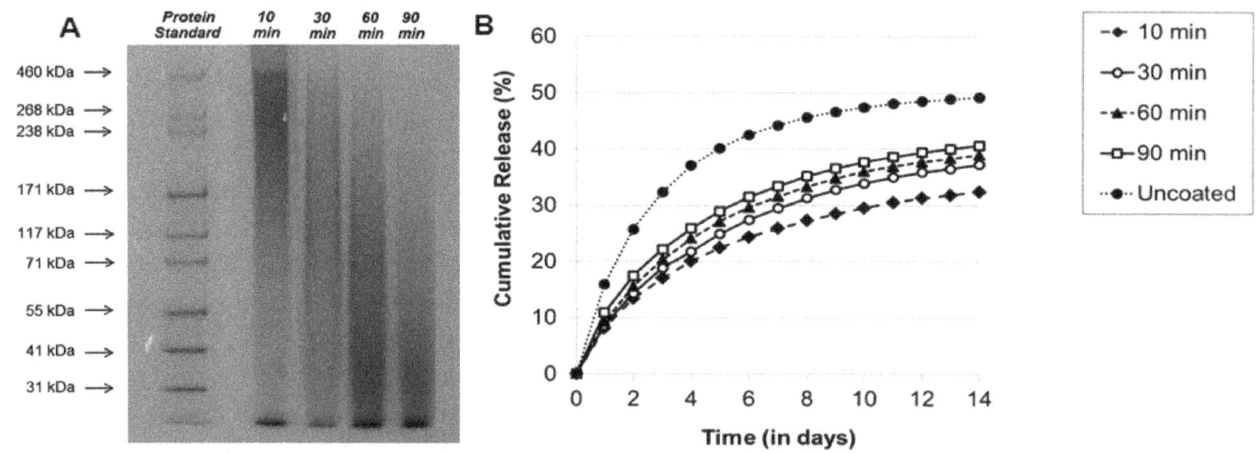

Figure 5. (**A**) SDS-PAGE analysis of silk with different degumming times (10 min, 30 min, 60 min and 90 min); (**B**) Cumulative release of rifampicin from silk gel films capped with a single layer of silk prepared using varied degumming times. (Reproduced with permission from Reference [27], John Wiley and Sons).

4.2. Nanoparticle Size

The drug load and release efficiency of protein nanoparticles can be largely influenced by the size distribution. Particle size is an important factor associated with biocompatibility [92]. By altering the nanoparticle size and controlling the size distribution, nanoparticles have the ability to penetrate the physiological barrier, which can affect the release efficiency and therapeutic impact [93]. In addition, synthesizing nanoparticles below their critical size can induce their magnetic (superparamagnetic) properties, which can be potentially used as an attractive drug-delivery vehicle for tumor cure [94–96]. In a report by Lu et al. [97], the group showed how mesoporous silica nanoparticles (MSNs) of about 50 nanometers could maximize cellular. This size factor can also be applied to magnetic particles delivered by biopolymers [98,99], as shown in Figure 6A, and the relationship between the magnetic coercivity and the particle size is shown in Figure 6B. While increasing the size of the particles, the distribution of nanoparticles circulated to the liver and spleen would increase [97]. Particle size can also affect the efficiency of nanoparticles extravasated from the vasculature. Therefore, maintaining good control of the nanoparticles size can overcome limits to certain tissue or organ where the traditional drug-delivery method cannot access, especially for the brain system.

The focus of osteoinductive biomaterials for bone tissue-engineering applications has recently been directed towards composite components that facilitate biomaterial integration, bone repair, and regeneration. Foo et al. have designed and developed a novel bioactive material that combines silk fibroin proteins with silica particles [100]. This unusual pairing can restore tissue structure and function at the implanted site by providing immediate structural support while remaining flexible. Unlike hydroxyapatite (HA) minerals which lack biological activity and low durability, silica is osteoinductive and has a morphological structure that can bear the load of hard tissue. Mieszawska et al. investigated the effect of silk-silica composites with human mesenchymal stem cells (hMSCs) subjected to osteogenic differentiation [101]. The study showed stimulated osteogenic cell growth and gene expression. With the addition of silk, smaller and more uniform silk-silica composites could be prepared with a diameter of 24 nm to 2 μm. This synergistic effect can decrease the size and amount of silica content used toward bone tissue regeneration.

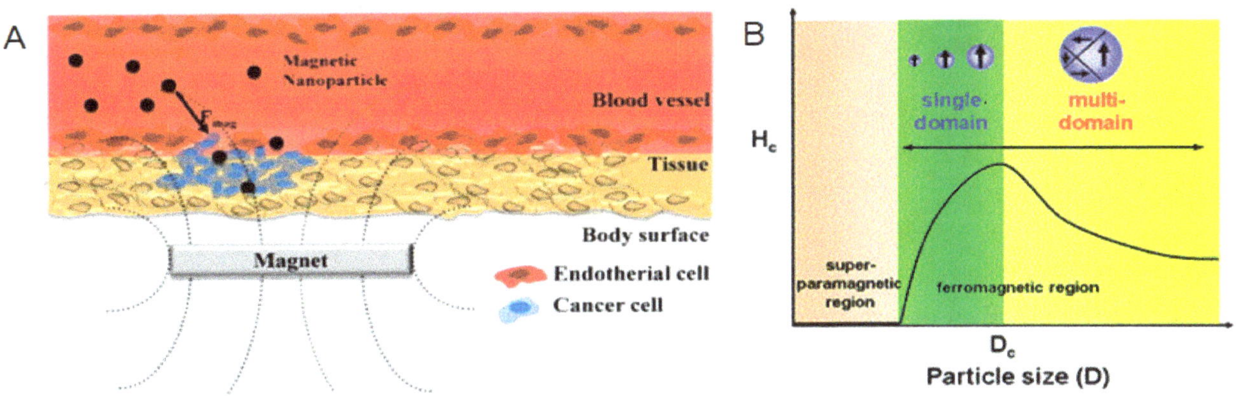

Figure 6. (**A**) Schematic of a magnetic nanoparticle-based drug-delivery system; (**B**) Plot of the magnetic coercivity (Hc) vs. the size of particle for drug delivery. (Reproduced with permission from Reference [98], Elsevier, and Reference [99], The Royal Society of Chemistry).

4.3. Morphology and Shape

Nanoparticle morphology and shape are important factors that influence the drug-delivery efficiency. Nanoparticles can take various form of morphology from a simple sphere, rod, or sheet to wormlike structures through different chemical and physical fabrication processes, as shown in Figure 7 [102–104]. The drug-release efficiency can be controlled by changing the geometry, coating thickness, porosity, or manipulating the crystallinity of the protein drug carriers [27]. Studies have been conducted to tailor the particle morphology through changing the monomer ratios of the copolymers and the pH of the solvent. Almería et al. [105] have controlled different morphologies of PLGA microparticles using an electrospray drying method. The morphology of the drug carrier particles were characterized by scanning electron microscopy (SEM) and transmission electron microscopy (TEM). To show how particle shape can affect the orientation, Champion et al. [106] illustrated that flexible disk-shaped red blood cells with a diameter less than 10 μm could pass through the spleen. However, if spherical-shaped nanoparticles were used, a diameter less than 200 nm could be used to pass through the spleen avoiding contact forces along vessel walls and other flow properties [106]. To achieve higher drug loading and eluting, drug-delivery vehicles can also be modified to possess large pore volumes and surface areas. For efficient drug delivery, a structure's height, diameter and thickness and its ultimate shape should be studied to better tailor drug-release efficacy.

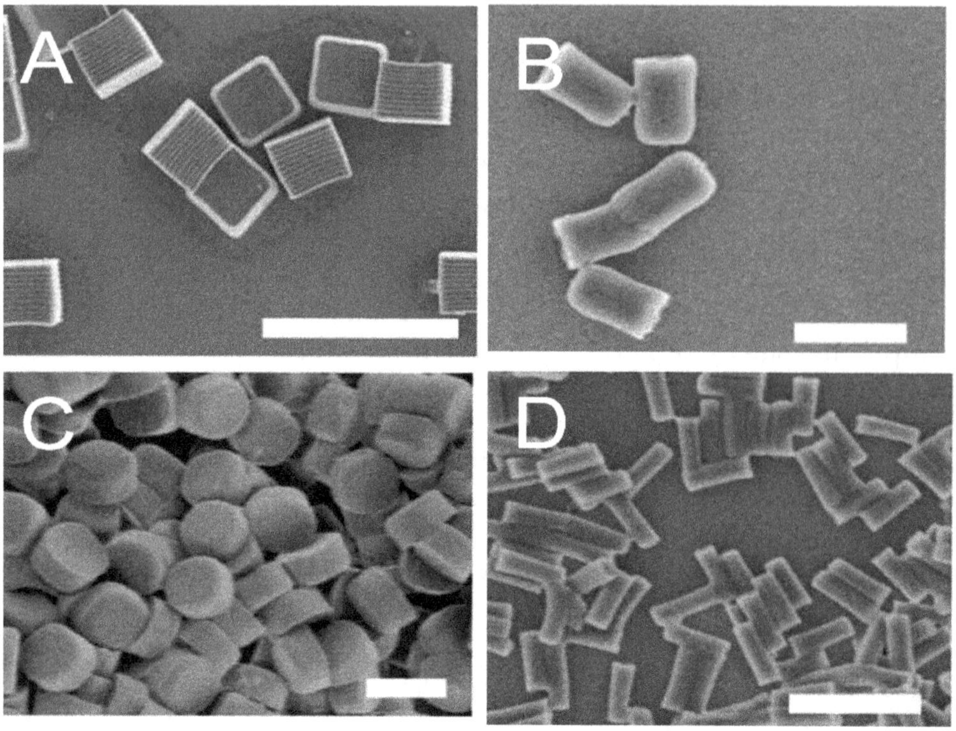

Figure 7. Micrographs of PRINT particles varying in both size and shape. The scale bars for (**A**) is 20 μm; (**B–D**) is 1 μm.

4.4. Porosity

Altering the porosity of a material is a common way to control drug delivery. Since surface area and permeability play an important part in drug-delivery vehicles, both the drug-loading capacity and release rate are directly associated with the porosity, pore size and pore interconnectivity of the material. Increasing the porosity percentage can enhance degradation and increase drug release in a polymer matrix, largely by the surface area to volume ratio. In order to achieve rapid drug delivery with a low percentage of pores, Itokazu et al. [107] developed an antibiotic-loaded hydroxyapatite ceramic scaffold with uniformly accessible pores, interlinked pore system, and enlarged macropores. Scaffold porosity may play an important role in determining drug-release kinetics [108,109].

5. Biomedical Applications

5.1. Bone Healing

Bone is an area of concentrated cellular and molecular organization, and any damage to the bone is considered a bone injury [110]. Bone tissue is capable of reconstruction following the time of injury. However, conditions exist such as osteoporosis resulting in weakened and brittle bones. Furthermore, bone is an area difficult to treat with drugs requiring heavy blood circulation [22]. The protein materials listed above with the various forms have been widely used to aid in bone healing. By providing access to drugs, stimuli, and other substances, protein-based drug delivery is part of the future of bone repair and bone strengthening.

For example, ELP depots can provide drug delivery not easily reached through blood circulation [22]. With a long half-life, the depots can be sustained for an extended period of time. These depots act as reservoirs of drugs and other substances favorable to treatment. The depots would be comprised of drug-loaded nanoparticles [22]. Taking advantage of the long half-life, the ELP depots can remain until sufficient drug has been released to induce adequate healing.

Collagen-based microparticles can also be employed for use in bone tissue regeneration [111]. To determine applicability, collagen-composite microparticle-based scaffolds were compared with non-collagen containing scaffolds [111] to demonstrate the statistical differences between the collagen and non-collagen models regarding degradation, cytocompatibility, porosity, and Young's modulus. Furthermore, new studies are being conducted to incorporate growth factors, antimicrobial substances, and other materials with collagen-based microparticles to heighten bone regeneration capabilities [111].

Silk, too, can be employed for bone tissue repair [112]. Silk scaffolds, similar to collagen, have the mechanical stability to be loaded into high-stress areas, such as bone. In contrast to collagen, the mechanical strength of bone can be achieved by silk materials without the need to chemically crosslink the proteins, lowering the probability of cellular toxicity, inflammatory response, and other undesired effects [112]. A study involved loading silk scaffolds with aspirin and using controlled drug release to determine the rate of skull tissue regeneration has been conducted in mice [14]. Silk and silk-composite scaffolds were tested, both showing effective drug release and tissue regeneration in vivo.

5.2. *Antibiotic Release*

Antibiotics date back to the early 1940s. The development of penicillin during this time revolutionized the world of medicine. One major area of study is the development of antibiotics with less bacterial resistance. However, another area of focus, administration, must not be overlooked [15]. There are areas of the body, such as bone and eyes, to which it is harder to administer antibiotics. Drug-loaded protein materials can aid in administering to rather difficult areas. Due to their tunable properties, drug release can be controlled in a substance that can match the mechanical properties and stress of natural tissue in those environments.

Drug-loaded silk films, microspheres, and hydrogels have all been shown to release penicillin and ampicillin tests proving in vivo efficacy in a murine infected wound model. Silk nanoparticles, in particular, have been shown to have high effectiveness when used in conjunction with metallic implants [113]. Several issues can arise when metallic and metal-based implants are first inserted. These include bacterial infection, inflammation, and implant loosening [114]. Titanium is a typical metal used in metal and metallic implants. A recent study infused silk nanoparticles with the antibiotic gentamicin [114]. The particles were then coated a titanium surface in an in vitro study. Over an 18-day period, the drug-loaded silk nanoparticles showed more efficient bacteria inhibition when compared to pure titanium [113].

Collagen hydrogels are also applicable for the sustained delivery of antibiotics [15]. For example, patented formulations for collagen hydrogels has been used to substitute daily eye drop administration [15]. Antibiotics or other drugs were first solidified into eye drop gels. By controlling biodegradation rate of collagen network, the gel can remain until the necessary dosages have been administered [15].

5.3. *Diabetes*

Diabetes is a condition that affects the way one's body reacts to insulin [115]. The most common forms of diabetes are type 1 and type 2. Type 1 diabetes indicates the pancreas's inability to produce a sufficient amount of insulin. As a result, patients must administer external insulin frequently. Type 2 diabetes is the most common form of diabetes, affecting 85–90% of diabetes patients [115]. This type of diabetes indicates insulin resistance or reduced insulin secretion with insulin resistance [115]. By 2025, diabetes is predicted to have affected 280 million patients worldwide [115]. As such, advances in treating diabetes are currently under heavy research. Improving drug release while reducing the frequency of administrations through, for example, protein materials, is within the realm of possibility.

Insulin is the key to aiding diabetes patients in reducing blood glucose levels. For about 80 years, hypodermic injections of insulin have been the standard method of insulin delivery. However, insulin activity is lost in the blood within 2–3 h. Preparing insulin bonded with silk nanoparticles increased the half-life by about 2.5 times more than pure insulin [43]. Crystalline silk nanoparticles were covalently bonded to insulin, showing high recovery from insulin-silk systems (>90%) [43].

ELP depots can also be used for diabetes treatment and complications from diabetes [116]. Treatment can be observed without having the depot directly in the disease site. Drugs for type 2 diabetes, such as glucagon-like peptide 1 (GLP-1), have potential therapeutic effects but require many administrations [22]. Due to the relatively quick degradation of GLP-1, an ELP-GLP-1 fusion depot was fabricated to provide a long-term and sustained admission of the drug [22]. This medication can be genetically fused to ELP molecules with arginine residues before the proteolytic cleavage of the arginine residues release the GLP-1 peptide drugs.

5.4. Cancer Treatment

Cancer is a disease that affects the formation of cells. It causes out-of-control cell growth, resulting in tumor build-up. Cancer has become one of the leading causes of death since the turn of the century. Administration of cancer-fighting drugs is an attractive area of study. The nature of cancer typically requires frequent administration, numerous clinical visits, and multiple procedures for drug administration. As a result, studies have turned to proteins for alternatives to the regular visits and administrations. Elastin and silk-based materials show potential in remedying such issues.

ELPs have tunable phase transition (temperature control), making them ideal for local and sustained drug delivery [22]. Cancerous tumors, for example, require prolonged drug delivery for treatment. Therefore, ELP depots were used for radiation therapy of cancerous tumors [22]. Adjusting ELP properties such as injection concentration and composition further optimized the depot for cancer treatment.

Silk nanoparticles can also be loaded with drugs such as curcumin and injected locally to areas with cancer cells. In vitro testing, for example, showed the killing of breast cancer cells over an eight-day period using drug-loaded silk nanoparticles [28]. Another study used desolvation to produce silk nanoparticles [28]. These particles improved the delivery of doxorubicin, a drug commonly used in chemotherapy, to the cancerous site [28].

5.5. Other Potential Applications

5.5.1. Neuroinflammation

Neuroinflammation is inflammation of the nervous tissue, resulting from brain injury, strokes, intracerebral hemorrhages, and other traumatic events [116]. Anti-inflammatory drugs are best administered locally. Using temperature-triggered ELP aggregation of nanoparticle depots can significantly decrease the loss of drug to circulation, optimizing the drug's contact to the site of inflammation [22].

5.5.2. Wound Healing

Surface wounds typically require disinfecting before covering with a bandage. Some injuries, however, require additional drugs for full treatment. Silk films have been tested for drug delivery and covering on skin surface [117]. In one study, silk and gelatin mixture was used in an in vitro test using rats [117]. Polyethylene glycol was added to the blend to reduce degradation speed. The result was promising, healing the wound in one week after the release of all of the drug loaded into the protein-composite film [117].

5.5.3. Corneal Regeneration

Corneal disease is the leading cause of blindness. The only widely accepted and effective treatment method is keratoplasty, a transplant from a healthy, human donor. With the shortage of donor tissue, the increasing demand for corneal graft replacements have made allogenic and synthetic materials the gold standard [118]. Although allogenic materials have excellent mechanical and physiological properties, their applicability is limited by quality-donor corneal graft availability, immunological rejection, and the risk of carrying viruses [18]. To address the shortages, synthetic-based polymers were developed. They are usually easy to process, modify and fabricate into any shape or structure to satisfy the patients' specifications. Nevertheless, synthetic keratoprostheses still require donor corneal tissue and can lead to other complications such as corneal melting, inflammation, necrosis, scarring, uveitis, and endophthalmitis [17]. To avoid the high costs of pre-transplant screening for transmissible pathogens and serious complications from a donor-derived infection in tissue banking, protein-based polymers, such as collagen, elastin, and silk proteins, can provide an excellent substitute for corneal regeneration [18]. To achieve key mechanical and physiological functions, Ghezzi et al. fabricated a three-dimensional (3D) silk culture system that closely resembled the native corneal stroma tissue [17]. As designed, the group showed seamless host-graft integration, cell organization and tissue regeneration in the stacked silk protein films after implantation. Protein-based polymer materials possess both physical and biofunctional properties needed to promote cell adhesion and cell proliferation as well as facilitate tissue repair.

6. Conclusions

Although the topic of controlled-release drug delivery is not new, advances in materials science have allowed for a diverse repertoire of new drug developments. Admission of such drugs can be achieved through various polymers and other materials. Synthetic polymers introduce the issue of biocompatibility, resulting in extensive testing to prove compatibility. Usage of various naturally occurring proteins and composites of such proteins show promise in improving drug delivery. Although biocompatibility must still be established, using naturally occurring proteins can minimize biocompatibility issues. Some drugs, for example, can also make use of the composition of the proteins used, binding to the amino acid components of the material.

This review focused on the properties and prospect of protein materials such as silk, collagen, elastin, and keratin. Each can be processed into various forms (microparticles, hydrogels, microneedles, etc.) to suit the application better. As research continues, more fabrication methods will arise, resulting in new diseases to be treated using proteins. Of course, there are still many challenges to be met. Some drugs, for example, may require development under high temperatures, which would denature proteins. In time, these challenges will be faced and overcome by fabricating thermally stable protein-composite materials. In time, development of other proteins with proven biomedical use can be adapted to drug-release applications. In time, the field will continue to grow, opening more avenues of research, more opportunities to fight disease, and more achievements in the area of science.

Acknowledgments: The authors would like to thank Maria Torculas for the initial support and assistance with this work. This study was supported by Rowan University Seed Research Grants, and New Jersey Health Foundation research program (PC111-17). Xiao Hu is also supported by the NSF Materials Eng. & Processing program (CMMI-1561966).

Author Contributions: Dave Jao, Ye Xue, Jethro Medina and Xiao Hu wrote the review paper together. All authors contributed equally to this work.

References

1. Bae, K.H.; Lee, F.; Xu, K.; Keng, C.T.; Tan, S.Y.; Tan, Y.J.; Chen, Q.; Kurisawa, M. Microstructured dextran hydrogels for burst-free sustained release of pegylated protein drugs. *Biomaterials* **2015**, *63*, 146–157. [CrossRef] [PubMed]
2. Peng, Z.; Li, S.; Han, X.; Al-Youbi, A.O.; Bashammakh, A.S.; El-Shahawi, M.S.; Leblanc, R.M. Determination of the composition, encapsulation efficiency and loading capacity in protein drug delivery systems using circular dichroism spectroscopy. *Anal. Chim. Acta* **2016**, *937*, 113–118. [CrossRef] [PubMed]
3. Hubbell, J.A.; Chilkoti, A. Nanomaterials for drug delivery. *Science* **2012**, *337*, 303–305. [CrossRef] [PubMed]

4. Garrait, G.; Beyssac, E.; Subirade, M. Development of a novel drug delivery system: Chitosan nanoparticles entrapped in alginate microparticles. *J. Microencapsul.* **2014**, *31*, 363–372. [CrossRef] [PubMed]
5. Paliwal, R.; Palakurthi, S. Zein in controlled drug delivery and tissue engineering. *J. Control. Release* **2014**, *189*, 108–122. [CrossRef] [PubMed]
6. Ferraro, V.; Anton, M.; Santé-Lhoutellier, V. The "sisters" α-helices of collagen, elastin and keratin recovered from animal by-products: Functionality, bioactivity and trends of application. *Trends Food Sci. Technol.* **2016**, *51*, 65–75. [CrossRef]
7. Rosenholm, J.M.; Meinander, A.; Peuhu, E.; Niemi, R.; Eriksson, J.E.; Sahlgren, C.; Lindén, M. Targeting of porous hybrid silica nanoparticles to cancer cells. *ACS Nano* **2008**, *3*, 197–206. [CrossRef] [PubMed]
8. Brennan, D.A.; Jao, D.; Siracusa, M.C.; Wilkinson, A.R.; Hu, X.; Beachley, V.Z. Concurrent collection and post-drawing of individual electrospun polymer nanofibers to enhance macromolecular alignment and mechanical properties. *Polymer* **2016**, *103*, 243–250. [CrossRef]
9. Van Herwaarden, S.; Iervolino, E.; Van Herwaarden, F.; Wijffels, T.; Leenaers, A.; Mathot, V. Design, performance and analysis of thermal lag of the ufs1 twin-calorimeter chip for fast scanning calorimetry using the mettler-toledo flash dsc 1. *Thermochim. Acta* **2011**, *522*, 46–52. [CrossRef]
10. Lee, J.W.; Park, J.-H.; Prausnitz, M.R. Dissolving microneedles for transdermal drug delivery. *Biomaterials* **2008**, *29*, 2113–2124. [CrossRef] [PubMed]
11. Lee, H.-J.; Ahn, S.-H.; Kim, G.H. Three-dimensional collagen/alginate hybrid scaffolds functionalized with a drug delivery system (dds) for bone tissue regeneration. *Chem. Mater.* **2011**, *24*, 881–891. [CrossRef]
12. Cilurzo, F.; Selmin, F.; Aluigi, A.; Bellosta, S. Regenerated keratin proteins as potential biomaterial for drug delivery. *Polym. Adv. Technol.* **2013**, *24*, 1025–1028. [CrossRef]
13. Srinivasan, B.; Kumar, R.; Shanmugam, K.; Sivagnam, U.T.; Reddy, N.P.; Sehgal, P.K. Porous keratin scaffold–promising biomaterial for tissue engineering and drug delivery. *J. Biomed. Mater. Res. Part B Appl. Biomater.* **2010**, *92*, 5–12. [CrossRef] [PubMed]
14. Zhang, J. Mesoporous bioglass/silk fibroin scaffolds as a drug delivery system: Fabrication, drug loading and release in vitro and repair calvarial defects in vivo. *J. Wuhan Univ. Technol.-Mater. Sci. Ed.* **2014**, *29*, 401–406. [CrossRef]
15. Friess, W. Collagen–biomaterial for drug delivery. *Eur. J. Pharm. Biopharm.* **1998**, *45*, 113–136. [CrossRef]
16. Rafat, M.; Li, F.; Fagerholm, P.; Lagali, N.S.; Watsky, M.A.; Munger, R.; Matsuura, T.; Griffith, M. Peg-stabilized carbodiimide crosslinked collagen–chitosan hydrogels for corneal tissue engineering. *Biomaterials* **2008**, *29*, 3960–3972. [CrossRef] [PubMed]
17. Ghezzi, C.E.; Marelli, B.; Omenetto, F.G.; Funderburgh, J.L.; Kaplan, D.L. 3D functional corneal stromal tissue equivalent based on corneal stromal stem cells and multi-layered silk film architecture. *PLoS ONE* **2017**, *12*. [CrossRef] [PubMed]
18. Zhao, X.; Song, W.; Liu, S.; Ren, L. Corneal regeneration by utilizing collagen based materials. *Sci. China Chem.* **2016**, *59*, 1548–1553. [CrossRef]
19. Almine, J.F.; Bax, D.V.; Mithieux, S.M.; Nivison-Smith, L.; Rnjak, J.; Waterhouse, A.; Wise, S.G.; Weiss, A.S. Elastin-based materials. *Chem. Soc. Rev.* **2010**, *39*, 3371–3379. [CrossRef] [PubMed]
20. Barenghi, R.; Beke, S.; Romano, I.; Gavazzo, P.; Farkas, B.; Vassalli, M.; Brandi, F.; Scaglione, S. Elastin-coated biodegradable photopolymer scaffolds for tissue engineering applications. *BioMed Res. Int.* **2014**. [CrossRef] [PubMed]
21. Chilkoti, A.; Christensen, T.; MacKay, J.A. Stimulus responsive elastin biopolymers: Applications in medicine and biotechnology. *Curr. Opin. Chem. Biol.* **2006**, *10*, 652–657. [CrossRef] [PubMed]
22. MacEwan, S.R.; Chilkoti, A. Applications of elastin-like polypeptides in drug delivery. *J. Control. Release* **2014**, *190*, 314–330. [CrossRef] [PubMed]
23. Annabi, N.; Mithieux, S.M.; Camci-Unal, G.; Dokmeci, M.R.; Weiss, A.S.; Khademhosseini, A. Elastomeric recombinant protein-based biomaterials. *Biochem. Eng. J.* **2013**, *77*, 110–118. [CrossRef] [PubMed]
24. Zhou, M.; Shmidov, Y.; Matson, J.B.; Bitton, R. Multi-scale characterization of thermoresponsive dendritic elastin-like peptides. *Colloids Surf. B Biointerfaces* **2017**, *153*, 141–151. [CrossRef] [PubMed]
25. Mobini, S.; Solati-Hashjin, M.; Peirovi, H.; Osman, N.A.A.; Gholipourmalekabadi, M.; Barati, M.; Samadikuchaksaraei, A. Bioactivity and biocompatibility studies on silk-based scaffold for bone tissue engineering. *J. Med. Biol. Eng.* **2013**, *33*, 207–214. [CrossRef]
26. Vollrath, F.; Porter, D. Spider silk as archetypal protein elastomer. *Soft Matter* **2006**, *2*, 377–385. [CrossRef]

27. Pritchard, E.M.; Hu, X.; Finley, V.; Kuo, C.K.; Kaplan, D.L. Effect of silk protein processing on drug delivery from silk films. *Macromol. Biosci.* **2013**, *13*, 311–320. [CrossRef] [PubMed]
28. Seib, F.P.; Kaplan, D.L. Silk for drug delivery applications: Opportunities and challenges. *Isr. J. Chem.* **2013**, *53*, 756–766. [CrossRef]
29. Kaplan, D.L.; Meinel, L. Silk-Based Drug Delivery System. Available online: https://www.google.com/patents/US20130195831 (accessed on 8 May 2017).
30. Teulé, F.; Miao, Y.-G.; Sohn, B.-H.; Kim, Y.-S.; Hull, J.J.; Fraser, M.J.; Lewis, R.V.; Jarvis, D.L. Silkworms transformed with chimeric silkworm/spider silk genes spin composite silk fibers with improved mechanical properties. *Proc. Natl. Acad. Sci. USA* **2012**, *109*, 923–928. [CrossRef] [PubMed]
31. Xia, X.-X.; Qian, Z.-G.; Ki, C.S.; Park, Y.H.; Kaplan, D.L.; Lee, S.Y. Native-sized recombinant spider silk protein produced in metabolically engineered escherichia coli results in a strong fiber. *Proc. Natl. Acad. Sci. USA* **2010**, *107*, 14059–14063. [CrossRef] [PubMed]
32. Qin, G.; Hu, X.; Cebe, P.; Kaplan, D.L. Mechanism of resilin elasticity. *Nat. Commun.* **2012**. [CrossRef] [PubMed]
33. Li, L.; Tong, Z.; Jia, X.; Kiick, K.L. Resilin-like polypeptide hydrogels engineered for versatile biological function. *Soft Matter* **2013**, *9*, 665–673. [CrossRef] [PubMed]
34. McGann, C.L.; Levenson, E.A.; Kiick, K.L. Resilin-based hybrid hydrogels for cardiovascular tissue engineering. *Macromol. Chem. Phys.* **2013**, *214*, 203–213. [CrossRef] [PubMed]
35. Sousa, F.; Luzardo-Álvarez, A.; Blanco-Méndez, J.; Martín-Pastor, M. Nmr techniques in drug delivery: Application to zein protein complexes. *Int. J. Pharm.* **2012**, *439*, 41–48. [CrossRef] [PubMed]
36. Bouman, J.; Belton, P.; Venema, P.; van der Linden, E.; de Vries, R.; Qi, S. Controlled release from zein matrices: Interplay of drug hydrophobicity and ph. *Pharm. Res.* **2016**, *33*, 673–685. [CrossRef] [PubMed]
37. Nonthanum, P.; Lee, Y.; Padua, G.W. Effect of γ-zein on the rheological behavior of concentrated zein solutions. *J. Agric. Food Chem.* **2012**, *60*, 1742–1747. [CrossRef] [PubMed]
38. Ramshaw, J.A.; Werkmeister, J.A.; Glattauer, V. Collagen-based biomaterials. *Biotechnol. Genet. Eng. Rev.* **1996**, *13*, 335–382. [CrossRef] [PubMed]
39. Lickorish, D.; Ramshaw, J.A.; Werkmeister, J.A.; Glattauer, V.; Howlett, C.R. Collagen–hydroxyapatite composite prepared by biomimetic process. *J. Biomed. Mater. Res. Part A* **2004**, *68*, 19–27. [CrossRef] [PubMed]
40. Sionkowska, A.; Kozłowska, J. Properties and modification of porous 3-d collagen/hydroxyapatite composites. *Int. J. Biol. Macromol.* **2013**, *52*, 250–259. [CrossRef] [PubMed]
41. Sell, S.A.; McClure, M.J.; Garg, K.; Wolfe, P.S.; Bowlin, G.L. Electrospinning of collagen/biopolymers for regenerative medicine and cardiovascular tissue engineering. *Adv. Drug Deliv. Rev.* **2009**, *61*, 1007–1019. [CrossRef] [PubMed]
42. Lee, J.; Macosko, C.W.; Urry, D.W. Swelling behavior of γ-irradiation cross-linked elastomeric polypentapeptide-based hydrogels. *Macromolecules* **2001**, *34*, 4114–4123. [CrossRef]
43. Yan, H.-B.; Zhang, Y.-Q.; Ma, Y.-L.; Zhou, L.-X. Biosynthesis of insulin-silk fibroin nanoparticles conjugates and in vitro evaluation of a drug delivery system. *J. Nanoparticle Res.* **2009**, *11*, 1937–1946. [CrossRef]
44. Srokowski, E.M.; Woodhouse, K.A. Development and characterisation of novel cross-linked bio-elastomeric materials. *J. Biomater. Sci. Polym. Ed.* **2008**, *19*, 785–799. [CrossRef] [PubMed]
45. Cappello, J.; Textor, G.; Bauerle, B. Bioresorption of implanted protein polymer films controlled by adjustment of their silk/elastin block lengths. In *Industrial Biotechnological Polymers*; Technomic Publishing Company: Lancaster, UK, 1995; pp. 249–256.
46. Nowatzki, P.J.; Tirrell, D.A. Physical properties of artificial extracellular matrix protein films prepared by isocyanate crosslinking. *Biomaterials* **2004**, *25*, 1261–1267. [CrossRef]
47. Huang, L.; McMillan, R.A.; Apkarian, R.P.; Pourdeyhimi, B.; Conticello, V.P.; Chaikof, E.L. Generation of synthetic elastin-mimetic small diameter fibers and fiber networks. *Macromolecules* **2000**, *33*, 2989–2997. [CrossRef]
48. Lee, J.; Macosko, C.W.; Urry, D.W. Elastomeric polypentapeptides cross-linked into matrixes and fibers. *Biomacromolecules* **2001**, *2*, 170–179. [CrossRef] [PubMed]
49. Tachibana, A.; Kaneko, S.; Tanabe, T.; Yamauchi, K. Rapid fabrication of keratin–hydroxyapatite hybrid sponges toward osteoblast cultivation and differentiation. *Biomaterials* **2005**, *26*, 297–302. [CrossRef] [PubMed]

50. Sierpinski, P.; Garrett, J.; Ma, J.; Apel, P.; Klorig, D.; Smith, T.; Koman, L.A.; Atala, A.; Van Dyke, M. The use of keratin biomaterials derived from human hair for the promotion of rapid regeneration of peripheral nerves. *Biomaterials* **2008**, *29*, 118–128. [CrossRef] [PubMed]
51. Apel, P.J.; Garrett, J.P.; Sierpinski, P.; Ma, J.; Atala, A.; Smith, T.L.; Koman, L.A.; Van Dyke, M.E. Peripheral nerve regeneration using a keratin-based scaffold: Long-term functional and histological outcomes in a mouse model. *J. Hand Surg.* **2008**, *33*, 1541–1547. [CrossRef] [PubMed]
52. Aboushwareb, T.; Eberli, D.; Ward, C.; Broda, C.; Holcomb, J.; Atala, A.; Van Dyke, M. A keratin biomaterial gel hemostat derived from human hair: Evaluation in a rabbit model of lethal liver injury. *J. Biomed. Mater. Res. Part B Appl. Biomater.* **2009**, *90*, 45–54. [CrossRef] [PubMed]
53. Tanabe, T.; Okitsu, N.; Tachibana, A.; Yamauchi, K. Preparation and characterization of keratin–chitosan composite film. *Biomaterials* **2002**, *23*, 817–825. [CrossRef]
54. Zoccola, M.; Aluigi, A.; Vineis, C.; Tonin, C.; Ferrero, F.; Piacentino, M.G. Study on cast membranes and electrospun nanofibers made from keratin/fibroin blends. *Biomacromolecules* **2008**, *9*, 2819–2825. [CrossRef] [PubMed]
55. Li, L.; Teller, S.; Clifton, R.J.; Jia, X.; Kiick, K.L. Tunable mechanical stability and deformation response of a resilin-based elastomer. *Biomacromolecules* **2011**, *12*, 2302. [CrossRef] [PubMed]
56. Renner, J.N.; Cherry, K.M.; Su, R.S.-C.; Liu, J.C. Characterization of resilin-based materials for tissue engineering applications. *Biomacromolecules* **2012**, *13*, 3678–3685. [CrossRef] [PubMed]
57. Straley, K.S.; Heilshorn, S.C. Independent tuning of multiple biomaterial properties using protein engineering. *Soft Matter* **2009**, *5*, 114–124. [CrossRef]
58. Koria, P.; Yagi, H.; Kitagawa, Y.; Megeed, Z.; Nahmias, Y.; Sheridan, R.; Yarmush, M.L. Self-assembling elastin-like peptides growth factor chimeric nanoparticles for the treatment of chronic wounds. *Proc. Natl. Acad. Sci. USA* **2011**, *108*, 1034–1039. [CrossRef] [PubMed]
59. Gellynck, K.; Verdonk, P.C.; Van Nimmen, E.; Almqvist, K.F.; Gheysens, T.; Schoukens, G.; Van Langenhove, L.; Kiekens, P.; Mertens, J.; Verbruggen, G. Silkworm and spider silk scaffolds for chondrocyte support. *J. Mater. Sci. Mater. Med.* **2008**, *19*, 3399–3409. [CrossRef] [PubMed]
60. Huemmerich, D.; Slotta, U.; Scheibel, T. Processing and modification of films made from recombinant spider silk proteins. *Appl. Phys. A Mater. Sci. Proc.* **2006**, *82*, 219–222. [CrossRef]
61. Hermanson, K.D.; Huemmerich, D.; Scheibel, T.; Bausch, A.R. Engineered microcapsules fabricated from reconstituted spider silk. *Adv. Mater.* **2007**, *19*, 1810–1815. [CrossRef]
62. Lammel, A.; Schwab, M.; Hofer, M.; Winter, G.; Scheibel, T. Recombinant spider silk particles as drug delivery vehicles. *Biomaterials* **2011**, *32*, 2233–2240. [CrossRef] [PubMed]
63. Lai, H.-M.; Padua, G.W. Properties and microstructure of plasticized zein films. *Cereal Chem.* **1997**, *74*, 771–775. [CrossRef]
64. Liu, X.; Sun, Q.; Wang, H.; Zhang, L.; Wang, J.-Y. Microspheres of corn protein, zein, for an ivermectin drug delivery system. *Biomaterials* **2005**, *26*, 109–115. [CrossRef] [PubMed]
65. Yao, C.; Li, Y.; Wu, F. Zein nanofibrous membranes as templates for biomineralization of hydroxyapatite crystallites. *Polym. Compos.* **2013**, *34*, 1163–1171. [CrossRef]
66. Li, Y.; Yao, C. Mineralization of hydroxyapatite crystallites on zein microspheres. *Polym. Compos.* **2012**, *33*, 961–966. [CrossRef]
67. Wang, X.; Yucel, T.; Lu, Q.; Hu, X.; Kaplan, D.L. Silk nanospheres and microspheres from silk/pva blend films for drug delivery. *Biomaterials* **2010**, *31*, 1025–1035. [CrossRef] [PubMed]
68. Gil, C.S.; Gil, V.S.; Carvalho, S.M.; Silva, G.R.; Magalhães, J.T.; Oréfice, R.L.; Mansur, A.; Mansur, H.S.; Patricio, P.S.; Oliveira, L.C. Recycled collagen films as biomaterials for controlled drug delivery. *New J. Chem.* **2016**, *40*, 8502–8510. [CrossRef]
69. Sahiner, M.; Alpaslan, D.; Bitlisli, B.O. Collagen-based hydrogel films as drug-delivery devices with antimicrobial properties. *Polym. Bull.* **2014**, *71*, 3017–3033. [CrossRef]
70. Mwangi, T.K.; Bowles, R.D.; Tainter, D.M.; Bell, R.D.; Kaplan, D.L.; Setton, L.A. Synthesis and characterization of silk fibroin microparticles for intra-articular drug delivery. *Int. J. Pharm.* **2015**, *485*, 7–14. [CrossRef] [PubMed]
71. Zhao, Z.; Li, Y.; Xie, M.-B. Silk fibroin-based nanoparticles for drug delivery. *Int. J. Mol. Sci.* **2015**, *16*, 4880–4903. [CrossRef] [PubMed]

72. Ciofani, G.; Genchi, G.G.; Guardia, P.; Mazzolai, B.; Mattoli, V.; Bandiera, A. Recombinant human elastin-like magnetic microparticles for drug delivery and targeting. *Macromol. Biosci.* **2014**, *14*, 632–642. [CrossRef] [PubMed]
73. Yamada, M.; Hori, A.; Sugaya, S.; Yajima, Y.; Utoh, R.; Yamato, M.; Seki, M. Cell-sized condensed collagen microparticles for preparing microengineered composite spheroids of primary hepatocytes. *Lab Chip* **2015**, *15*, 3941–3951. [CrossRef] [PubMed]
74. Joscelyne, S.M.; Trägårdh, G. Membrane emulsification—A literature review. *J. Membr. Sci.* **2000**, *169*, 107–117. [CrossRef]
75. Numata, K.; Yamazaki, S.; Naga, N. Biocompatible and biodegradable dual-drug release system based on silk hydrogel containing silk nanoparticles. *Biomacromolecules* **2012**, *13*, 1383–1389. [CrossRef] [PubMed]
76. Ita, K. Transdermal delivery of drugs with microneedles—Potential and challenges. *Pharmaceutics* **2015**, *7*, 90–105. [CrossRef] [PubMed]
77. Sivamani, R.K.; Stoeber, B.; Wu, G.C.; Zhai, H.; Liepmann, D.; Maibach, H. Clinical microneedle injection of methyl nicotinate: Stratum corneum penetration. *Skin Res. Technol.* **2005**, *11*, 152–156. [CrossRef] [PubMed]
78. Tsioris, K.; Raja, W.K.; Pritchard, E.M.; Panilaitis, B.; Kaplan, D.L.; Omenetto, F.G. Fabrication of silk microneedles for controlled-release drug delivery. *Adv. Funct. Mater.* **2012**, *22*, 330–335. [CrossRef]
79. Singaravelu, S.; Ramanathan, G.; Raja, M.; Nagiah, N.; Padmapriya, P.; Kaveri, K.; Sivagnanam, U.T. Biomimetic interconnected porous keratin–fibrin–gelatin 3d sponge for tissue engineering application. *Int. J. Biol. Macromol.* **2016**, *86*, 810–819. [CrossRef] [PubMed]
80. Li, Q.; Zhu, L.; Liu, R.; Huang, D.; Jin, X.; Che, N.; Li, Z.; Qu, X.; Kang, H.; Huang, Y. Biological stimuli responsive drug carriers based on keratin for triggerable drug delivery. *J. Mater. Chem.* **2012**, *22*, 19964–19973. [CrossRef]
81. Han, S.; Ham, T.R.; Haque, S.; Sparks, J.L.; Saul, J.M. Alkylation of human hair keratin for tunable hydrogel erosion and drug delivery in tissue engineering applications. *Acta Biomater.* **2015**, *23*, 201–213. [CrossRef] [PubMed]
82. Chen, Y.; Youn, P.; Furgeson, D. Thermo-targeted drug delivery of geldanamycin to hyperthermic tumor margins with diblock elastin-based biopolymers. *J. Control. Release* **2011**, *155*, 175–183. [CrossRef] [PubMed]
83. Dash, B.C.; Mahor, S.; Carroll, O.; Mathew, A.; Wang, W.; Woodhouse, K.A.; Pandit, A. Tunable elastin-like polypeptide hollow sphere as a high payload and controlled delivery gene depot. *J. Control. Release* **2011**, *152*, 382–392. [CrossRef] [PubMed]
84. Kim, M.S.; Lee, D.-W.; Park, K.; Park, S.-J.; Choi, E.-J.; Park, E.S.; Kim, H.R. Temperature-triggered tumor-specific delivery of anticancer agents by crgd-conjugated thermosensitive liposomes. *Colloids Surf. B Biointerfaces* **2014**, *116*, 17–25. [CrossRef] [PubMed]
85. Barbaresso, R.C.; Rău, I.; Zgârian, R.G.; Meghea, A.; Ghica, M.V. Niflumic acid-collagen delivery systems used as anti-inflammatory drugs and analgesics in dentistry. *C. R. Chim.* **2014**, *17*, 12–17. [CrossRef]
86. Wu, H.; Liu, S.; Xiao, L.; Dong, X.; Lu, Q.; Kaplan, D.L. Injectable and ph-responsive silk nanofiber hydrogels for sustained anticancer drug delivery. *ACS Appl. Mater. Interfaces* **2016**, *8*, 17118–17126. [CrossRef] [PubMed]
87. Pritchard, E.M.; Kaplan, D.L. Silk fibroin biomaterials for controlled release drug delivery. *Expert Opin. Drug Deliv.* **2011**, *8*, 797–811. [CrossRef] [PubMed]
88. Wilz, A.; Pritchard, E.M.; Li, T.; Lan, J.-Q.; Kaplan, D.L.; Boison, D. Silk polymer-based adenosine release: Therapeutic potential for epilepsy. *Biomaterials* **2008**, *29*, 3609–3616. [CrossRef] [PubMed]
89. Pandit, M.; Sagar, A.J.; Rao, M.N. Studies on silk fibroin. I. Molecular weight, sedimentation coefficient, viscosity and optical rotation of silk fibroin from carbonate-extracted silk fiber. *Archiv. Biochem. Biophys.* **1972**, *149*, 259–268. [CrossRef]
90. Yamada, H.; Nakao, H.; Takasu, Y.; Tsubouchi, K. Preparation of undegraded native molecular fibroin solution from silkworm cocoons. *Mater. Sci. Eng. C* **2001**, *14*, 41–46. [CrossRef]
91. Fang, J.-Y.; Chen, J.-P.; Leu, Y.-L.; Wang, H.-Y. Characterization and evaluation of silk protein hydrogels for drug delivery. *Chem. Pharm. Bull.* **2006**, *54*, 156–162. [CrossRef] [PubMed]
92. Tang, F.; Li, L.; Chen, D. Mesoporous silica nanoparticles: Synthesis, biocompatibility and drug delivery. *Adv. Mater.* **2012**, *24*, 1504–1534. [CrossRef] [PubMed]
93. Brannon-Peppas, L.; Blanchette, J.O. Nanoparticle and targeted systems for cancer therapy. *Adv. Drug Deliv. Rev.* **2004**, *56*, 1649–1659. [CrossRef] [PubMed]

94. Widder, K.J.; Senyei, A.E.; Scarpelli, D.G. Magnetic microspheres: A model system for site specific drug delivery in vivo. *Exp. Biol. Med.* **1978**, *158*, 141–146. [CrossRef]
95. Alexiou, C.; Arnold, W.; Klein, R.J.; Parak, F.G.; Hulin, P.; Bergemann, C.; Erhardt, W.; Wagenpfeil, S.; Luebbe, A.S. Locoregional cancer treatment with magnetic drug targeting. *Cancer Res.* **2000**, *60*, 6641–6648. [PubMed]
96. Mody, V.V.; Cox, A.; Shah, S.; Singh, A.; Bevins, W.; Parihar, H. Magnetic nanoparticle drug delivery systems for targeting tumor. *Appl. Nanosci.* **2014**, *4*, 385–392. [CrossRef]
97. Lu, F.; Wu, S.H.; Hung, Y.; Mou, C.Y. Size effect on cell uptake in well-suspended, uniform mesoporous silica nanoparticles. *Small* **2009**, *5*, 1408–1413. [CrossRef] [PubMed]
98. Park, J.H.; Saravanakumar, G.; Kim, K.; Kwon, I.C. Targeted delivery of low molecular drugs using chitosan and its derivatives. *Adv. Drug Deliv. Rev.* **2010**, *62*, 28–41. [CrossRef] [PubMed]
99. Jun, Y.-W.; Choi, J.-S.; Cheon, J. Heterostructured magnetic nanoparticles: Their versatility and high performance capabilities. *Chem. Commun.* **2007**, 1203–1214. [CrossRef] [PubMed]
100. Foo, C.W.P.; Patwardhan, S.V.; Belton, D.J.; Kitchel, B.; Anastasiades, D.; Huang, J.; Naik, R.R.; Perry, C.C.; Kaplan, D.L. Novel nanocomposites from spider silk–silica fusion (chimeric) proteins. *Proc. Natl. Acad. Sci. USA* **2006**, *103*, 9428–9433.
101. Mieszawska, A.J.; Fourligas, N.; Georgakoudi, I.; Ouhib, N.M.; Belton, D.J.; Perry, C.C.; Kaplan, D.L. Osteoinductive silk–silica composite biomaterials for bone regeneration. *Biomaterials* **2010**, *31*, 8902–8910. [CrossRef] [PubMed]
102. Cai, Q.; Luo, Z.-S.; Pang, W.-Q.; Fan, Y.-W.; Chen, X.-H.; Cui, F.-Z. Dilute solution routes to various controllable morphologies of mcm-41 silica with a basic medium. *Chem. Mater.* **2001**, *13*, 258–263. [CrossRef]
103. Gratton, S.E.; Ropp, P.A.; Pohlhaus, P.D.; Luft, J.C.; Madden, V.J.; Napier, M.E.; DeSimone, J.M. The effect of particle design on cellular internalization pathways. *Proc. Natl. Acad. Sci. USA* **2008**, *105*, 11613–11618. [CrossRef] [PubMed]
104. Chun, A.L. Nanoparticles: Shape also matters. *Nat. Nanotechnol.* **2008**. [CrossRef]
105. Almería, B.; Deng, W.; Fahmy, T.M.; Gomez, A. Controlling the morphology of electrospray-generated plga microparticles for drug delivery. *J. Colloid Interface Sci.* **2010**, *343*, 125–133. [CrossRef] [PubMed]
106. Champion, J.A.; Katare, Y.K.; Mitragotri, S. Particle shape: A new design parameter for micro- and nanoscale drug delivery carriers. *J. Control. Release* **2007**, *121*, 3–9. [CrossRef] [PubMed]
107. Itokazu, M.; Yang, W.; Aoki, T.; Ohara, A.; Kato, N. Synthesis of antibiotic-loaded interporous hydroxyapatite blocks by vacuum method and in vitro drug release testing. *Biomaterials* **1998**, *19*, 817–819. [CrossRef]
108. Kundu, B.; Soundrapandian, C.; Nandi, S.K.; Mukherjee, P.; Dandapat, N.; Roy, S.; Datta, B.K.; Mandal, T.K.; Basu, D.; Bhattacharya, R.N. Development of new localized drug delivery system based on ceftriaxone-sulbactam composite drug impregnated porous hydroxyapatite: A systematic approach for in vitro and in vivo animal trial. *Pharm. Res.* **2010**, *27*, 1659–1676. [CrossRef] [PubMed]
109. Horcajada, P.; Serre, C.; Vallet-Regí, M.; Sebban, M.; Taulelle, F.; Férey, G. Metal–organic frameworks as efficient materials for drug delivery. *Angew. Chem.* **2006**, *118*, 6120–6124. [CrossRef]
110. Athanasou, N.A. Pathology of bone injury. *Diagn. Histopathol.* **2009**, *15*, 437–443. [CrossRef]
111. Zugravu, M.V.; Smith, R.A.; Reves, B.T.; Jennings, J.A.; Cooper, J.O.; Haggard, W.O.; Bumgardner, J.D. Physical properties and in vitro evaluation of collagen–chitosan–calcium phosphate microparticle-based scaffolds for bone tissue regeneration. *J. Biomater. Appl.* **2012**. [CrossRef] [PubMed]
112. Wenk, E.; Merkle, H.P.; Meinel, L. Silk fibroin as a vehicle for drug delivery applications. *J. Control. Release* **2011**, *150*, 128–141. [CrossRef] [PubMed]
113. Sharma, S.; Bano, S.; Ghosh, A.S.; Mandal, M.; Kim, H.-W.; Dey, T.; Kundu, S.C. Silk fibroin nanoparticles support in vitro sustained antibiotic release and osteogenesis on titanium surface. *Nanomed. Nanotechnol. Biol. Med.* **2016**, *12*, 1193–1204. [CrossRef] [PubMed]
114. Chen, Q.; Thouas, G.A. Metallic implant biomaterials. *Mater. Sci. Eng. R: Rep.* **2015**, *87*, 1–57. [CrossRef]
115. Donath, M.Y.; Shoelson, S.E. Type 2 diabetes as an inflammatory disease. *Nat. Rev. Immunol.* **2011**, *11*, 98–107. [CrossRef] [PubMed]
116. Chow, J.P.; Simionescu, D.T.; Warner, H.; Wang, B.; Patnaik, S.S.; Liao, J.; Simionescu, A. Mitigation of diabetes-related complications in implanted collagen and elastin scaffolds using matrix-binding polyphenol. *Biomaterials* **2013**, *34*, 685–695. [CrossRef] [PubMed]

117. Alam, A.M.; Shubhra, Q.T. Surface modified thin film from silk and gelatin for sustained drug release to heal wound. *J. Mater. Chem. B* **2015**, *3*, 6473–6479. [CrossRef]
118. Salehi, S.; Fathi, M.; Javanmard, S.H.; Bahners, T.; Gutmann, J.S.; Ergün, S.; Steuhl, K.P.; Fuchsluger, T.A. Generation of pgs/pcl blend nanofibrous scaffolds mimicking corneal stroma structure. *Macromol. Mater. Eng.* **2014**, *299*, 455–469. [CrossRef]

3

Ethylcellulose–A Pharmaceutical Excipient with Multidirectional Application in Drug Dosage Forms Development

Katarzyna Wasilewska and Katarzyna Winnicka *

Department of Pharmaceutical Technology, Medical University of Bialystok, Mickiewicza 2c, 15-222 Bialystok, Poland; katarzyna.wasilewska@umb.edu.pl

* Correspondence: kwin@umb.edu.pl

Abstract: Polymers constitute the most important group of excipients utilized in modern pharmaceutical technology, playing an essential role in the development of drug dosage forms. Synthetic, semisynthetic, and natural polymeric materials offer opportunities to overcome different formulative challenges and to design novel dosage forms for controlled release or for site-specific drug delivery. They are extensively used to design therapeutic systems, modify drug release, or mask unpleasant drug taste. Cellulose derivatives are characterized by different physicochemical properties, such as swellability, viscosity, biodegradability, pH dependency, or mucoadhesion, which determine their use in industry. One cellulose derivative with widespread application is ethylcellulose. Ethylcellulose is used in pharmaceutical technology as a coating agent, flavoring fixative, binder, filler, film-former, drug carrier, or stabilizer. The aim of this article is to provide a broad overview of ethylcellulose utilization for pharmaceutical purposes, with particular emphasis on its multidirectional role in the development of oral and topical drug dosage forms.

Keywords: ethylcellulose; polymeric material; cellulose derivative; pharmaceutical excipient

---

1. Introduction

Modern pharmaceutical technology could not exist without polymers, which play an integral role in the advancement of drug delivery (e.g., by providing controlled release of therapeutic agents, masking bitter taste of drugs, or serving as carriers in targeted therapy). They have a wide range of physicochemical characteristics according to their molecular weight and configuration. Therefore, polymers approved for use in medicines are receiving considerable attention as essential excipients in the development of different drug dosage forms. Cellulose derivatives are an important group among the most commonly used polymers in pharmaceutical technology. Cellulose is one of the most abundant polymers in nature. It is produced by photosynthesis and constitutes a basic plant component. It is a linear polymer composed of glucopyranose residues, where the units are connected by 1,4-β-glycosidic bonds. It is a tasteless and odorless component with fibrous structure that is practically insoluble both in cold and hot water. Among the cellulose modifiers, its esters and ethers are of practical importance. Cellulose-based biomaterials are widely utilized as biocompatible templates for designing novel drug delivery systems with a wide range of pharmaceutical applications via different routes and pharmacotherapeutic purposes [1–4].

Ethylcellulose (EC), an ethyl ether of cellulose, is a free-flowing, white to light-tan powder prepared from wood pulp or cotton that is used in pharmaceutical manufacturing industries. The European Pharmacopoeia (Ph. Eur.) and United States Pharmacopoeia (USP) monographs describe EC as partially O-ethylated cellulose [5–7]. EC with ethoxyl substitution molecular formula is $C_{12}H_{23}O_6(C_{12}H_{22}O_5)nC_{12}H_{23}O_5$, where n can vary in order to provide a wide variety of molecular weights, which affect its properties. It is insoluble at any pH that occurs in organisms, but it undergoes swelling in the presence of gastric juice [3,4]. There is very limited data detailing possible side effects of EC, hence it is generally regarded as safe (GRAS) and included in the US Food and Drug Administration (FDA) Inactive Ingredients database as well as in the Canadian List of Acceptable Non-medicinal Ingredients to be utilized in oral capsules, suspensions, tablets, topical emulsions, and vaginal or ocular preparations. In contrast to other polymers which are insoluble in the gastrointestinal tract (e.g., nitrocellulose, cellulose acetate, Eudragit RL, or Eudragit RS), EC is characterized as a non-ionic material, having the advantage of being non-reactive. Moreover, safety data on utilizing cellulose acetate and methacrylic acid copolymers in pediatric preparations are limited, while EC is clinically tested and approved for use in pediatric formulations. EC is also allowed for use in non-parenteral medicines licensed in Europe. The polymer is accepted for use as a food additive because it is a non-calorific and metabolically inert substance following oral consumption. As EC is not considered to be a health hazard, the World Health Organisation (WHO) has not specified its acceptable daily intake [4,8,9]. According to the intended use, the commercially available EC can be classified in two categories of products: industrial grade and pharmaceutical grade. For the pharmaceutical grade, the quality standard should meet USP, Ph. Eur., Chinese Pharmacopoeia, and Japanese Pharmacopoeia standards [6,7,10,11].

2. Physicochemical Characteristics of EC

The polymer is obtained by synthesis (etherification) through the substitution of the cellulose hydroxyl groups with ethoxyl ones. The chemical reaction involves cellulose dissolution in sodium hydroxide aqueous solution, which leads to degradation of the cellulose's molecular structure. This results in the formation of an alkali cellulose and exposure of the cellulose hydroxyl group for reaction. Afterwards, ethyl chloride gas is added to the reaction medium, leading to bonding with the alkalized cellulose. EC, sodium chloride, and water are formed (Figure 1) [1–5].

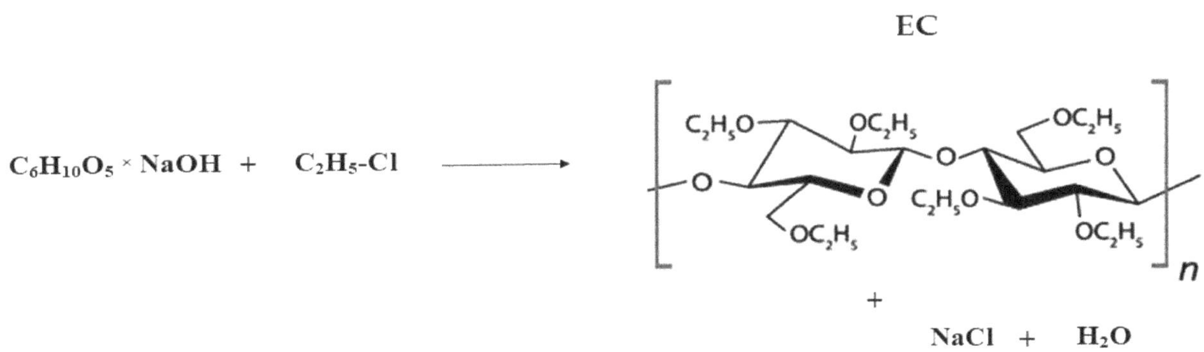

Figure 1. Schematic illustration of ethylcellulose (EC) obtainment.

EC contains 44–51% ethoxyl groups (-OC_2H_5) and is composed of β-anhydroglucose units joined together via acetal linkage. EC is a biocompatible, non-allergenic, nonirritant, colorless, odorless, and tasteless hydrophobic polymer soluble in a wide variety of organic solvents (alcohols, ketones, and polycyclic aromatic hydrocarbons), but does not dissolve in water, glycerin, or propylene glycol. EC that contains no less than 46.5% of ethoxyl groups is freely soluble in chloroform, ethanol, ethyl acetate, methanol, and toluene. EC is compatible with a wide array of excipients and most of the plasticizers used in pharmaceutical formulations, and therefore can be well mixed with many softeners, oils, and waxes (dibutyl phthalate, diethyl phthalate, dibutyl sebacate, triethyl citrate, tributyl citrate, acetylated monoglyceride, butyl and glycol esters of fatty acids, refined mineral oils, oleic acid, stearic acid, stearyl alcohol, castor oil). It shows incompatibilities with paraffin and microcrystalline wax. EC exhibits a high degree of stability within pH 3–11, making it useful both in acidic and alkaline mixtures. EC is also slightly hygroscopic, absorbing very little water from humid air or during immersion. In addition, it can form tough and tensile films and maintains flexibility even at low temperatures. It possesses good thermal stability and low ash content when burning [1,3–5].

The physical characteristic of EC types and their performance depends on the degree of etherification or substitution (ethoxyl content), molecular uniformity, and molecular weight of the cellulosic backbone. Solubility in organic solvents is achieved with degree of substitution (DS) values between 2.2 and 2.6. A range of commercial products is available with a degree of substitution between 2.15 and 2.60, corresponding to a range of ethoxyl contents from 43% to 50%. At low DS values (0.8–1.3), the replacement of some of the hydroxyl groups by ethoxyl groups reduces the hydrogen bonding across the cellulosic chains to such an extent that the material is soluble in water. Further replacement of hydroxyl groups by the less polar and more hydrocarbon ethoxyl groups increases the water resistance. Fully etherified EC is soluble only in non-polar solvents [1–5].

The molecular weight can be regulated by controlled degradation of the alkali cellulose in the presence of air. This can be done either before or during etherification. The molecular weight of commercial grades is usually expressed indirectly as viscosity. The completely etherified material with a degree of substitution of 3 has an ethoxyl content of 54.88%. The viscosities are determined using a capillary viscometer and recorded in millipascal-seconds (mPa·s) or centipoise (cP) synonymous for a 5% *w/w* solution in toluene/ethanol solvent mixture (80:20), being determined at 25 °C and expressed in mPa·s. For each viscosity grade of EC, the pharmacopoeial specification allows variation of 80–120% within the stated nominal viscosity (depending on manufacturer). Several types of EC (e.g., Ethocel™ 4, Ethocel™ 10, and Ethocel™ 45) differ in the length of the polymer chains, the rate of dissolution, and the viscosity of their solutions. The mechanical properties are largely determined by chain length; softening point, hardness, water absorption, and solubility are rather more influenced by the degree of substitution [1–5,12,13].

EC viscosities increase with the increase in the polymeric backbone chain length. The impact of EC molecular weight variation (measured by viscosity) on the drug release was determined by Mehta et al. Metoprolol was selected as a model drug that is highly soluble in water and acetaminophen as one with low aqueous solubility. Drug-layered sugar spheres were coated with EC of different viscosity grades at varying coating weight gains, and their drug release profiles were determined. The study revealed that viscosity variation within the manufacturer's specifications of EC (Ethocel™ 10, 20, and 100 cP) had a minimal effect on release of model drugs. Acetaminophen multiparticulates exhibited slower drug release and longer lag time when compared to the metoprolol beads. The obtained results can be associated with the lower aqueous solubility of acetaminophen compared to metoprolol. Based on the study, it was concluded that all grades of EC were suitable for organic solvent coating of extended release barrier membrane multiparticulates [14]. In another study, sustained-release metformin hydrochloride nanoparticulate systems were developed, and the effect of different viscosity EC grades on their in vitro characteristics was investigated. The sustainability of EC was enhanced by the increase in its apparent viscosity—the EC with higher viscosity grade sustained metformin release more efficiently [15].

3. Pharmaceutical Characteristics of EC

EC has been widely used in the pharmaceutical industry for decades, being utilized in oral and topical pharmaceutical formulations for various purposes. It has the potential to modulate and improve the physiological performance of drug dosage forms because of its hydrophobic nature and swelling capacity. The main goal of EC utilization is the development of drug dosage forms with modified release (MR), as EC ensures drug dissolution in the entire gastrointestinal tract, providing constant drug concentration and eliminating the necessity of taking several doses a day, hence improving pharmacotherapeutic effectiveness. Because it is an inert hydrophobic polymer and possesses properties such as lack of toxicity, stability during storage, and good compressibility, it is suitable for designing sustained-release preparations [1–5,16]. EC provides the formation of hydrophobic coatings, filaments, or backing layers; masks unpleasant medicine tastes; creates matrices and nanostructures for the preparation of bioactive materials or is used as an encapsulation excipient for the preparation of sustained-release microparticles; and serves as moisture protector or binder. It can also be used as a dispersing, stabilizing, and water-retaining agent to prevent drugs from getting wet and to promote the safe storage of drugs. Shell tablets can be obtained by suspending drug in the gastrointestinally insoluble carrier. EC has also been used as a matrix in the preparation of both water-soluble and sparingly water-soluble drugs using solid dispersion technique. It is ubiquitously utilized as a coating material in sustained-release preparations due to its film-forming properties and good mechanical strength. Also, in the coating context, its important feature is insolubility at any physiological pH. However, the polymer exhibits swelling in the presence of gastric juice, making it permeable for water and permitting extended modified drug release [4,17–22]. EC-coated beads have also demonstrated the ability to absorb pressure and hence protect the coating from fracture during compression. Drug release from EC-based film coatings depends on the coating level, drug solubility, and the form in which the polymer is applied in the coating process (e.g., as powder, aqueous dispersion, or organic solution). It is also common to employ blending polymers to get suitable and desired results, as using a single polymer may not give the desired drug release profile. Owing to its hydrophobic properties, EC reduces the penetration of water into the solid polymeric matrix, hence reducing drug release [4,23].

EC can be found in different forms, such as powders with various viscosity grades or aqueous dispersions. Examples of organic solids are Ethocel™ or Aqualon™, and aqueous dispersions include Surelease®, Aquacoat® ECD, Aquarius™ Control ECD, and AshaKote® (Table 1, Figure 2) [12,24–28]. Commercially available types of EC (e.g., Ethocel™ 4, Ethocel™ 10, and Ethocel™ 45) differ in the length of the polymer chains, the rate of dissolution, molecular weights, and hence the viscosity of their solutions (ranging from 3 to 110 mPa·s) [12].

Table 1. Characteristics of commercially available EC *.

Organic EC products
Ethocel™
Available in many varieties that differ in grade and viscosity (e.g., Ethocel™ Standard Grade 4 Premium, 7 Premium, 10 Premium, 20 Premium, 45 Premium, 100 Premium). Ethocel™ are white to light-tan granular powders in physical appearance with bulk density and specific gravity of about 0.4 g/cm^3 and 1.12–1.15 g/cm^3 respectively and glass transition temperatures range between 129 and 133 °C. They dissolve in a wide range of solvents such as aliphatic alcohols, chlorinated solvents, and natural oils. They are practically insoluble in glycerin, propylene glycol, and water. Films made from Ethocel™ are tough, with high tensile strength and high flexibility even at low temperatures. They can be combined with water soluble polymers such as methylcellulose and hypromellose (HPMC) in aqueous coating liquids. They are characterized by thermoplastic nature and ability to soften at 135–160 °C which makes them versatile in pharmaceutical hot melt extrusion processes. They ensure desired drug release properties and improved bioavailability of especially poorly soluble drugs [12].
Aqualon™ ethylcellulose
During preparation, the substitution of ethoxyl groups is controlled to obtain commercially useful range of 48–52% ethoxyl (or 2.3–2.6 ethoxyl groups out of a theoretical maximum of 3.0) per anhydroglucose unit. Over this ethoxyl range, Aqualon™ ethylcellulose is classified into three ethoxyl types: N (low substitution), T (mid substitution), and X (high substitution). The improved compressible grade (Aqualon™ T10) was developed with optimized compactability (high ethoxyl content and low viscosity) and good powder flow. The grades of Aqualon™ ethylcellulose are compliant with the monograph requirements of the United States Pharmacopoeia (USP) and the European Pharmacopoeia (Ph. Eur.) [24].
Aqueous dispersion of ethylcellulose

Table 1. *Cont.*

Surelease®
Surelease® is a family of fully formulated, aqueous dispersion products which constitute plasticized aqueous dispersions of EC with 25% (*w/w*) solid content available in four types: E-7-19029, E-7-19030, E7-19040, E-7-19050. They are plasticized (depending on type) with dibutyl sebacate (3.5%-E-7-19029, E-7-19030) and oleic acid (1.9%-E7-19040). Surelease® is produced in the following steps: EC is blended with plasticizer, then extruded and melted. The molten plasticized EC is then directly emulsified in ammoniated water in a high-shear mixing device under pressure. Ammonium oleate is formed in situ in order to stabilize and form the dispersion of plasticized EC particles. Then, purified water is added to achieve the final solids content. Applications of Surelease® include beads and particles coating, matrix granulation (the dispersion can be used as a binder in wet granulation for the production of free-flowing granules, which can subsequently be compressed into tablets), taste-masking coating, or nutritional enteric coating [25].
Aquacoat® ECD
It contains primarily EC with a surfactant and a stabilizer from the emulsion stage (sodium lauryl sulfate (SLS) and cetyl alcohol (CA)). Depending on type it consists of EC (24.5–29.5%), CA (1.7–3.3%), and SLS (0.9–1.7%). Traces of dimethylopolysiloxane to enhance foaming during distillation may also be present. EC is dissolved in a water-immiscible organic solvent with CA addition as a dispersion stabilizer. The solution is then emulsified into an aqueous SLS solution. The resulting crude emulsion is homogenized to yield a submicron emulsion which is then distilled to remove the organic solvent and water to yield a solid dispersion. EC is present in the dispersion as spherical particles in the size range of 0.1–0.3 µm. It exists as a milky white liquid with the characteristic odor of EC. Product does not contain plasticizer. Recommended plasticizers include dibutyl sebacate, acetylated monoglycerides, triacetin or glyceryl triacetate, acetyltriethyl citrate, and triethyl citrate. It is used for the aqueous film coating of solid dosage forms to extend drug release, taste mask, or to protect against moisture [26].

* The table presents examples of selected, most commonly used, products.

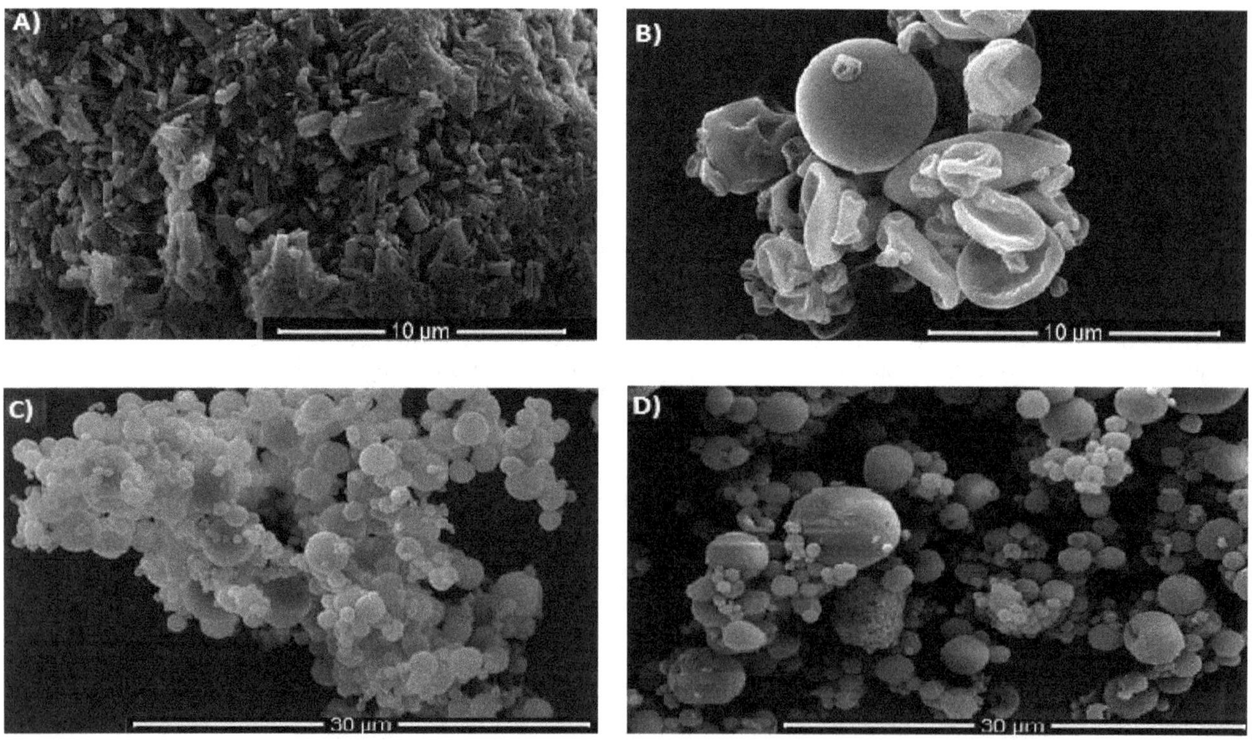

Figure 2. SEM pictures of (**A**) EC in powder form; (**B**) spray-dried ethanolic solution of EC (inlet temperature 65 °C, aspirator flow 98%, feed flow 3.5 mL/min); (**C**) spray-dried Surelease®; and (**D**) spray-dried Aquacoat™ ECD-30 (author's pictures under magnification 10,000× (**A**,**B**); 5000× (**C**,**D**)).

4. Applicability of EC in Pharmaceutical Formulations

4.1. EC as An MR Coating Material in Oral Delivery Systems

Because of EC's potential to modify drug release, it is widely studied as a coating agent. EC as release retardant was employed in a once-a-day sustained-release system of tacrolimus. The pellets were coated with EC using a fluid bed granulator. Drug release was markedly impeded by the outer EC-based coating layer, displaying about 60% drug release after 8 h, regardless of the acidity of the medium. It was assessed that there were no statistical differences between the obtained pellets and the marketed sustained-release capsules (Advagraf®) [29,30]. Shah et al. developed a multiunit formulation for the colon-targeted delivery of metronidazole using EC and Eudragit® S 100 as coating polymers to prevent initial drug release in the gastric region (Figure 3). Cores of mini tablets containing drug were prepared using suitable swelling agents to provide pH-sensitive pulsatile drug delivery [31].

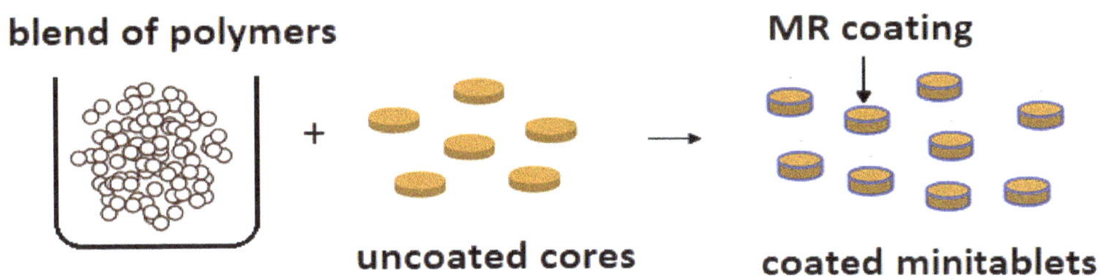

Figure 3. Schematic illustration of coated modified release (MR) minitablets.

A double-layer coated colon-specific drug delivery system was developed by Kim et al. The system consisted of a chitosan-based polymeric subcoating of the core tablet (containing citric acid for microclimate acidification), followed by an enteric EC coating. The system showed drug release in a controlled manner by inhibiting drug release in the stomach and intestine, but releasing the drug gradually in the colon [32]. The example of utilizing EC as a release-retarding coating is a commercially available preparation called Micro-K® in hard gelatin capsules, containing small crystalline particles of potassium chloride (KCl). Each crystal of KCl is microencapsulated by a patented process with an insoluble EC polymeric coating which functions as a semi-permeable membrane ensuring controlled release of K^+ and Cl^- ions. Fluids pass through the membranes and gradually dissolve KCl within the microcapsules. As a result, drug slowly diffuses outward through the membrane over an 8–10 h period [33,34]. Another example is Theo-24®—the first commercial product for 24-h theophylline therapy launched on the market. The technology utilized in the formulation uses a chemical timing complex (protected by patent) to produce very small theophylline-coated beads that provide dependable zero-order controlled drug release. Tiny spheres of a sugar and starch blend form the core of the beads. The core is first coated with theophylline and then with a timing complex utilizing EC. The resulting beads are put into capsules. When the capsule dissolves in the gastrointestinal tract, the insoluble coating on the bead slowly erodes. The drug, which is highly soluble, moves through the coating. In the core, the starch swells and pushes the drug out while the dissolving sugar also helps carry the drug through the chemical timing complex, which results in a constant release [33,35].

Matrix tablets of hydrochlorothiazide were coated with an insoluble barrier membrane using aqueous EC coating (Surelease®) and HPMC-based Opadry® as a pore former, at 85:15 *w/w* ratio. The combination of barrier membrane and hydrophilic matrix system was utilized as a strategy to modulate drug diffusion from hydrophilic matrices and to reduce the overall variability in release [36]. The aims of another study were to control the release of a water-soluble theophylline from mini matrices made of HPMC by applying an EC film coating (Surelease®) and to assess coating load on release rates. At low coating weight gains, tablets released the entire drug within 0.5 h, while at high coating weight gains only a very small amount (<5%) of drug was released after 12 h [17].

EC has found its application as a coating material in commercially available modern MR solid dosage forms (Diffucaps, DiffCORE™, SODAS®, or Geomatrix® systems). It is also used in medicines dedicated to patients suffering from ADHD: Adzenys XR®-ODT and Cotempla® XR-ODT [16,33,37–42]. Diffucaps are a multiparticulate system, where drug profiles are created by layering a drug onto a neutral core (e.g., sugar spheres, crystals, or granules) followed by the application of a rate-controlling functional EC membrane. Such a system is applied in Metadate CD® capsules (Figure 4) [16,37].

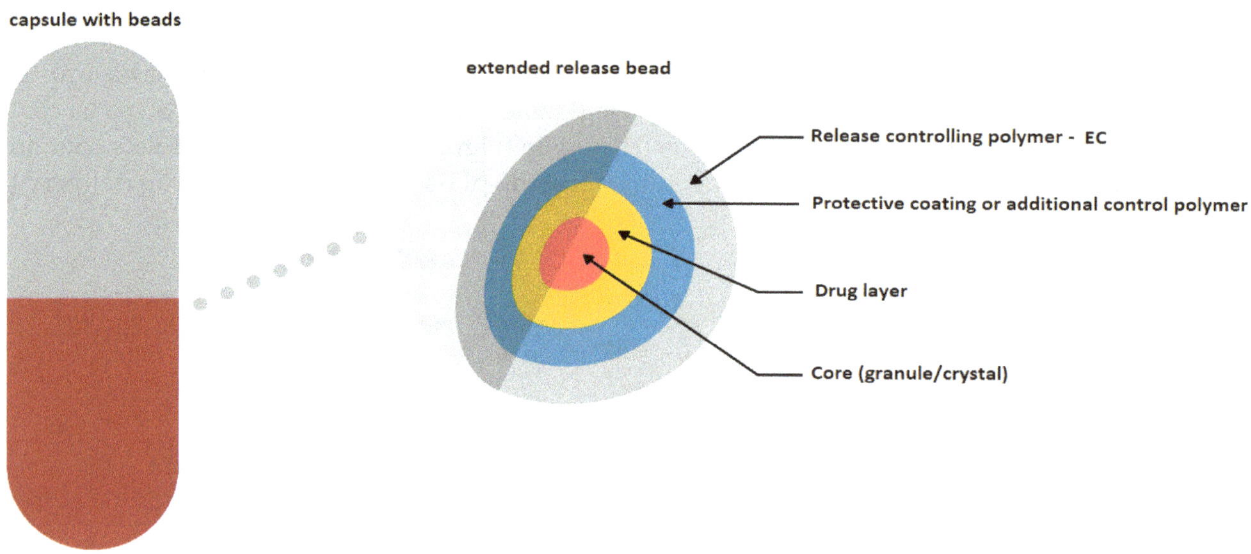

Figure 4. Schematic illustration of Diffucaps system in a Metadate CD® capsule.

Another example of an EC-coating-based oral system is DiffCORE™ (Lamictal® XR) (Figure 5). DiffCORE™ is a technology developed to achieve extended release by delivering drug from a tablet core through one or several apertures in an impermeable coat made of EC. The technology combines the use of apertures that are mechanically drilled into functional film-coated tablets (on both faces of the tablet's structure) with a polymer coating that controls the mechanism of diffusion. This combination is designed to ensure the dissolution rate of drug over a period of approximately 12–15 h [16,38].

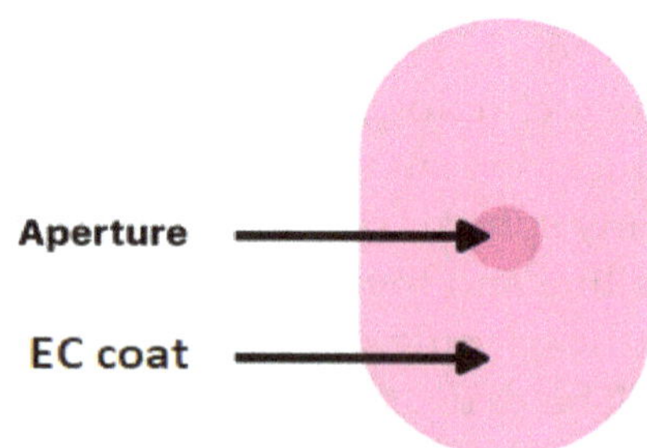

Figure 5. Schematic illustration of DiffCORE™ system.

Adzenys® XR-ODT and Cotempla® XR-ODT are examples of orally disintegrating tablets which dissolve quickly in the mouth, maintaining extended drug release along gastrointestinal tract. The technology utilized in the medicines uses two different types of particles (in different ratios depending on the formulation): immediate release and extended release. Two different polymer coatings are applied to the extended release beads: interior polymer coating as diffusion barrier (EC) and pH-dependent exterior polymer coating (methacrylic acid) (Figure 6) [16,41,42].

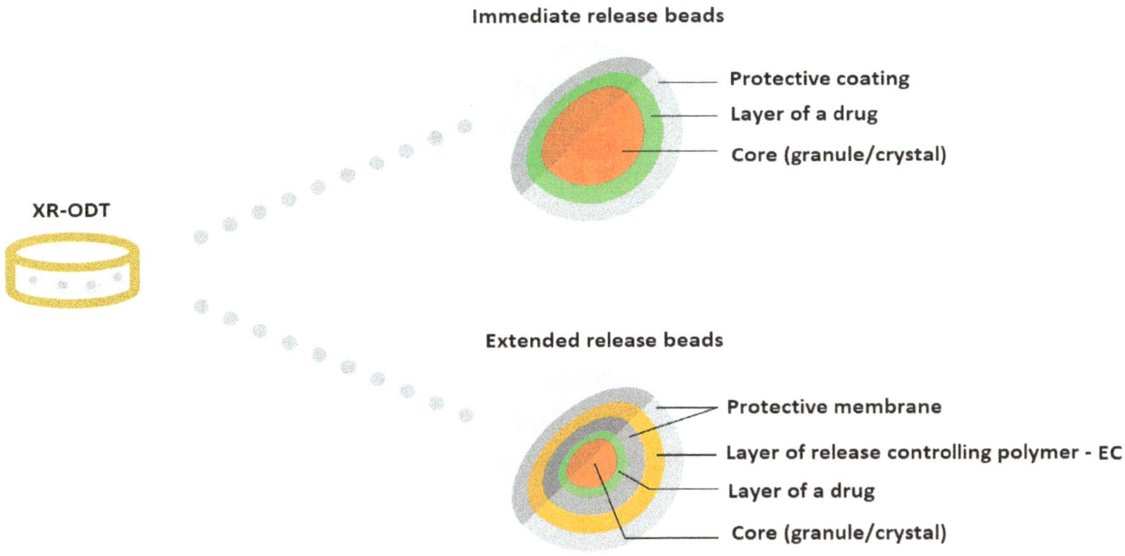

Figure 6. Schematic illustration of XR-ODT system.

Inderal® LA, long-acting capsules with propranolol, uses polymer-coated controlled diffusion technology to achieve 12 h release of drug for hypertension treatment. Inderal® LA consists of small spheroids placed in a gelatin capsule. Each spheroid containing propranolol and a microcrystalline cellulose is coated with a porous membrane made of a mixture of EC, HPMC, and plasticizer [33,43]. Dilacor XR® is a one-per-day oral formulation of diltiazem provided in capsule. The capsules contain degradable, controlled-release tablets designed based on Geomatrix® technology to release diltiazem over a 24 h period. Geomatrix™ is a patented controlled-release system incorporated in the tablets. Each capsule contains multiple extended-release diltiazem tablets, consisting of two inactive surfaces sandwiched around the drug core (made of HPMC and hydrogenated castor oil) swellable in an aqueous medium. The inactive surfaces are composed of a methylcellulose–EC combination. The drug is released as a result of the swelling of the core, which acts as a drug reservoir. Controlled release of diltiazem begins within 1 h, with maximum plasma concentrations being achieved 4–6 h after administration. The inactive surfaces hydrate at a rate much slower than the core, thus regulating the drug release and assuring constant 24 h medicine delivery (Figure 7) [33,44].

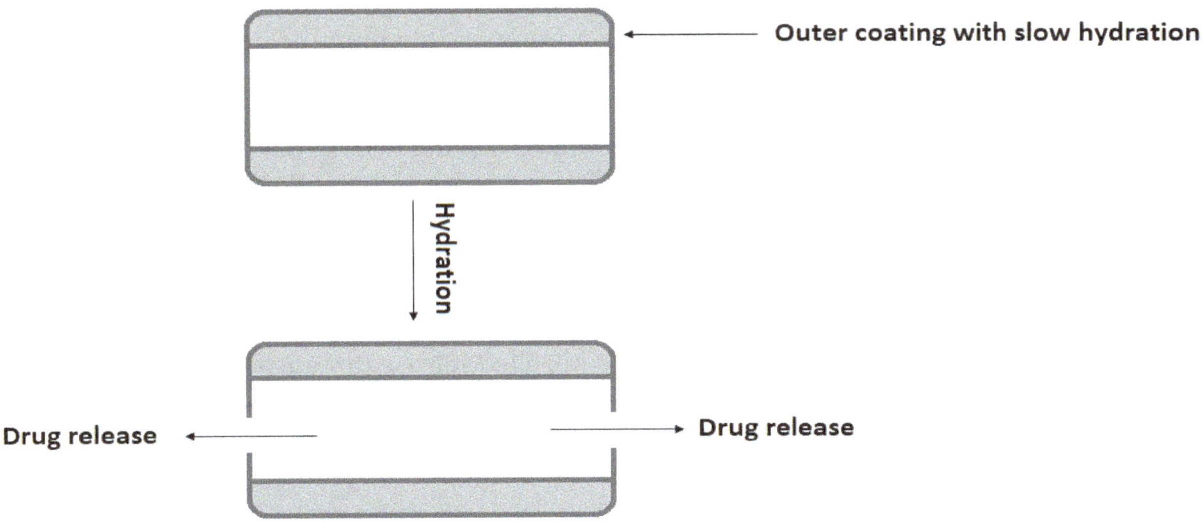

Figure 7. Schematic illustration of drug release from Geomatrix™ system modified from Wan et al. [33].

An interesting example of applying EC as a coating is SODAS® (Spheroidal Oral Drug Absorption System), utilized in Cardizem® CD. The medicine is formulated as capsules and consists of two populations of sustained-release beads that differ only by the thickness of the polymer (EC) surrounding them. The EC membrane contains added water-soluble polymers which dissolve and create pores in the membrane. The polymer beads release 40% of the total diltiazem amount in the first 12 h (Figure 8) [33,39,40,45].

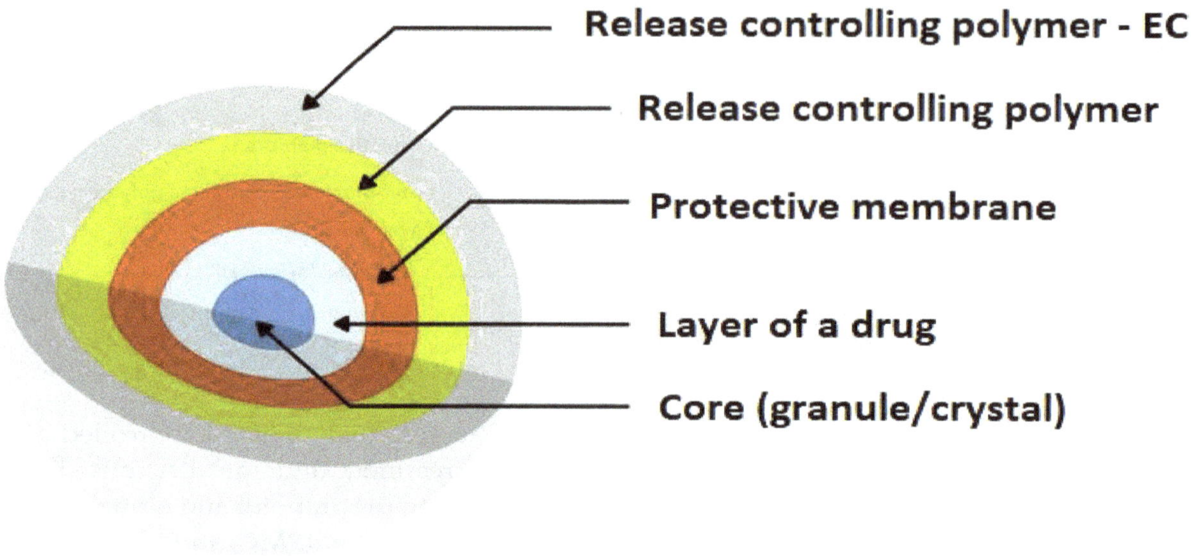

Figure 8. Scheme illustration of SODAS® delivery system modified from Elan drug technologies [39].

Core elements of drugs coated with a water-insoluble polymer such as EC offer reduced dissolution profiles, and as a consequence provide a taste-masking effect [46,47]. EC was used as taste-masking agent for quinine, utilizing a spray drying method. The obtained results showed that the quinine dissolution rate was altered, the bitter taste of quinine was successfully masked, and its intestinal absorption was simultaneously controlled [48]. EC for taste-masking purposes was tested in organic (Ethocel™) and aqueous form (Surelease®). To determine whether the designed particles effectively masked the bitter taste of rupatadine fumarate, three independent methods were used: a human taste panel, an in vitro release test conducted in conditions mimicking the oral cavity environment, and an electronic taste sensing system (electronic tongue). It was clearly confirmed that particles formulated from aqueous dispersions of EC provided a very effective taste-masking barrier [49]. Evaluation of the use of Surelease® as a barrier membrane coating with pediatric precedence of use on the taste-masking of immediate-release acetaminophen granules was also conducted. The dissolution profiles of obtained granules were successfully modified using a Surelease® and Opadry® blend as a barrier membrane, providing slow initial drug release [50]. Another study concerned the development of orally disintegrating caffeine citrate tablets utilizing hot melt extrusion technology (EC was used as a polymeric taste-masking carrier) [51]. EC was also applied as a taste-masking and release-slowing agent to develop a gabapentin nanosponge-based controlled release dry suspension for pediatric use, using the suspension layering technique [52].

Utilizing of EC as release modifier in marketed oral formulations is presented in Table 2.

Table 2. Examples of commercially available oral solid dosage forms with EC as release modifier.

Product (Manufacturer)	Drug	Dosage Form	EC Role	Reference
Aciphex® Sprinkle™ (Eisai Management Co., Ltd.)	rabeprazole	granules in capsule	coating, delayed release	[53]
Adzenys XR-ODT™ (Neos Therapeutics)	amphetamine	extended release orally disintegrating tablet with beads	coating, extended release	[41]
Advagraf XL™	tacrolimus	capsules	extended release	[30]
Cotempla XR-ODT® (Neos Therapeutics)	methylphenidate	extended release orally disintegrating tablet with beads	coating, extended release	[42]
Cardizem CD® (Abbot Laboratories)	diltiazem	tablets in capsule	coating, extended release	[45]
Dilacor XR® (Actavis Pharma, Inc.)	diltiazem	tablets in capsule	extended release	[44]
Dilatrate-SR (Epic Pharma, LLC)	diltiazem	beads in capsule	extended release	[54]
Durlaza (New Haven Pharmaceuticals, Inc.)	acetylsalicylic acid	capsules	extended release	[55]
Enjuvia (Teva Pharmaceuticals USA, Inc.)	estrogens	coated tablets	extended release	[56]
Entocort EC *(Astra Zeneca)*	budesonide	coated granules in capsules	sustained release	[57]
Inderal® LA (Wyeth Pharmaceuticals, Inc.)	propranolol	granules in capsules	coating, extended release	[43]
Levbid® (Mylan Pharmaceuticals Inc.)	hyoscyamine	tablets	extended release	[58]
Metadate CD® (UCB Manufacturing, Inc.)	methylphenidate	granules in capsule	coating, extended release	[37]
Micro-K® (KV Pharmaceutical)	potassium	microcapsules in capsules	coating, extended release	[34]
Lamictal® XR (GSK)	lamotrigine	tablets	coating, extended release	[38]
Orfiril Long (Desitin Arzneimittel GmbH)	natrii valproas	minitablets	extended release	[59]
Palladone *(PF Laboratories Inc.)*	hydromorphone	capsules	extended release	[60]
Pentasa® (Ferring GmbH)	mesalamine	granules	prolonged release	[61]
Qsymia® (Vivus, Inc.)	phentermine, topiramate	capsules	extended release	[62]
Tegretol® XL (Novartis)	carbamazepine	tablets	matrix, extended release	[63]
Theo-24® (UCB Pharma, Inc.)	theophylline	beads in capsule	coating, extended release	[35]
Trokendi XR™ (Catalent Pharma Solutions)	topiramate	capsules	extended release	[64]

4.2. EC as a Sustained Release Material in Topical Delivery Systems

The utilization of EC to obtain a sustained release profile is also exploited in preparations for external use (e.g., transungual, ocular, vaginal, or transdermal). Successful topical therapy depends on effective drug release and penetration into the objective area, which can be achieved using an adequately developed drug dosage form [1–5,65]. EC can be applied in transungual delivery systems as a release modifier and a biocompatible agent ensuring optimal viscosity of the formulation. An isotretinoin nail lacquer intended for the treatment of nail psoriasis was developed, and its penetration efficiency across the nail plate was accessed. Lacquer with EC (at 6% concentration) possessed improved handling characteristics and enhanced drug distribution across the nail [66]. Another study documented an antifungal nail lacquer with miconazole developed with 0.5% EC which extended drug release up to 48 h [67]. Šveikauskaitė et al. studied naftifine hydrochloride release from experimental nail lacquer formulations obtained from EC and Eudragit. By using microcalorimetry they revealed possible interactions between naftifine and EC [68].

Eye administration is a demanding issue in pharmaceutical technology, and to enhance ocular bioavailability, sustained-release drug dosage forms such as hydrogels, inserts, contact lenses, or minitablets are designed. Among the materials employed in developing ophthalmic formulations, EC can be utilized as a polymer extending drug release [69] (Table 3).

Reports have also documented the application of EC as matrix material for transdermal patches for systemic delivery, showing desired permeation enhancement and flexibility [1–5]. Interestingly, EC has also been indicated in the formulation of a transdermal spray with clotrimazole to improve drug transport through the skin up to 12 h and to promote its in vivo antifungal activity [70].

Table 3 presents literature examples of EC utilization in ocular and transdermal drug delivery systems.

Table 3. Examples of ocular and transdermal delivery systems based on EC.

Drug Dosage Form	Active Substance	Used Excipients	EC Role	Reference
		Ocular formulations		
ocular inserts	brimonidine	sodium alginate, EC	hydrophobic, sustained release coating	[71]
ocular inserts	ciprofloxacin	gelatin, EC	rate-controlling, increasing residence time membrane	[72]
ocular insert	acyclovir	sodium alginate, EC	rate-controlling membrane	[73]
in situ ophthalmic hydrogel	besifloxacin	sodium alginate, xanthan gum, EC	increase the pre-corneal residence time	[74]
minitablet	ciprofloxacin	HPMC, sodium carboxymethyl cellulose, EC, hydroxyethyl cellulose, carbopol	sustained release	[75]
		Transdermal formulations		
transdermal patch	amlodipine	EC	sustained release	[76]
transdermal patch	flurbiprofen	EC, propylene glycol, dibutyl phthalate	constant drug release	[77]
transdermal delivery system	topiramate	EC, povidone, Eudragit L 100, carbopol	extended release	[78]
transdermal patch	dexibuprofen	EC, povidone, di-N-butyl phthalate	matrix formation	[79]
transdermal patch	centchroman	EC, polydimethylsiloxane, propylene glycol, Di-n-butyl-phthalate	Film-forming polymer	[80]

4.3. EC-Based Solid Dispersions

In preparation of MR dosage forms, the concepts of solid dispersions and drug incorporation in an insoluble EC carrier have been also explored [81–85]. Tsunashima et al. aimed to prepare MR formulation of tacrolimus to achieve both an extended release profile and improved drug solubility. Extended release solid dispersions of tacrolimus were successfully prepared via the solvent evaporation method using EC and HPMC as polymeric materials [82]. Sadeghi et al. compared characteristics of EC matrices prepared from solid dispersion systems with those prepared from a physical mixture of drug and polymer. Sodium diclofenac was used as a model drug. It was shown that matrices prepared from physical mixtures were harder than those prepared from solid dispersion systems, and their release rates were considerably faster. In the solid dispersion system, drug particles were incorporated in an EC matrix, which caused a great delay in drug diffusion through the polymer and made diffusion a rate-retarding process in the drug release mechanism [83]. Evaluation of the release mechanism of a poorly water-soluble drug (indomethacin) from extended-release solid dispersion systems with EC and HPMC was performed by Ohara et al. The dissolution behavior of indomethacin depended on the structures of EC–HPMC matrices and showed pH dependency—the drug dissolution rate was slower in an acidic environment than in a neutral one. The obtained results revealed that hydrophobic interaction between indomethacin and EC occurred under lower pH and strongly delayed the dissolution rate of the drug [84]. Sustained-release solid dispersions with EC and Eudragit RSPO were designed to control the release of verapamil hydrochloride. Solid dispersions obtained by a simple solvent evaporation technique and physical mixture formulations were compressed to tablets. The in vitro drug release study revealed that solid dispersions containing a combination of EC and Eudragit RSPO extended the release rate for 20 h compared to the physical mixtures at the same ratio, and that the release of verapamil from tablets containing solid dispersion could be effectively controlled [85].

4.4. EC-Based Micro- and Nanocarriers

A common approach to modifying drug release is preparing polymeric micro- or nanocarriers which contain drug enclosed in the polymer shell or incorporated in the polymer matrix (Figure 9). Micro- and nanoparticles have gained significant interest for their use in various drug formulations not only to sustain drug release, but also in order to improve bioavailability, decrease side effects, or increase drug stability [86]. An extended-release oral flexible tablet (ER-OFT) formulation was developed using carbamazepine as model drug for pediatric and geriatric compliance. Microparticles of carbamazepine were prepared using EC as a matrix polymer and HPMC as a hydrophilic pore former utilizing a high-shear granulator fitted with an atomizing spray system. Granulation of carbamazepine and EC with ethanolic binder solution resulted in obtaining microparticles with 16 h extended release [87]. EC microparticles can be formulated using a variety of techniques: interfacial and in situ polymerization, coacervation phase separation, spray drying, spray congealing, or by rotary fluidization bed granulator method [88].

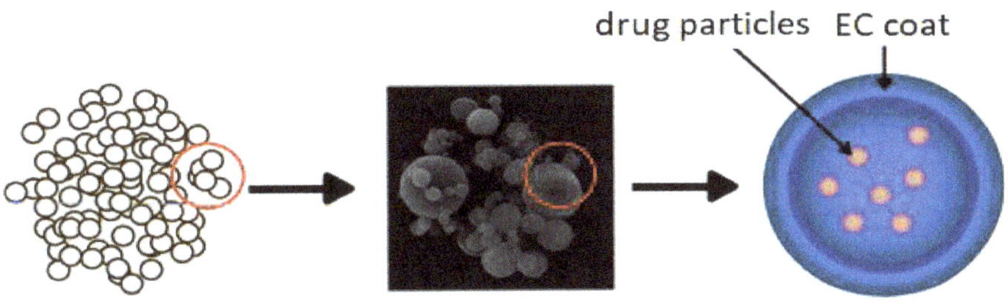

Figure 9. Schematic illustration of microparticles as a drug delivery system.

As the extreme acidic environment of the stomach contributes to poor success in the treatment of *Helicobacter pylori* infections, Pan-In et al. encapsulated clarithromycin into particles made of pH-resistant polymer (i.e., EC). Nanoparticles were prepared via a simple anti-solvent particle induction method [89]. Similarly, EC nanocomposites containing rifampicin obtained by supercritical anti-solvent process prolonged drug release and increased its bioavailability [90]. Interestingly, EC was also tested as a carrier for protecting the L-alanyl-L-glutamine peptide and simultaneously providing its prolonged release [91].

Shankar et al. formulated EC microparticles for the vaginal delivery of metronidazole by thermal change method [92]. EC was also utilized in the development of nanoparticles for the topical delivery of corticosteroids [93] or to modulate the release and reduce the ulcerogenicity of piroxicam after oral administration [93]. A reduction of 66% in mean ulcer index was observed, indicating that the obtained particles had a significant potential of offsetting deleterious side effects common in piroxicam use [94]. Similarly, as etoricoxib has many side effects when taken orally, EC nanoparticles produced by a nanoprecipitation technique were designed. Etoricoxib-loaded EC nanoparticles for local drug delivery in arthritis provided sustained drug release, thereby improving patient compliance [95]. Interestingly, nanocapsules of beclomethasone were prepared for pulmonary delivery using EC as a protective polymer. They were characterized by delayed drug photodegradation, prolonged drug release without burst effect, and insignificant cytotoxic effect [96].

EC can also be utilized to prepare sustained-release oral liquids, such as syrup with hydrocodone and chlorpheniramine (Tussionex®) or suspension with mirabegron based on ion-exchange technology [97–99].

Maulavi et al. tested EC-based-microparticles-laden hydrogel contact lenses to provide the sustained ocular delivery of timolol. Prototype poly(hydroxyethyl methacrylate) hydrogel contact lenses improved drug bioavailability due to the increase in ocular residence time [100]. Timolol-encapsulated EC nanoparticles lenses for controlled sustained ocular drug delivery were also evaluated in vivo using rabbits. Nanoparticles were prepared by a double emulsion method and incorporated into acrylate hydrogel, then implanted in hydrogel contact lenses. They exhibited extended timolol release and an intra-ocular pressure lowering effect for 192 h in rabbits without significant ocular complications [101].

Application of EC microparticles containing naproxen to textile materials was studied by Arici et al. Microparticles were prepared by spray-drying using an aqueous EC dispersion and applied to orthopedic support materials. Since these materials are used for traumatic irritations, over-forced ligaments and tendons, and specific problems of various joints, it was concluded that they can serve as potential drug delivery systems [102].

Another approach to obtaining microcarriers is microsponge development. Microsponges are novel drug delivery systems, which ensure effective sustained drug release. They possess unique properties including self-sterilizability, due to the minimal pore size which does not allow bacteria to enter and contaminate the formulation. Microsponges can entrap drugs up to three times their weight due to their very high porosity. EC is utilized as a foundation material for microsponges and for microsponge engineering due to its nonirritating, nontoxic, and nonallergic nature [103–105]. Bothiraja et al. focused on the development of an EC microsponge gel as a topical carrier for the controlled release and cutaneous drug deposition of eberconazole. The microsponges were prepared using the quasi emulsion solvent diffusion method. An in vivo skin deposition study demonstrated higher retention in the stratum corneum layer as compared with commercial cream with eberconazole [106]. Jelvehgari et al. developed a microsponge delivery system to facilitate the topical delivery of benzyl peroxide. As benzyl peroxide has many side effects when applied per se in gel form, such a delivery system to the skin could reduce those effects while reducing its percutaneous absorption [107]. EC was also utilized to prepare microsponges to overcome problems connected with the poor water solubility, low stability, and high volatility of tea tree oil. Microsponges loaded with tea tree oil were prepared using EC and polyvinyl alcohol and incorporated into carbopol gel [108]. Another study describes the development of the topical delivery of oxybenzone—one of the most widely used chemical filters found in commercial sunscreens—using a microsponge-loaded gel. As the ingredient can cause dermatitis and skin irritation, oxybenzone-loaded microsponges were successfully formulated by a quasi emulsion solvent diffusion method with EC utilization. It was shown that controlled release of oxybenzone from the microsponge structures and barrier effect of gel resulted in prolonged retention with reduced permeation, reduced irritation, and enhanced sun protection factor [109]. The aim of another study was to develop a sustained-release delivery system of tacrolimus, formulated using a microsponge base, employing EC and xanthan gum by modified double emulsification techniques [110]. EC microsponges can be designed for ocular delivery; acetazolamide formulated in a microsponges–Pluronic F-127 in situ gel was characterized by improved therapeutic efficacy and reduced systemic side effects of oral acetazolamide. The obtained formulation showed higher therapeutic efficacy compared to free drug in gel [111].

EC has also been studied as a material for nanofibers, which possess a broad range of new applications in pharmaceutical technology [112]. Over the past years, electrospinning has been attractive as a simple, reproducible, versatile, and cost-effective technique for nanofiber production. Electrospun nanofibers have been extensively used for different biomedical applications, including wound dressing, tissue engineering, and drug delivery. The fiber morphology can be manipulated by changing the solvent ratio, resulting in a decreased fiber diameter. Membranes made of EC nanofibers possess good physical properties and are characterized by beneficial air permeability [113,114]. Drug delivery rate is affected by the polymer type, fiber diameter, and drug concentration in the fiber [114,115]. EC as a filament-forming matrix was tested in ketoprofen nanofiber delivery systems designed by triaxial electrospinning [116]. EC was also utilized for creating a 5-fluorouracil loaded core for the fabrication of electrospun fibers [117] and in preparing water-stable composite nanofibers loaded with indomethacin with a sustained, diffusion-controlled release profile [118]. The inclusion of EC as a matrix former improved mechanical properties of the entire delivery system [118]. Another study employed blend fibers of poly(N-vinylcaprolactam) and EC with the aim of developing thermoresponsive sustained release formulations fabricated by twin-jet electrospinning containing ketoprofen. The obtained fibers were largely smooth and homogeneous, and the addition of a drug did not affect their morphology [115]. Additionally, Liu et al. reported that nanofibers obtained by electrospinning using blends of EC and gelatin were characterized by fine morphology and possessed improved thermal stability [119].

4.5. EC in Mucoadhesive Delivery Systems

In the development of dosage forms applied on mucous membranes, the selection of suitable polymers with adhesive properties is a crucial issue. Polymers that are bioadhesive and do not dissolve before releasing the incorporated drug are highly appreciated for sustain drug release. As a water-insoluble polymer, EC is often used as backing membrane for its film-forming property, low water permeability, drug impermeability, and moderate flexibility. It possesses bioadhesive properties, however lesser than Carbopol and chitosan [120]. Bagul et al. evaluated the in vitro mucoadhesive strength of various polymers and reported the following ascending order for force of adhesion expressed in Newtons (N): gelatin (1.42) < gum dammar (1.47) < gum copal (1.52) < ethyl cellulose (1.60) < sodium alginate (1.71) < xanthan gum (1.81) < chitosan (1.91) < HPMC (2.25) < carbopol (2.40) [120].

EC forms a hydrophobic network when the mixture comes into contact with water, resulting in sustained drug release. The utilization of EC as a single polymer or in conjunction with other adjuvants in the preparation of film-like drug carriers is well documented. Drug-loaded EC films are characterized by good adhesion, mechanical strength, and sustained release profile. They provide a flexible diffusion barrier and its properties can be changed by the amount of pore-forming agent, film thickness, and EC molecular weight [1,3–5]. Abruzzo et al. designed buccal films for propranolol administration. A polymeric layer was prepared by casting and drying with polyvinylpyrrolidone or polyvinylalcohol and the addition of gelatin or chitosan. EC was employed to formulate a second layer was applied onto the primary one in order to obtain prolonged drug delivery, increase adhesion, and mask the drug's bitter taste [121]. A bilayer mucoadhesive buccal film containing a combination of ornidazole and dexamethasone was prepared using solvent casting to treat oral ulcers, with EC utilized as a backing layer. The formulation showed favorable swelling characteristics, and both drugs were released at 95% after 4 h [122]. EC was also applied for the preparation of allantoin-loaded films for the management of dry mouth syndrome. The findings revealed that the produced films were functional, mucoadhesive, flexible, and stable, with the potential for treating various intraoral diseases [123]. EC-based mucoadhesive buccal films containing fluticasone formulated by solvent casting technique showed acceptable physicochemical properties, homogenous drug distribution, adequate mucoadhesion time, moderate swelling, and sustained drug release up to 12 h [124]. The objective of another study was to develop a two-layered buccal mucoadhesive system consisting of a highly water-soluble drug (i.e., risedronate). Varied concentrations of chitosan, HPMC, and EC acting as an impermeable backing membrane ensuring sustained release were tested. The obtained systems showed good swelling and mucoadhesive characteristics, with 90–100% drug release within 8–12 h [125]. EC, as a biocompatible backing layer, was also utilized in the development of mucoadhesive bi-layered strips used in dental treatment for the controlled delivery of lidocaine [126]. EC dissolved in N-methyl pyrrolidone was successfully used as a polymeric matrix for the in situ forming gel (with doxycycline, metronidazole, and benzyl peroxide) as dosage form applied in periodontal pocket in periodontitis treatment. It turned out that increasing the amount of EC increased the viscosity of system while still exhibiting Newtonian flow and simultaneously decreasing the release of drug [127]. Another prolonged-release mucoadhesive gel containing metronidazole for periodontal application was developed basing on a mixture of glycerylmonooleate and EC. EC reduced the initial metronidazole release and significantly sustained its release profile [128]. Pathak et al. developed a mucoadhesive coating for fluconazole tablets for oral thrush treatment. EC coating reduced fluconazole permeation through the buccal mucosa, thereby ensuring high local drug concentration and faster provision of the fluconazole minimum inhibitory concentration in the oral cavity [129].

5. Conclusions

EC is a water-insoluble cellulose derivative with attractive features such as biocompatibility, gastroresistance, and degradation to non-toxic and readily excreted products. It is extensively utilized in pharmaceutical technology. It is generally recognized as safe to use, even in pediatric therapy. EC is easy to process alone or with the addition of other excipients (e.g., plasticizers or other polymers). Considering its multifunctional properties, EC is being widely exploited in oral and topical drug dosage forms. EC's main advantage is its ability to modify the release of the drug, which allows for the creation of controlled delivery systems—the unique tailored carriers for many pharmaceuticals. EC-based materials are widely utilized as matrices for designing novel drug delivery systems with a wide range of applications.

Author Contributions: Conceptualization, K.W. (Katarzyna Wasilewska) and K.W. (Katarzyna Winnicka); Formal Analysis, K.W. (Katarzyna Winnicka); Resources, K.W. (Katarzyna Wasilewska); Data Curation, K.W. (Katarzyna Wasilewska); Writing—Original Draft Preparation, K.W. (Katarzyna Wasilewska); Writing—Review and Editing, K.W. (Katarzyna Wasilewska) and K.W. (Katarzyna Winnicka); Visualization, K.W. (Katarzyna Wasilewska); Supervision, K.W. (Katarzyna Winnicka); Project Administration, K.W. (Katarzyna Wasilewska); Funding Acquisition, K.W. (Katarzyna Wasilewska) and K.W. (Katarzyna Winnicka).

Acknowledgments: We are grateful to the Editors for the permission to reprint selected figures from our previous publication (Reference number 15): Trofimiuk, M.; Wasilewska, K.; Winnicka, K. How to modify drug release in paediatric dosage forms? Novel technologies and modern approaches with regard to children's population. *Int. J. Mol. Sci.* **2019**, 29. We are thankful to Anna Basa (Institute of Chemistry, University of Białystok, Poland) for preparing SEM pictures (Inspect™S50, FEI Company, Hillsboro, OR, USA).

References

1. Qiu, Y.; Lee, P.I. Rational design of oral modified-release drug delivery systems. In *Developing Solid Oral Dosage Forms. Pharmaceutical Theory and Practice*, 2nd ed.; Qui, Y., Zhang, G.G.Z., Mantri, R.V., Chen, Y., Yu, L., Eds.; Academic Press: Cambridge, MA, USA, 2017; pp. 1127–1160.
2. FDA. Available online: https://www.fda.gov/downloads/Drugs/.../UCM291010.pdf (accessed on 20 July 2019).
3. Rathbone, M.J.; Hadgraft, J.; Roberts, M.S.; Lane, M.E. *Modified-Release Drug Delivery Technology*, 2nd ed.; Informa Healthcare: London, UK, 2008; Volume 2.
4. Rowe, R.C.; Sheskey, P.J.; Quinn, M.E. *Handbook of Pharmaceutical Excipients*, 6th ed.; Pharmaceutical Press: London, UK; Chicago, IL, USA; Washington, DC, USA, 2009; pp. 262–267.
5. Ethyl Cellulose. Available online: https://pubchem.ncbi.nlm.nih.gov/compound/24832091#section=Probable-Routes-of-Human-Exposure (accessed on 21 July 2019).
6. *The European Pharmacopoeia*, 9th ed.; Council of Europe: Strasburg, France, 2016.
7. *The United States Pharmacopeia and National Formulary (USP41-NF 36)*; Pharmacopeia Convention: Rockville, MD, USA, 2018; Volume 2.
8. FDA Inactive Ingredients Database. Available online: https://search.fda.gov/search?utf8=%E2%9C%93&affiliate=fda1&query=ethylcellulose&commit=Search (accessed on 20 July 2019).
9. Canadian List of Acceptable Non-Medicinal Ingredients. Available online: https://www.canada.ca/en/health-canada/services/drugs-health-products/natural-non-prescription/applications-submissions/product-licensing/compendium-monographs.html (accessed on 20 July 2019).
10. *The Pharmacopoeia of the People's Republic of China 2015 Edition*; The Stationery Office: London, UK, 2015.
11. *The Japanese Pharmacopoeia, Seventeenth Edition (JP17)*; The Ministry of Health, Labour and Welfare: Tokyo, Japan, 2016.
12. Ethocel, Colorcon. Available online: https://www.pharma.dupont.com/pharmaceutical-products/ethocel.html (accessed on 20 July 2019).
13. Brydson, J.A. *Plastics Materials*, 6th ed.; Butterworth-Heinemann: Oxford, UK, 1995.
14. Mehta, R.; Teckoe, J.; Schoener, C.; Workentine, S.; Ferrizzi, D.; Rajabi-Siahoboomi, A. Investigation into effect of ethylcellulose viscosity variation on the drug release of metoprolol tartrate and acetaminophen extended release multiparticulates—Part I. *AAPS PharmSciTech* **2016**, *17*, 1366–1375. [CrossRef]
15. Lokhande, A.B.; Ravindra, S.M.; Jitendra, D.K.; Naik, B. Influence of different viscosity grade ethylcellulose polymers on encapsulation and in vitro release study of drug loaded nanoparticles metformin. *J. Pharm. Res.* **2013**, *5*, 414–420.
16. Trofimiuk, M.; Wasilewska, K.; Winnicka, K. How to modify drug release in paediatric dosage forms? Novel technologies and modern approaches with regard to children's population. *Int. J. Mol. Sci.* **2019**, *20*, 3200. [CrossRef]
17. Hamedelniel, E.I.; Bajdik, J.; Pintye-Hódi, K. Optimization of preparation of matrix pellets containing ethylcellulose. *Chem. Eng. Process.* **2010**, *49*, 120–124. [CrossRef]
18. Mallipeddi, R.; Saripella, K.K.; Neau, S.H. Use of fine particle ethylcellulose as the diluent in the production of pellets by extrusion-spheronization. *SPJ.* **2014**, *22*, 360–371. [CrossRef]
19. Grund, J.; Koerber, M.; Walther, M.; Bodmeier, R. The effect of polymer properties on direct compression and drug release from water-insoluble controlled release matrix tablets. *Int. J. Pharm.* **2014**, *469*, 94–101. [CrossRef]
20. Cifuentes, C.; Aguilar-de-Leyva, A.; Rajabi-Siahboomi, A.R.; Caraballo, I. Critical points in ethylcellulose matrices: Influence of the polymer, drug and filler properties. *Acta Pharm.* **2013**, *63*, 115–129. [CrossRef]
21. Bruschi, M. *Strategies to Modify Drug Release from Pharmaceutics Systems*, 1st ed.; Woodhead Publishing: Cambridge, UK, 2015; pp. 87–119.
22. Mehta, R.Y.; Missaghi, S.; Tiwari, S.B.; Rajabi-Siahboomi, A.R. Application of ethylcellulose coating to hydrophilic matrices: A strategy to modulate drug release profile and reduce drug release variability. *AAPS Pharm. Sci. Tech.* **2014**, *15*, 1049–1059. [CrossRef]
23. Pawar, A.; Deepak, V.B.; Vineeta, V.K.; Vilasrao, J.K. Advances in pharmaceutical coatings. *Int. J. Chem. Tech. Res.* **2010**, *1*, 733–737.
24. Aqualon, Ashland. Available online: https://www.ashland.com/industries/pharmaceutical/oral-soliddose/aqualon-ethylcellulose (accessed on 20 July 2019).

25. Surelease, Colorcon. Available online: https://www.colorcon.com/products-formulation/all-products/film-coatings/sustained-release/surelease (accessed on 20 July 2019).
26. Aquacoat, ECD. Available online: http://www.fmcbiopolymer.com/Pharmaceutical/Products/Aquacoat.aspx (accessed on 20 July 2019).
27. Aquarius, Ashland. Available online: https://www.ashland.com/file_source/Ashland/links/PTR-112_Aquarius_Control_ECD_reconstitution_instructions.pdf (accessed on 20 July 2019).
28. AshaKote, Ashaland. Available online: http://www.ashacel.com/AshaKote.PDF (accessed on 20 July 2019).
29. Shin, T.H.; Ho, M.J.; Kim, S.R.; Im, S.H.; Kim, C.H.; Lee, S.; Kang, M.J.; Choi, Y.W. Formulation and in vivo pharmacokinetic evaluation of ethyl cellulose-coated sustained release multiple-unit system of tacrolimus. *Int. J. Biol. Macromol.* **2018**, *1*, 544–550. [CrossRef]
30. Full Prescribing Information Advagraf®. Available online: https://www.ema.europa.eu/en/documents/product-information/advagraf-epar-product-information_en.pdf (accessed on 20 July 2019).
31. Shah, N.; Sharma, O.P.; Mehta, T.; Amin, A. Design of experiment approach for formulating multi-unit colon-targeted drug delivery system: In vitro and in vivo studies. *Drug Dev. Ind. Pharm.* **2016**, *42*, 825–835. [CrossRef]
32. Kim, M.S.; Yeom, D.W.; Kim, S.R.; Yoon, H.Y.; Kim, C.H.; Son, H.Y.; Kim, J.H.; Lee, S.; Choi, Y.W. Development of a chitosan based double layer-coated tablet as a platform for colon-specific drug delivery. *Drug Des. Devel. Ther.* **2017**, *11*, 45–57. [CrossRef]
33. Wan, H.; Park, K. *Oral Controlled Release Formulation Design and Delivery. Theory to Practice*; Wiley: Hoboken, NJ, USA, 2010.
34. Full Prescribing Information Micro-K™. Available online: https://www.rxlist.com/micro-k-drug.htm (accessed on 20 July 2019).
35. Full Prescribing Information Theo-24®. Available online: https://www.drugs.com/dosage/theo-24.html (accessed on 20 July 2019).
36. Mohamed, F.A.; Roberts, M.; Seton, L.; Ford, J.L.; Levina, M.; Rajabi-Siahboomi, A.R. Film-coated matrix mini-tablets for the extended release of a water-soluble drug. *Drug Dev. Ind. Pharm.* **2015**, *41*, 623–630. [CrossRef]
37. Full Prescribing Information Metadate CD®. Available online: https://www.accessdata.fda.gov/drugsatfda_docs/label/2009/021259s021lbl.pdf (accessed on 20 July 2019).
38. Full Prescribing Information Lamictal®XR. Available online: https://www.fda.gov/downloads/drugs/developmentapprovalprocess/developmentresources/ucm215664.pdf (accessed on 20 July 2019).
39. Venkata, P.D.B. Spheroidal oral drug absorption system (SODAS). *J. Glob. Pharma Technol.* **2011**, *3*, 1–5.
40. Elan Drug Technologies. Spheroidal Drug Absorption System (SODAS®). Available online: http://www.elandrugtechnologies.com/oral_controlled_release/sodas (accessed on 20 July 2019).
41. Full Prescribing Information Adzenys XR-ODT®. Available online: https://www.accessdata.fda.gov/drugsatfda_docs/label/2017/204326s002lbl.pdf (accessed on 20 July 2019).
42. Full Prescribing Information Cotempla XR-ODT®. Available online: https://www.accessdata.fda.gov/drugsatfda_docs/label/2017/205489s000lbl.pdf (accessed on 20 July 2019).
43. Full Prescribing Information Inderal® LA. Available online: https://www.accessdata.fda.gov/drugsatfda_docs/label/2011/016418s080,016762s017,017683s008lbl.pdf (accessed on 20 July 2019).
44. Full Prescribing Information Dilacor-XR®. Available online: https://www.drugs.com/pro/dilacor-xr.htmlDilcaor (accessed on 20 July 2019).
45. Full Prescribing Information Cardizem® CD. Available online: https://www.accessdata.fda.gov/drugsatfda_docs/label/2010/020062s040lbl.pdf (accessed on 20 July 2019).
46. Amelian, A.; Winnicka, K. Polymers in pharmaceutical taste masking applications. *Polimery* **2017**, *6*, 417–496. [CrossRef]
47. Faisal, W.; Farag, F.; Abdellatif, A.A.H.; Abbas, A. Taste masking approaches for medicines. *Curr. Drug Deliv.* **2018**, *15*, 167–185. [CrossRef]
48. Taki, M.; Tagami, T.; Ozeki, T. Preparation of polymer-blended quinine nanocomposite particles by spray drying and assessment of their instrumental bitterness-masking effect using a taste sensor. *Drug. Dev. Ind. Pharm.* **2017**, *43*, 715–722. [CrossRef]

49. Wasilewska, K.; Szekalska, M.; Ciosek-Skibinska, P.; Lenik, J.; Jacyna, J.; Markuszewski, M.; Winnicka, K. Ethylcellulose in organic solution or aqueous dispersion form in designing taste-masked microparticles by the spray drying technique with a model bitter drug: Rupatadine fumarate. *Polymers* **2019**, *11*, 522. [CrossRef]
50. Ito, D.; Tackoe, J.; Rajabi-Siahboomo, A. Investigation of Taste Masking Performance of an Aqueous Ethylcellulose Dispersion (Surelease®) on Acetaminophen Granules. Poster (AAPS 2013). Available online: https://www.colorcon.com/products-formulation/all-products/download/311/552/34?method=view (accessed on 20 July 2019).
51. Pimparade, M.B.; Morott, J.T.; Park, J.B.; Kulkarni, V.I.; Majumdar, S.; Murthy, S.N.; Lian, Z.; Pinto, E.; Bi, V.; Durig, T.; et al. Development of taste masked caffeine citrate formulations utilizing hot melt extrusion technology and in vitro-in vivo evaluations. *Int. J. Pharm.* **2015**, *20*, 167–176. [CrossRef]
52. Rao, M.R.; Bhingole, R.C. Nanosponge-based pediatric-controlled release dry suspension of gabapentin for reconstitution. *Drug. Dev. Ind. Pharm.* **2015**, *41*, 2029–2036. [CrossRef]
53. Full Prescribing Information Aciphex®Sprinkle™. Available online: https://www.accessdata.fda.gov/drugsatfda_docs/label/2014/020973s035204736s005lbl.pdf (accessed on 20 July 2019).
54. Full Prescribing Information Dilatrate-SR. Available online: https://www.drugs.com/pro/dilatrate-sr.html (accessed on 20 July 2019).
55. Full Prescribing Information Durlaza. Available online: https://www.drugs.com/pro/durlaza.html (accessed on 20 July 2019).
56. Full Prescribing Information Enjuvia. Available online: https://www.drugs.com/pro/enjuvia.html (accessed on 20 July 2019).
57. Full Prescribing Information Entocort EC. Available online: https://www.drugs.com/pro/entocort-ec.html (accessed on 20 July 2019).
58. Full Prescribing Information Levbid®. Available online: https://www.rxlist.com/levbid-extended-release-drug.htm#indications (accessed on 20 July 2019).
59. Orfiril Long Minitablets Information. Available online: https://ec.europa.eu/health/documents/community-register/2018/20180531140837/anx_140837_en.pdf (accessed on 20 July 2019).
60. Full Prescribing Information Palladone. Available online: https://www.drugs.com/pro/palladone.html (accessed on 20 July 2019).
61. Full Prescribing Information Pentasa. Available online: https://www.accessdata.fda.gov/drugsatfda_docs/label/2018/020049s031lbl.pdf (accessed on 20 July 2019).
62. Full Prescribing Information Qsymia. Available online: https://www.drugs.com/qsymia.html (accessed on 20 July 2019).
63. Full Prescribing Information Tegretol®-XR. Available online: https://www.accessdata.fda.gov/drugsatfda_docs/label/2009/016608s101,018281s048lbl.pdf (accessed on 20 July 2019).
64. Full Prescribing Information Trokendi XR. Available online: https://www.drugs.com/pro/trokendi-xr.html (accessed on 20 July 2019).
65. Kathe, K.; Kathpalia, H. Film forming systems for topical and transdermal drug delivery. *Asian J. Pharm. Sci.* **2017**, *12*, 487–497. [CrossRef]
66. Joshi, M.; Sharma, V.; Pathak, K. Matrix based system of isotretinoin as nail lacquer to enhance transungal delivery across human nail plate. *Int. J. Pharm.* **2015**, *478*, 268–277. [CrossRef] [PubMed]
67. Vipin, K.V.; Sarath, C.C.; Ann, R.A.; Premaletha, K.; Muriakose, M.R. Formulation and evaluation of an antifungal nail lacquer for onychomycosis. *Br. Biomed. Bull.* **2014**, *2*, 242–248.
68. Šveikauskaitė, I.; Briedis, V. Effect of film-forming polymers on release of naftifine hydrochloride from nail lacquers. *Int. J. Polym. Sci.* **2017**, *1*, 7. [CrossRef]
69. Baranowski, P.; Karolewicz, B.; Gajda, M.; Pluta, J. Ophthalmic drug dosage forms: Characterisation and research methods. *Sci. World J.* **2014**, *2014*, 1–14. [CrossRef]
70. Paradkar, M.; Thakkar, V.; Soni, T.; Gandhi, T.; Gohel, M. Formulation and evaluation of clotrimazole transdermal spray. *Drug Dev. Ind. Pharm.* **2015**, *41*, 1718–1725. [CrossRef]
71. Goudanavar, P.; Ambhore, N.; Hiremath, D.; Udupi, R. Comparative evaluation of polymer combination in the design of brimonidine tartrate ocular inserts. *Indian Drugs* **2012**, *49*, 30–35.
72. Mundada, A.S.; Shrikhande, B.K. Design and evaluation of soluble ocular drug insert for controlled release of ciprofloxacin hydrochloride. *Drug Dev. Ind. Pharm.* **2006**, *32*, 443–448. [CrossRef]

73. Khan, S.; Ali, A.; Singhavi, D.; Yeole, P. Preparation of ophthalmic insert of acyclovir using ethylcellulose rate-controlling membrane. *J. Appl. Ther. Res.* **2008**, *6*, 19–24.
74. Kala, S.; Gurudiwn, P.; Juyal, D. Formulation and evaluation of besifloxacin loaded in situ gel for ophthalmic delivery. *UKJPB.* **2018**, *6*, 36–40. [CrossRef]
75. Mortazavi, S.A.; Jaffariazar, Z.; Damercheli, E. Formulation and in-vitro evaluation of ocular ciprofloxacin-containing minitablets prepared with different combinations of carbopol 974P and various cellulose derivatives. *IJPR.* **2010**, *9*, 107–114. [PubMed]
76. John, L.; Kumar, A.; Samuel, S. Formulation and evaluation of amlodipine transdermal patches using ethyl cellulose. *Int. Res. J. Pharm.* **2013**, *4*, 84–88. [CrossRef]
77. Idrees, A.; Rahman, N.U.; Javaid, Z.; Kashif, M.; Aslam, I.; Abbas, K.; Hussain, T. In vitro evaluation of transdermal patches of flurbiprofen with ethyl cellulose. *Acta Pol. Pharm.* **2014**, *71*, 287–295. [PubMed]
78. Cherukuri, S.; Ba, U.R. Formulation and evaluation of transdermal drug delivery of topiramate. *Int. J. Pharm. Investig.* **2017**, *7*, 10–17. [PubMed]
79. Akhlaq, M.; Arshad, M.S.; Mudassir, A.M.; Hussain, A.; Kucuk, I.; Haj-Ahmad, R.; Rasekh, M.; Ahmad, Z. Formulation and evaluation of anti-rheumatic dexibuprofen transdermal patches: A quality-by-design approach. *J. Drug. Targ.* **2016**, *24*, 603–612. [CrossRef]
80. Gupta, V.; Singh, S.; Srivarstava, M.; Ahmad, H.; Pachauri, S.D.; Khandelwal, K.; Dwivedi, P.; Dwivedi, A.K. Effect of polydimethylsiloxane and ethylcellulose on in vitro permeation of centchroman from its transdermal patches. *Drug Deliv.* **2016**, *23*, 113–122. [CrossRef]
81. Huang, Y.; Dai, W.G. Fundamental aspects of solid dispersion technology for poorly soluble drugs. *Acta Pharm. Sin. B* **2014**, *4*, 18–25. [CrossRef]
82. Tsunashima, D.; Yamashita, K.; Ogawara, K.; Sako, K.; Higaki, K. Preparation of extended release solid dispersion formulations of tacrolimus using ethylcellulose and hydroxypropylmethylcellulose by solvent evaporation metod. *J. Pharm. Pharmacol.* **2016**, *68*, 316–323. [CrossRef]
83. Sadeghi, F.; Garekani, H.A.; Sadeghi, R. Comparison of ethylcellulose matrix characteristics prepared by solid dispersion technique or physical mixing. *Daru J. Fac. Pharm.* **2012**, *11*, 27–34.
84. Ohara, T.; Kitamura, S.; Kitagawa, T.; Terada, K. Dissolution mechanism of poorly water-soluble drug from extended release solid dispersion system with ethylcellulose and hydroxypropylmethylcellulose. *Int. J. Pharm.* **2005**, *302*, 95–102. [CrossRef]
85. Samba, M.; Kumawat, M.; Sambamoorthly, U. Formulation of sustain release solid dispersion of verapamil hydrochloride using ethyl cellulose and Eudragit RSPO. *Int. J. Pharm. Pharm. Sci.* **2011**, *3*, 116–122.
86. Singh, M.N.; Hemant, K.S.Y.; Ram, M.; Shivakumar, H.G. Microencapsulation: A promising technique for controlled drug delivery. *Res. Pharm. Sci.* **2010**, *5*, 65–77. [PubMed]
87. Chandrasekaran, P.; Kandasamy, R. Solid oral flexible formulations for pediatric and geriatric patients: Age-appropriate formulation platforms. *Indian J. Pharm. Sci.* **2018**, *80*, 14–25. [CrossRef]
88. Murtaza, G. Ethylcellulose microparticles: A review. *Acta Pol. Pharm.* **2012**, *69*, 11–22.
89. Pan-In, P.; Banlunara, W.; Chaichanawongsaroj, N.; Wanichwecharungruang, S. Ethyl cellulose nanoparticles: Clarithomycin encapsulation and eradication of *H. pylori*. *Carbohydr. Polym.* **2014**, *109*, 22–27. [CrossRef]
90. Djerafi, R.; Swanepoel, A.; Crampon, C.; Kalombo, L.; Labuschagne, P.; Badens, E.; Masmoudi, Y. Supercritical antisolvent co-precipitation of rifampicin and ethyl cellulose. *Eur. J. Pharm. Sci.* **2017**, *102*, 161–171. [CrossRef]
91. Villa Nova, M.; Gonçalves Mde, C.; Nogueira, A.C.; Herculano Lda, S.; Medina, A.N.; Bazotte, R.B.; Bruschi, M.L. Formulation and characterization of ethylcellulose microparticles containing L-alanyl-L-glutamine. *Drug Dev. Ind. Pharm.* **2014**, *40*, 1308–1317. [CrossRef]
92. Shankar, N.B.; Kumar, R.P.; Kumar, N.U.; Brata, B.B. Development and characterization of bioadhesive gel of microencapsulated metronidazole for vaginal use. *Iran J. Pharm. Res.* **2010**, *9*, 209–219.
93. Balzus, B.; Sahle, F.F.; Hönzke, S.; Gerecke, C.; Schumacher, F.; Hedtrich, S.; Kleuser, B.; Bodmeier, R. Formulation and ex vivo evaluation of polymeric nanoparticles for controlled delivery of corticosteroids to the skin and the corneal epithelium. *Eur. J. Pharm. Biopharm.* **2017**, *115*, 122–130. [CrossRef]
94. El-Habashy, S.E.; Allam, A.N.; El-Kamel, A.H. Ethyl cellulose nanoparticles as a platform to decrease ulcerogenic potential of piroxicam: Formulation and in vitro/in vivo evaluation. *Int. J. Nanomed.* **2016**, *11*, 2369–2380.

95. Begum, N.; Sailaja, A.K. Formulation and evaluation of Cox-2 inhibitor (etoricoxib) loaded ethyl cellulose nanoparticles for topical drug delivery. *Nano. Biomed. Eng.* **2018**, *10*, 1–9.
96. Chassot, J.M.; Ribas, D.; Silveira, E.F.; Grünspan, L.D.; Pires, C.C.; Farago, P.V.; Braganhol, E.; Tasso, L.; Cruz, L. Beclomethasone dipropionate-loaded polymeric nanocapsules: Development, in vitro cytotoxicity, and in vivo evaluation of acute lung injury. *J. Nanosci. Nanotechnol.* **2015**, *15*, 855–864. [CrossRef] [PubMed]
97. Tussionex®Drug Information: Description, User Reviews, Drug Side Effects, Interactions—Prescribing Information. Available online: https://www.rxlist.com/tussionex-drug.htm (accessed on 20 July 2019).
98. Kasashima, Y.; Uchida, S.; Yoshihara, K.; Yasuji, T.; Sako, K.; Namiki, N. Oral sustained-release suspension based on a lauryl sulfate salt/complex. *Int. J. Pharm.* **2016**, *30*, 677–683. [CrossRef] [PubMed]
99. Singh, I.; Rehni, A.K.; Kalra, R.; Joshi, G.; Kumar, M.; Aboul-Enein, H.Y. Ion exchange resins: Drug delivery and therapeutic applications. *FABAD J. Pharm. Sci.* **2007**, *32*, 91–100.
100. Maulvi, F.A.; Soni, T.G.; Shah, D.O. Extended release of timolol from ethyl cellulose microparticles laden hydrogel contact lenses. *Open Pharm. Sci.* **2015**, *2*, 1–12. [CrossRef]
101. Maulvi, F.A.; Lakdawala, D.H.; Shaikh, A.A.; Desai, A.R.; Choksi, H.H.; Vaidya, R.J.; Ranch, K.M.; Koli, A.R.; Vyas, B.A.; Shah, D.O. In vitro and in vivo evaluation of novel implantation technology in hydrogel contact lenses for controlled drug delivery. *J. Control Release* **2016**, *226*, 47–56. [CrossRef]
102. Arici, M.; Topbas, O.; Karavana, S.Y.; Ertan, G.; Sariisik, M.; Ozturk, C. Preparation of naproxen-ethyl cellulose microparticles by spray drying technique and their application to textile materials. *J. Microencapsul.* **2014**, *31*, 654–666. [CrossRef]
103. Patel, S.; Patel, H.; Seth, A. Microsponge drug delivery system: An overview. *JGPT.* **2010**, *2*, 1–9.
104. Aloorkar, N.; Kulkarni, A.; Ingale, D.; Patil, R. Microsponges as innovative drug delivery systems. *Int. J. Pharm. Sci. Nanotechnol.* **2012**, *5*, 1597–1606.
105. Kappor, D.; Patel, M.; Vyas, R.; Lad, C.; Tyagi, B. A review on microsponge drug delivery system. *JDDT.* **2014**, *4*, 29–35. [CrossRef]
106. Bothiraja, C.; Gholap, A.D.; Shaikh, K.S.; Pawar, A.P. Investigation of ethyl cellulose microsponge gel for topical delivery of eberconazole nitrate for fungal therapy. *Ther. Deliv.* **2014**, *5*, 781–794. [CrossRef] [PubMed]
107. Jelvehgari, M.; Siahi-Shadbad, M.R.; Azarmi, S.; Martin, G.P.; Nokhodchi, A. The microsponge delivery system of benzoyl peroxide: Preparation, characterization and release studies. *Int. J. Pharm.* **2006**, *308*, 124–132. [CrossRef] [PubMed]
108. Yadav, E.; Rao, R.; Kumar, S.; Mahant, S.; Vohra, P. Microsponge based gel of tea tree oil for dermatological microbial infections. *Nat. Prod. J.* **2018**, *8*, 1. [CrossRef]
109. Pawar, A.P.; Gholap, A.P.; Kuchekar, A.B.; Bothiraja, C.; Mali, A.J. Formulation and evaluation of optimized oxybenzone microsponge gel for topical delivery. *J. Drug. Deliv.* **2015**, 1–9. [CrossRef]
110. Zaman, M.; Qureshi, S.; Sultana, K.; Hanif, M.; Mahmood, A.; Shaheryar, Z.A.; Gulzar, F.; Barkat, K.; Abdel-Daim, M.M. Application of quasi-emulsification and modified double emulsification techniques for formulation of tacrolimus microsponges. *Int. J. Nanomed.* **2018**, *13*, 4537–4548. [CrossRef]
111. Obiedallah, M.M.; Abdel-Mageed, A.M.; Elfaham, T.H. Ocular administration of acetazolamide microsponges in situ gel formulations. *SPJ* **2018**, *6*, 909–920. [CrossRef]
112. Bharathala, S.; Sharma, P. Biomedical applications of nanoparticles. Recent Trends and Future Perspectives. In *Nanotechnology in Modern Animal Biotechnology*; Maurya, P.K., Singh, S., Eds.; Springer Singapore: Singapore, 2019; pp. 113–132.
113. Liu, M.; Zhang, Y.; Sun, S.; Khan, A.R.; Ji, J.; Yang, M.; Zhai, G. Recent advances in electrospun for drug delivery purpose. *J. Drug Target.* **2019**, *27*, 270–282. [CrossRef]
114. Goyal, R.; Macri, L.K.; Kaplan, H.M.; Kohn, J. Nanoparticles and nanofibers for topical drug delivery. *J. Control Release* **2016**, *28*, 77–92. [CrossRef]
115. Li, H.; Liu, K.; Williams, G.R.; Wu, J.; Wu, J.; Wang, H.; Niu, S.; Zhu, L.M. Dual temperature and pH responsive nanofiber formulations prepared by electrospinning. *Colloids Surf. B* **2018**, *171*, 142–149. [CrossRef]
116. You, D.G.; Li, X.Y.; Wang, X.; Yang, J.H.; Bligh, S.A.; Williams, G.R. Nanofibers fabricated using triaxial electrospinning as zero order drug delivery systems. *ACS Appl. Mater. Interfaces* **2015**, *7*, 18891–18897. [CrossRef]
117. Illangakoon, U.E.; Yu, D.G.; Ahmad, B.S.; Chatterton, N.P.; Williams, D.R. 5-Fluorouracil loaded Eudragit fibers prepared by electrospinning. *Int. J. Pharm.* **2015**, *495*, 895–902. [CrossRef] [PubMed]

118. Lu, H.; Wang, Q.; Li, G.; Qiu, Y.; Wei, Q. Electrospun water-stable zein/ethyl cellulose composite nanofiber and its drug release properties. *Mater. Sci. Eng. C Matter. Biol. Appl.* **2017**, *74*, 86–93. [CrossRef] [PubMed]
119. Liu, Y.; Deng, L.; Zhang, C.; Feng, F.; Zhang, H. Tunable physical properties of ethylcellulose/gelatin composite nanofibers by electrospinning. *J. Agric. Food Chem.* **2018**, *28*, 1907–1915. [CrossRef] [PubMed]
120. Bagul, U.; Gujar, K.; Dhat, S.; Aphale, S.; Bhavsar, M. In vitro study of mucoadhesive strength of polymers for mucoadhesive drug delivery systems. *Int. J. Curr. Pharm. Res.* **2009**, *1*, 42–46.
121. Abruzzo, A.; Nicoletta, F.P.; Dalena, F.; Cerchiara, T.; Luppi, B.; Bigucci, F. Bilayered buccal films as child-appropriate dosage form for systemic administration of propranolol. *Int. J. Pharm.* **2017**, *5*, 257–265. [CrossRef] [PubMed]
122. Zhang, C.; Liu, Y.; Li, W.; Gao, P.; Xiang, D.; Ren, X.; Liu, D. Mucoadhesive buccal film containing ornidazole and dexamethasone for oral ulcers: In vitro and in vivo studies. *Pharm. Dev. Technol.* **2019**, *24*, 118–126. [CrossRef] [PubMed]
123. Laffleur, F.; Krouská, J.; Tkacz, J.; Pekař, M.; Aghai, F.; Netsomboon, K. Buccal adhesive films with moisturizer-the next level for dry mouth syndrome? *Int. J. Pharm.* **2018**, *550*, 309–315. [CrossRef] [PubMed]
124. Ammar, H.O.; Ghorab, M.M.; Mahmoud, A.A.; Shahin, H.I. Design and in vitro/in vivo evaluation of ultra-thin mucoadhesive buccal film containing fluticasone propionate. *AAPS PharmSciTech.* **2017**, *18*, 93–103. [CrossRef]
125. Mukherjee, D.; Bharath, S. Design and characterization of double layered mucoadhesive system containing bisphosphonate derivative. *ISRN Pharm.* **2013**, *19*, 604690. [CrossRef]
126. Roh, J.; Han, M.; Kim, K.N.; Kim, K.M. The in vitro and in vivo effects of a fast-dissolving mucoadhesive bi-layered strip as topical anesthetics. *Dent. Mater. J.* **2016**, *35*, 601–605. [CrossRef]
127. Phaechamud, T.; Mahadlek, J. Solvent exchange-induced in situ forming gel comprising ethyl cellulose-antimicrobial drugs. *Int. J. Pharm.* **2015**, *494*, 381–392. [CrossRef] [PubMed]
128. Sallam, A.S.; Hamudi, F.F.; Khalil, E.A. Effect of ethylcellulose and propylene glycol on the controlled-release performance of glyceryl monooleate–mertronidazole periodontal gel. *Pharm. Dev. Technol.* **2015**, *20*, 159–168. [CrossRef] [PubMed]
129. Pathak, K.; Sharma, V.; Akhtar, N.; Rastogi, P. Localization of fluconazole in oral cavity by preferential coating of buccoadhesive tablet for treatment of oral thrush. *Int. J. Pharm. Invest.* **2016**, *6*, 106–115. [CrossRef] [PubMed]

4

Cell Theranostics on Mesoporous Silicon Substrates

Maria Laura Coluccio [1,†], Valentina Onesto [1,†], Giovanni Marinaro [2,3], Mauro Dell'Apa [4], Stefania De Vitis [1], Alessandra Imbrogno [5], Luca Tirinato [1], Gerardo Perozziello [1], Enzo Di Fabrizio [6], Patrizio Candeloro [1], Natalia Malara [1,*,‡] and Francesco Gentile [4,*,‡]

1 Department of Experimental and Clinical Medicine, University Magna Graecia, 88100 Catanzaro, Italy; coluccio@unicz.it (M.L.C.); valentina.onesto@unicz.it (V.O.); stefania.devitis24@gmail.com (S.D.V.); tirinato@unicz.it (L.T.); gerardo.perozziello@unicz.it (G.P.); patrizio.candeloro@unicz.it (P.C.)
2 Institute of Process Engineering, Technische Universität Dresden, 01069 Dresden, Germany; giovanni.marinaro@kaust.edu.sa
3 Institute of Fluid Dynamics, Helmholtz-Zentrum Dresden-Rossendorf (HZDR), 01328 Dresden, Germany
4 Department of Electrical Engineering and Information Technology, University Federico II, 80125 Naples, Italy; mauro.dellapa@gmail.com
5 Emerging Materials & Devices, Tyndall National Institute, Cork T12 R5CP, Ireland; alessandra.imbrogno@tyndall.ie
6 Department of Applied Science and Technology, Polytechnic University of Turin, 10129 Torino, Italy; enzo.difabrizio@polito.it
* Correspondence: nataliamalara@unicz.it (N.M.); francesco.gentile2@unina.it (F.G.)
† These authors contributed equally to this work.
‡ These two authors share senior authorship.

Abstract: The adhesion, proliferation, and migration of cells over nanomaterials is regulated by a cascade of biochemical signals that originate at the interface of a cell with a substrate and propagate through the cytoplasm to the nucleus. The topography of the substrate plays a major role in this process. Cell adhesion molecules (CAMs) have a characteristic size of some nanometers and a range of action of some tens of nanometers. Controlling details of a surface at the nanoscale—the same dimensional over which CAMs operate—offers ways to govern the behavior of cells and create organoids or tissues with heretofore unattainable precision. Here, using electrochemical procedures, we generated mesoporous silicon surfaces with different values of pore size (PS $\approx$ 11 nm and PS $\approx$ 21 nm), roughness (Ra $\approx$ 7 nm and Ra $\approx$ 13 nm), and fractal dimension (Df $\approx$ 2.48 and Df $\approx$ 2.15). Using electroless deposition, we deposited over these substrates thin layers of gold nanoparticles. Resulting devices feature (i) nanoscale details for the stimulation and control of cell assembly, (ii) arrays of pores for drug loading/release, (iii) layers of nanostructured gold for the enhancement of the electromagnetic signal in Raman spectroscopy (SERS). We then used these devices as cell culturing substrates. Upon loading with the anti-tumor drug PtCl (O,O′-acac)(DMSO) we examined the rate of adhesion and growth of breast cancer MCF-7 cells under the coincidental effects of surface geometry and drug release. Using confocal imaging and SERS spectroscopy we determined the relative importance of nano-topography and delivery of therapeutics on cell growth—and how an unbalance between these competing agents can accelerate the development of tumor cells.

Keywords: nanoporous silicon; gold nanoparticles; drug delivery; cancer cells; theranostics

1. Introduction

Tissue engineering is a combination of techniques and materials for the fabrication of scaffolds and devices that, interacting with the cells, can lead to the formation of an analogue of tissues and organs that can improve, assist, or replace those already existing in the human body [1–4]. The biomaterials to be used in tissue engineering should exhibit the most convenient combination of mechanical properties, macro-scale architecture, and nanoscale geometry, to influence the collective behavior of cells and induce cells to form efficient structures. Those structures should be biocompatible, energetically efficient, autonomous, computationally efficient, and should be organized in a way to optimize the exchange of biochemical signals, nutrients, and oxygen between the several different parts of the structures and the external environment [1,2,4,5]. Thus, an ideal scaffold should present details over different hierarchical length scales to enable cell colonization, migration, and organization, and should be preferentially porous to enable the transport of bio-molecules.

At the nanoscale, cell behavior is strongly influenced by their interaction with the surrounding microenvironment [6–11]. Nanomaterials can interact without intermediation with the those adhesion molecules (integrins, cadherins, selectins, the immunoglobulin superfamily of cell surface proteins) involved in several different cell functions, including recognition, binding, adhesion, migration, apoptosis, differentiation, survival, and transcription [7–9,11,12]. Due to this unmediated interaction, nanomaterials can be fine-tuned to manipulate cellular function [13]. Materials with a controlled design at the nanoscale have been demonstrated in applications such as stem cells differentiation [14], the activation of the immune synapse [15], the shaping and signaling in neuronal networks [16], cell adhesion [17–19] and growth [20,21], the manipulation and control of neural polarity [22]. While many of the reported works have focused on bi-dimensional geometries, recent advances in additive manufacturing technologies [23], such as light assisted photopolymerization techniques [24], stereolithography [25], digital light projection, and two-photon polymerization [26], allowed a smooth transition from a 2D to a 3D design of the intended nano-structures [27]. The resulting cell culture models have an increased degree of complexity, an increased number of degrees of freedom, and exhibit a more faithful adherence to the 3D complex architectures of cells in living tissue and organs. This in turn enables to reproduce with an increased level of fidelity the natural microenvironment of cells [28].

Nevertheless, despite important advances in the production of scaffolds for tissue engineering applications, the development of characterization techniques has lagged behind the progress of fabrication. Recently, the demand for new devices for the analysis of the behavior of cells at the length scale of cell receptor is increasing. Those devices may reveal the fundamental biological mechanisms behind cell adhesion, migration, and organization at the cell-adhesion-molecule level, disclosing precious information for those interested in designing the scaffolds in the most efficient way.

In this paper, we present a mesoporous silicon device with details over multiple scales for cell culture, growth, and assembly. The device is functionalized with gold nanoparticle clusters that can be exploited to amplify the Raman signal measured at the cell interface. Thanks to the pores in the silicon matrix, the device can release drugs, growth factors, or other biomolecules to the cells over time. Thus, the device combines the ability of a scaffold to support cell growth with the ability of a drug delivery system to vehicle active-molecules to the cells adhering to the scaffold. The gold nanoparticles on the device enable to examine the combined effects of surface nano-topography and the delivery of drugs on cell adhesion and proliferation. In experiments in which we put in culture cancerous MCF-7 cells on the device, we measured the simultaneous effect of the pore size and of the delivery of an anti-tumor drug on the adhesive and proliferation properties of cells. Moreover, using Raman spectroscopy and a multivariate analysis of data, we mapped the spatial distribution of receptors expressed over the cell surface, and correlated that distribution to the nanoscale architecture of the device. We found that cells exhibit an increased ability to grow and to form clusters on substrates with smaller pore size (PS $\approx$ 11 nm) and roughness ($R_a \approx 7$ nm), compared to substrates with larger pore size (PS $\approx$ 21 nm) and roughness (Ra $\approx$ 13 nm), in line with previous studies [29,30]. Both substrates deliver their payload efficiently, up to 10 days from the initial release, demonstrating high anti-cancer efficacy and killing up to 90% of cancerous cells on the smaller mesoporous substrate after 72 h from cell culture.

The multi-functional device that we developed can be used to evaluate the coincidental effects of (i) a timely administrated drug or nutrient and of the (ii) nanoscale characteristics of a surface on the efficacy of a therapeutic treatment, the functionalities of a scaffold, or a combination of the two. The device can be potentially used in applications that bridge traditional drug delivery, traditional tissue engineering and regenerative medicine, and diagnostics.

2. Methods

2.1. *Fabrication of Mesoporous Silicon Surfaces*

A detailed scheme of the fabrication of the Au-functionalized substrates is reported in Figure 1. Silicon substrates were electrochemically etched to obtain porous silicon. Porous silicon is a form of silicon with arrays of pores penetrating through its structure [31]. The average pore size (PS) determines the class of the porous silicon material: substrates with PS < 2 nm, 2 < PS < 50 nm, or PS > 50 nm are classified as nanoporous, mesoporous, macroporous silicon substrates, respectively [31]. In this work we produced mesoporous silicon substrates with two different non-overlapping values of pore size: MeP_1 silicon substrates with $PS_1 \approx 11$ nm and MeP_2 silicon substrates with $PS_2 \approx 21$ nm. We used P-type, 100 silicon wafers as a substrate. We cut the originating silicon wafers into regular square chips with a side of ≈1 cm. We then positioned the chips in an impermeable electrolytic cell where samples were exposed to a solution of hydrofluoric acid (HF) and ethanol or methanol, under the action of an external electric field [30]. As a result, hydrogen ions in solution were accelerated towards the silicon substrate etching the pores. Substrates with a different pore size were obtained by tuning the parameters of the technique: the intensity of etching current, the concentration of HF in solution, the type of neutral component in solution (ethanol or methanol), and the time of the process. MeP_1 silicon with an average pore size of PS ≈ 11 nm was obtained using a mixture of HF, D.I. (de-ionized) water and ethanol in a proportion of 1:1:1 in volume. In the process, a value of current density of I = 20 mA/cm^2 was applied for 5 min at 25 °C. MeP_2 silicon with an average pore size of PS ≈ 21 nm was obtained using a mixture of HF, D.I. water, and methanol in a proportion of 5:3:2 in volume. In the process, a value of current density of I = 4 mA/cm^2 was applied for 5 min at 25 °C. In all cases, the thickness of the porous layer is of some tens of micrometers. Since porous silicon is intrinsically hydrophobic [32], samples were oxidized in an oven at 200 °C for 2 h before use. The photoluminescence of mesoporous silicon was verified by imaging the light emission of the samples under UV radiation (365 nm).

2.2. *Electroless Deposition of Gold Nanoparticles Clusters*

Clusters of gold nanoparticles were deposited on the porous sample surface using electroless deposition techniques. In the technique, metal ions in solution are reduced on an autocatalytic surface to form solid deposits of that metal [33]. Following the methods reported in [34], we treated the porous silicon samples in a solution of HF and gold (III) chloride ($AuCl_3$) in a concentration of 0.15 M (HF) and 1 mM ($AuCl_3$) for 3 min at 50 °C. In solution, the ions of gold react with the exposed silicon surface yielding gold nanoparticles with an average particle size d ≈ 20 nm. Samples were then rinsed in D.I. water at room temperature for 30 s.

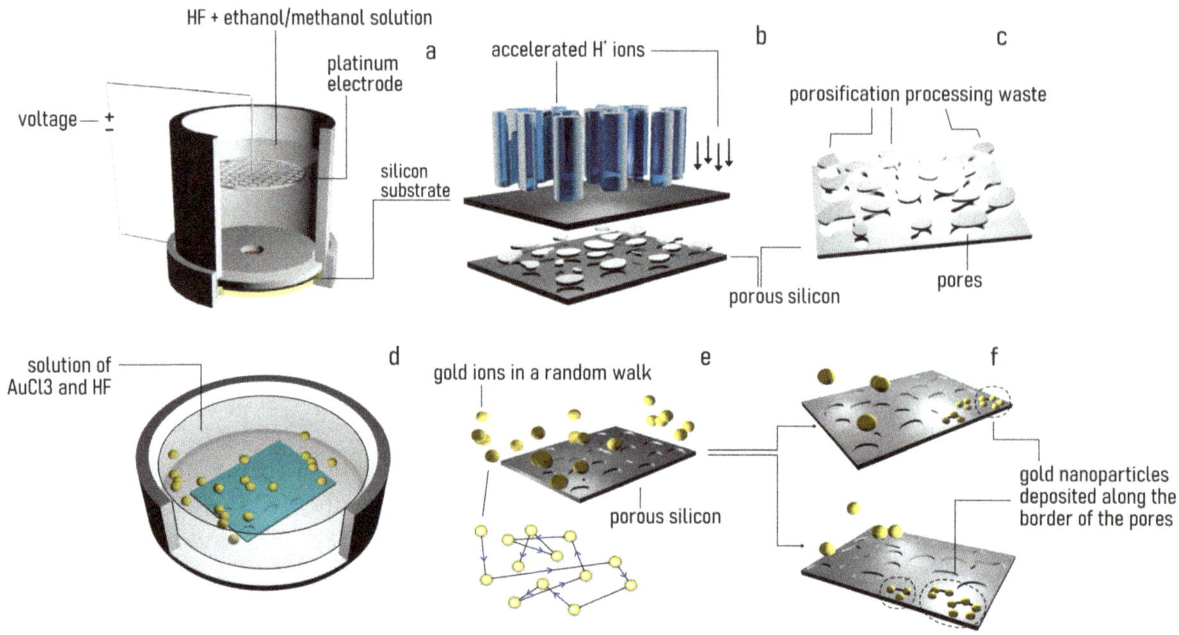

Figure 1. (**a**) An initial silicon chip of approximately 1 × 1 cm is electrochemical etched using a Teflon cell containing a solution of hydrofluoric acid (HF), D.I. (de-ionized) water, and methanol/ethanol in different ratios. (**b**) Upon activation of an external controlled voltage, positive ions in solution are accelerated towards the silicon substrate, creating pores within its structure. (**c**) Depending on the parameters of the process, including etching time, current and voltage intensity, and the concentration of the reagents in solution, one can obtain porous silicon surfaces with a tailored morphology. (**d**) The porous silicon sample is then placed in a baker along with a solution of hydrofluoric acid (HF) and gold(III) chloride ($AuCl_3$). (**e**) The resulting electroless process enables the deposition of gold ions in solution on the autocatalytic porous-silicon surface. (**f**) By varying the parameters of the electroless process, including temperature, concentration, and time, one can produce substrates with controlled gold-nanoparticles shape, size, and density.

2.3. *SEM Sample Characterization*

SEM (Scanning Electron Microscopy) analysis was conducted with a Zeiss GeminiSEM 500 at Dresden Center for Nanoanalysis (DCN), TU Dresden, Germany. Two types of porous silicon samples were analyzed: mesoporous 1 (MeP_1) and mesoporous 2 (MeP_2). Both samples were provided with and without gold nanoparticles deposited on their surface. Samples were fixed on stubs with a long pin and then mounted on a carousel 9 × 9 mm sample holder. In order to fix the samples, a small amount of silver paint was applied between the edge of the silicon substrate and the stub. A further copper lever was screwed in order to secure the sample on the stub. Several images of the samples were acquired in High Vacuum mode at 3 kV, a magnification factor of 300,000, and a working distance of about 3 mm with an InLens Detector (ZEISS) for secondary electrons. In order to reduce the drift, a frame integration (N = 14) was performed. In this way, every frame was scanned and averaged 14 times.

2.4. *AFM Sample Characterization*

Sample nanotopography was verified using atomic force microscopy (ICON Atomic Force Microscope, Bruker, Coventry, UK). We measured the surface profile over a sampling area of $1 \times 1\ \mu m^2$, in a dynamic tapping mode in air. All measurements were performed at room temperature. During image acquisition, the scan rate was fixed as 0.5 Hz, while images were discretized in 1024 × 1024 points. We used Ultra-sharp Si probes (ACLA-SS, AppNano, Mountain View, CA, USA) with a nominal tip radius less than 5 nm to assure high resolution. Multiple measurements were done in different scan directions to avoid artefacts. At least four images were recorded per sample to reduce uncertainty. After acquisition, images were analyzed using the methods developed in [17] to determine the average surface roughness (Ra) and fractal dimension (Df) for each sample.

2.5. Contact Angle Characterization of Samples

The wettability of the samples was verified using an automatic contact angle meter (KSV CAM 101, KSV Instruments Ltd., Helsinki, Finland). A drop of 5 μL of D.I. water was gently positioned on the sample surface at room temperature. After 5 s from deposition, the contact angle of the drop at the interface with the substrate was measured.

2.6. MCF-7 Cell Culture and Staining

Breast carcinoma MCF-7 cells were grown on the porous silicon surfaces. Cultures were carried out at 37 °C in a humidified 5% CO_2/air atmosphere in a Dulbecco's modified eagle's medium (DMEM, Euroclone) supplied with 10% heat-inactivated fetal bovine serum (Euroclone, Pero (Mi), Italy), streptomycin (0.2 mg/mL) and penicillin (200 IU/mL). When cells on the petri dishes reached 90% confluence, they were dissociated: medium was removed and MCF-7 were treated with a solution of 0.25% Trypsin-0.53mM EDTA (Euroclone) for about 5 min at 37 °C. Trypsin was deactivated by adding medium and completely removed after centrifugation of the cell suspension (1300 rpm, 5 min, 18 °C). Then, trypsin/growth medium solution was removed. Single sterilized porous Si wafer specimens with and without loaded drugs, having a size of around 15 × 15 mm, were individually placed into each well of a 6-well plate (Corning Incorporated) and washed with phosphate-buffered saline solution (PBS, Invitrogen). After that, cells were seeded in complete cell medium and cultured up to 15 days in a humidified incubator at 37 °C with 5% of CO_2. After the incubation period, cell culture medium was removed and the MCF-7 cells were washed twice in PBS, fixed with 4% PFA (paraformaldehyde), and left for 30 min at room temperature (RT). Subsequently, cells were washed twice in PBS and permeabilized with 0.05% triton (Invitrogen, Milano, Italy) for 5 min at RT. Fixed and permeabilized cells were stained with 100 μL DAPI (40, 6-Diamidino-2-phenylindole, Sigma Aldrich, Milano, Italy) solution for 10 min at 4 °C in dark environment. In the end, the DAPI solute ion was removed and each sample was washed with PBS. The total number of cells n_{tot} initially seeded in each well for incubation was approximately $n_{tot} \approx 10^5$. Cells were sub-confluent for the duration of the experiment. MCF-7 cells were chosen as a cell-model because they are characterized by a moderate expression of the integrins. As previously reported [35], the change in the intensity and type of expression of integrin is the basis of the cancer disease progression. Notably, MCF-7 are a secondary cell line. The choice of another cell line, perhaps a primary cell line, while could possibly enhance clustering, may not have—at the same time—the same effect on the expression of integrins in the system.

2.7. Imaging Cells on the Substrates

An inverted Leica TCS-SP2® laser scanning confocal microscopy (Wetzlar, Germany) system was used to image cells adhering on the substrates. All measurements were performed using ArUv laser (Leica, Wetzlar, Germany). The pinhole was set to ≈ 80 μm (1.5 Airy units) and the laser power to 80% of the maximum, these values of the parameters were maintained constant throughout each acquisition. Confocal images of blue (DAPI) fluorescence were acquired using a 405 nm excitation line and a 10× dry objective, so that several cells could be simultaneously imaged in the region of interest, that was of 1174 × 882 μm^2, resulting in a pixel size of ≈ 1.72 μm. For each substrate, a large number of images was taken for statistical analysis. Each image was averaged over four lines and 10 frames to reduce noise. Images were acquired with a resolution of 1024 × 768 pixels, and were exported to a computer for processing and analysis.

2.8. Image Analysis and Topological Characteristics of Cell Networks

Confocal images of cell nuclei stained with DAPI were analyzed with Matlab® to extract the cell positions. Images were preprocessed to enhance contrast and low-pass filtered to remove constant power additive noise. Each image was partitioned into k = k different segments (going gradually from bright, k = 1, to dark, k = k) by k-means segmentation algorithms [30]. The information content of the image was thus associated with a gray level k = t and all the segments brighter than a certain threshold t were considered as background and shifted to 0. The values of the remaining segments, representing the cells, were shifted to 1. After that, the resulting image (g) was downsampled: if f was the average operator, f was shifted over g by steps of size r, where r^2 was the expected area of a cell nucleus in pixels. The pixel intensity (ranging from 0 to 1) of the resulting image indicated the probability that a pixel is a cell. If this probability is greater than a threshold, that pixel is considered being a node of the graph in a bi-dimensional grid. At this point, the links between the nodes can be established using the Waxman model [36], according to which the probability $P(u,v)$ of being a connection between two nodes u and v exponentially decays with their Euclidean distance d. If L is the largest Euclidean distance:

$$P(u,v) = \alpha e^{-d(u,v)/\beta L} \tag{1}$$

where d is the Euclidean distance between nodes u and v, and L is the largest possible Euclidean distance between two nodes of the grid. In the equation, α and β are the Waxman model parameters. According to α and β, which have to be chosen between 0 and 1, the density of links in a graph changes. In particular, low values of these parameters result in a low number of connections. For our study, $\alpha = 1$ and $\beta = 0.025$. The probability P ranges between 0 (if the distance between the pair of nodes is ideally infinite) and 1 (if the distance between the pair of nodes is zero). The connectivity information of a graph is described in the adjacency matrix A. A is a square matrix in which each element a_{ij} indicates whether two nodes i and j are connected ($a_{ij} = 1$) or not ($a_{ij} = 0$). In the analysis, diagonal elements were all zero, since links from a node to itself were not allowed. Moreover, graphs were considered being undirected, so that information could bidirectionally flow from i to j. As a consequence A was symmetric and $a_{ij} = a_{ji}$. As the Euclidean distances d_{ij} in the networks were extracted, we could decide if a pair of nodes is connected by the subsequent formula

$$\alpha e^{-d_{i,j}/\beta L} - R \geq 0 \tag{2}$$

in which R is a constant that we chose as 0.1 so that the probability of being a connection is $P = 0.9$. Once established the connections between the nodes, the network parameters including clustering coefficient, characteristic path length, and small-world-ness can be extracted. The definition and significance of these terms may be found in influential textbooks [37] and papers [38–41]. Once obtained the Cc and Cpl values, we found a precise measure of 'small-world-ness', the 'small-world-ness' coefficient (SW), based on the trade-off between high local clustering and short path length as described in [42]:

$$\mathrm{SW} = \frac{Cc_{graph}}{Cc_{rand}} / \frac{Cpl_{graph}}{Cpl_{rand}} \tag{3}$$

where Cc_{graph} and Cpl_{graph} are the clustering coefficient and the characteristic path length of the graph G under study, and Cc_{rand} and Cpl_{rand} are the equivalent values for a random Erdös-Rényi graph with the same number of nodes and edges of G.

2.9. Raman Analysis of Samples

MCF-7 cells fixed on the Au-mesoporous sample surface were analyzed by a WITec Raman microscope Alpha300 AR equipped with a 50×/0.7 N.A. (Numerical Aperture) objective. The signal was excited by a 633 nm laser, set to a power of 1 mW. For each sample, SERS (Surface Enhanced Raman Spectroscopy) maps of a portion of a cell were acquired in the x-y plane with a 0.5 μm stepsize, with the aim to analyze the SERS spectra coming in particular from the cell membrane, searching the different biochemical composition of each point to evidence the possible presence of adhesion proteins [43]. The Raman spectra were collected in the spectral range from 700 to 3250 1/cm, with an integration time of 1 s.

2.10. Principal Components Analysis of Raman Spectra

Spectra were pre-processed to minimize the effect of the fluorescence of samples by normalization on the total spectrum area. A principal component analysis (PCA) and a clustering analysis were performed on the spectral collection to highlight the chemical differences between the membrane's points [44]. The first five principal components (PCs) accounted for nearly 90% of the total spectral variation and they were then used to implement the clustering analysis by the Kmean method, imposing a number of five classes. All the pre-processing steps, the PCA, and the clustering analysis were carried out using the free software package Raman Tool Set (available on http://ramantoolset.sourceforge.net).

2.11. UV Characterization of Drug Release

To assess the drug-delivery capability of the device we verified the release over time of the anti-tumor drug PtCl(O,O^-acac)(*DMSO*). PtCl(O,O′-acac)(*DMSO*) is a platinum(II) complex containing acetylacetonate (*acac*), characterized by a high toxicity both in immortalized cell lines, as human cervical carcinoma (HeLa) cells or human breast cancer (MCF-7) cells, and in primary cultured human breast epithelial cells [45]. In this work, we incubated the mesoporous silicon samples in 30 μM/50 μM solutions of PtCl(O,O′-acac)(DMSO) in D.I. water for 60 h to load the drug. The release kinetic was tested over time up to 15 days, by immersion of the loaded sample in DI water and monitoring the drug concentration at different time, through the analysis of drug in solution by a spectrophotometer UV/Vis (LAMBDA 25 UV/Vis PerkinElmer), after standard calibration procedures of the samples.

2.12. Statistical Analysis

Data in the article and in the figures are represented as mean ± standard deviation. We used a Student's *t*-test statistics (two-tailed, unpaired) to perform comparison between means of different groups, where we assumed that elements in each group are normally distributed. In performing the test, the null hypothesis is that the means between pairs of samples are equal. Everywhere in the text and the figures the difference between two subsets of data is considered statistically significant if the Student's *t*-test gives a significant level p (p value) less than 0.05.

3. Results

3.1. Producing Gold-Functionalized Mesoporous Surfaces

Using electrochemical etching techniques described in Section 2, we produced porous silicon surfaces. Tuning the parameters of the electrochemical etching, we obtained two different pore morphologies: (i) mesoporous silicon samples with a pore size that oscillates around the central value PS = 11 nm (MeP_1 silicon with a pore size in the lower nanometer range) and (ii) mesoporous silicon samples with an average pore size PS = 21 nm (MeP_2 silicon with a pore size in the higher nanometer range). Scanning electron micrographs (SEM) of MeP_1 and MeP_2 samples taken at different magnifications reveal the morphology of the porous surface at different scales (Figure 2a–f). Pores on the surface of MeP_1 silicon are less uniformly distributed, are less dense, and result in a porosity of the sample of about $P \approx 12\%$ (Figure 2a–c). The porosity or void fraction is a measure of the void spaces in a material, it is a fraction of the volume of voids over the total volume, expressed here as a percentage between 0% and 100%: it was calculated following the image analysis algorithms reported in the Supporting Information 1 of Supplementary Materials. Differently, pores on the surface of MeP_2 silicon are more uniform and are more densely packed compared to the pores found in the MeP_1 morphology: for this category, the porosity of the sample soars to $P \approx 40\%$ (Figure 2d–f).

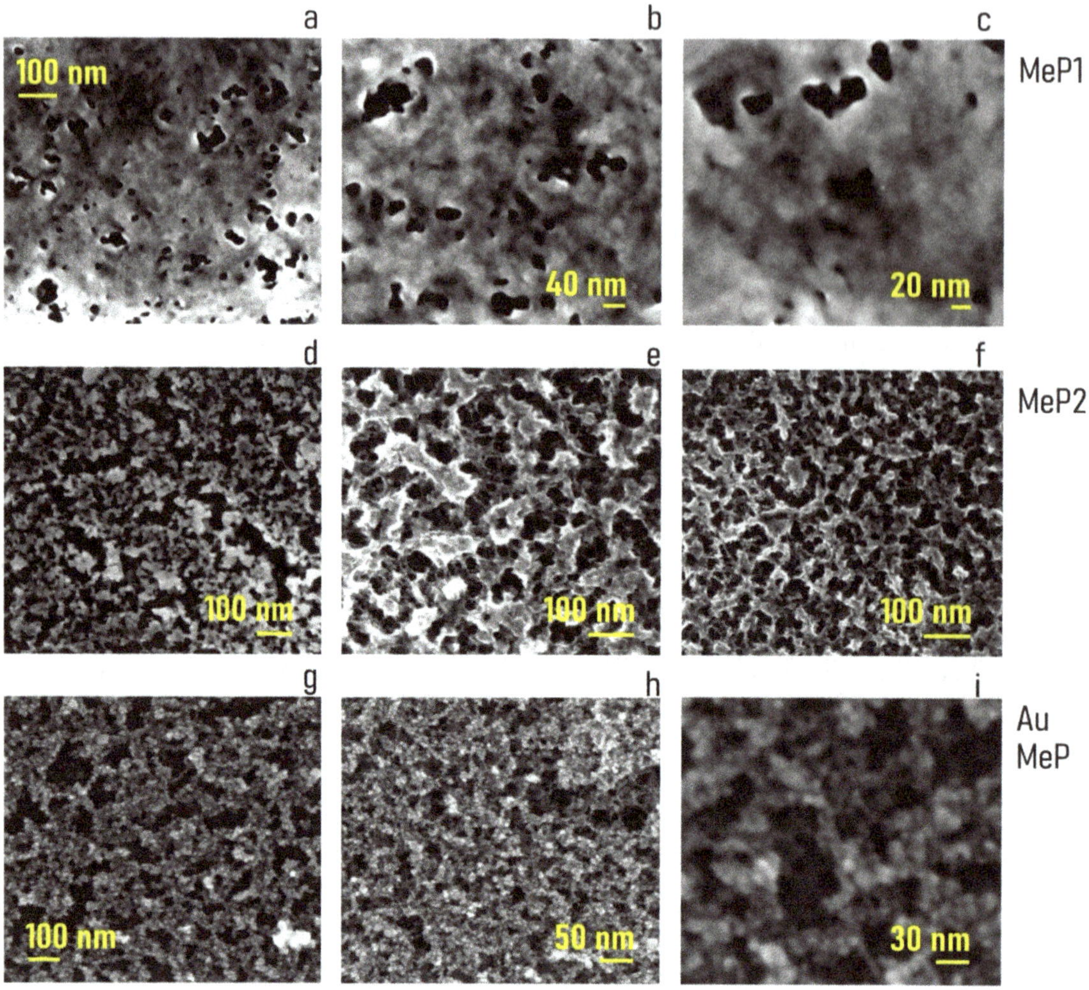

Figure 2. (**a–c**) SEM micrographs of MeP_1 substrates at different levels of magnification, the pores are less uniformly distributed over the sample surface with an average pore size of PS ≈ 11 nm. (**d–f**) SEM micrographs of MeP_2 substrates at different levels of magnification, the pores are uniformly distributed over the sample surface with an average pore size of PS ≈ 21 nm. (**g–i**) SEM micrographs of clusters of gold nanoparticles deposited over the porous sample surfaces, the particles follow the profile of the samples without occluding the pores, the average particle size is ≈8 nm.

Thus, the room potentially available to accommodate drugs or other molecules is significantly larger for MeP_2 silicon than for MeP_1 samples. After porosification, MeP_1 and MeP_2 samples were functionalized with gold nanoparticles using electroless deposition techniques. Electroless deposition is a technique that enables the reduction of metal ions on a solid surface as bulk metal without the application of external electric fields or forces [33]. Samples were treated with a solution of gold chloride and hydrofluoric acid for 3 min at 50 °C (Section 2). The process resulted in the homogeneous deposition of clusters of gold nanoparticles on the surface of the porous samples. SEM images of the sample surface (Figure 2d–f) and a convenient analysis of data (Supporting Information 2 of Supplementary Materials) indicate that the average diameter of the gold nanoparticles is $s_{np} = 8$ nm, with a small deviation around the mean $\sigma(s_{np}) \approx 1$ nm. In no case do the gold nanoparticles occlude the pores, therefore, preventing the correct release of drugs of molecules from the porous matrix. Porous surfaces functionalized with gold nanoparticle were verified using atomic force microscopy (AFM). AFM imaging enabled to resolve the structure of the samples at the nanoparticle level for both MeP_1 (Figure 3a) and MeP_2 (Figure 3c) silicon. Fast Fourier transform of AFM data enabled to derive the power spectrum associated to MeP_1 (Figure 3b) and MeP_2 (Figure 3d) silicon functionalized with gold. The power spectrum reports the change of information content as a change of size in a bi-logarithmic scale thus indicating how much of the originating complexity is maintained by changing the degree of detail of a surface [46]. Upon analysis of AFM data we found the values of roughness (Ra) and fractal dimension (Df) of the samples as $Ra^{MeP1} = 7 \pm 2$ nm and $Df^{MeP1} = 2.48 \pm 0.4$ for MeP_1, and $Ra^{MeP2} = 13 \pm 3$ nm and $Df^{MeP2} = 2.15 \pm 0.2$ for MeP_2 silicon. Thus MeP_1 samples exhibit values of roughness and fractal dimension larger than the corresponding values found for MeP_2 silicon. For comparison, nominally flat silicon surfaces, used as a control, have significantly smaller values of roughness ($Ra^{Si} = 1 \pm 0.1$ nm) and fractal dimension ($Df^{Si} = 2.1 \pm 0.2$) (Figure 3h). The luminescence properties of porous silicon samples were verified under UV light (Figure 3e). The intense luminescence emission from MeP_1 samples, compared to the low emission of MeP_2 and to the no-emission from simple silicon, indicates that MeP_1 samples may have—in the long tail of their pore size distribution—pores with a size smaller than 2 nm [31]. The wettability of mesoporous silicon samples was verified using contact angle measurements. Before oxidation, porous silicon samples as made exhibit a marked hydrophobicity with values of contact angles (CA) approaching 120 (Figure 3f). After treatment (Section 2), contact angle values measured on the sample surface shift to smaller values (CA $\approx$ 35°) typical of a hydrophilic surface.

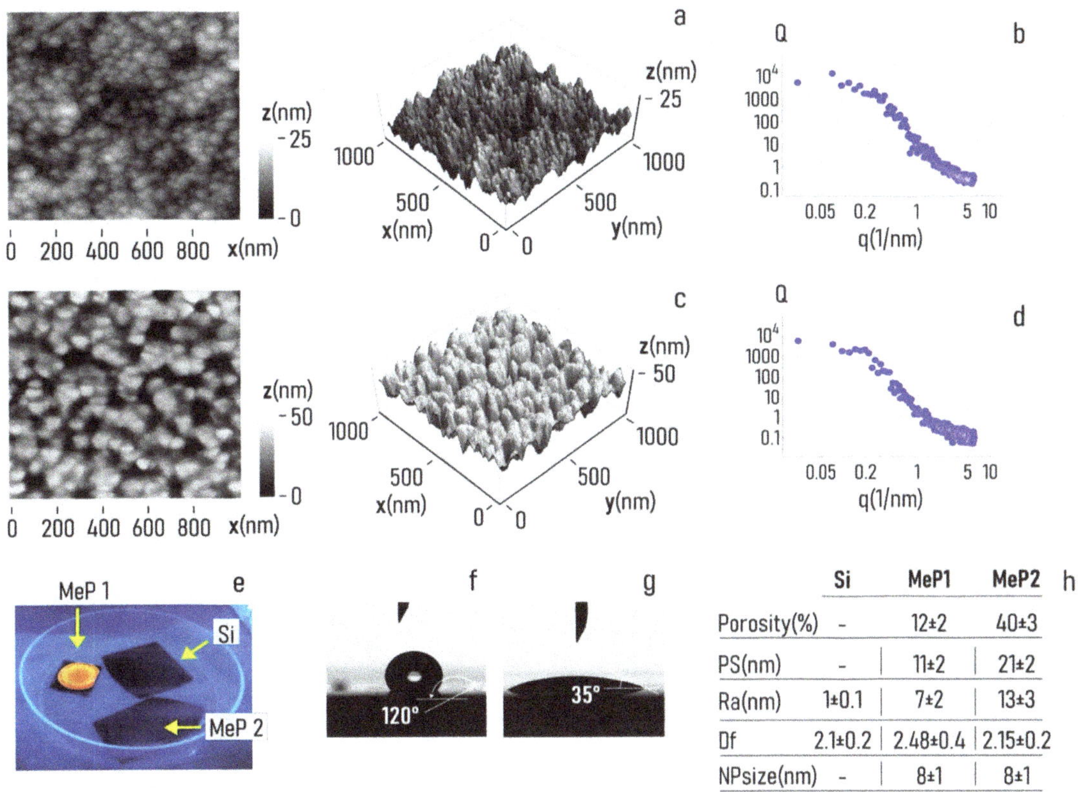

	Si	MeP1	MeP2
Porosity(%)	-	12±2	40±3
PS(nm)	-	11±2	21±2
Ra(nm)	1±0.1	7±2	13±3
Df	2.1±0.2	2.48±0.4	2.15±0.2
NPsize(nm)	-	8±1	8±1

Figure 3. (**a**) Atomic force microscopy (AFM) profile of MeP_1 substrates functionalized with gold nanoparticles imaged over a sampling area of 1 × 1 μm, the height values of the profile fall within the 0–25 nm range. (**b**) Power spectrum density function associated to the topography of the MeP_1 substrate, the slope of the function in the linear regime is indicative of the fractal dimension of the samples. (**c**) AFM profile of MeP_2 substrates functionalized with gold nanoparticles imaged over a sampling area of 1 × 1 μm, the height values of the profile fall within the 0–50 nm range. (**d**) Power spectrum density function associated to the topography of the MeP_2 substrate. (**e**) Luminescence of MeP_1 and MeP_2 samples under UV light, compared to the light emission of silicon. Contact angle of a drop of D.I. water measured on the porous surfaces before (**f**) and after (**g**) sample oxidation. (**h**) Values of porosity, pore size, roughness, fractal dimension, and characteristic size of the gold nanoparticles of the porous surfaces determined through analysis of SEM and AFM images of samples.

3.2. Controlling Cell Organization on Au-Mesoporous Silicon Surfaces

The substrates that we produced exhibit different values of pore size ($PS^{MeP1} \approx 11$ nm, $PS^{MeP2} \approx 21$ nm), gold nanoparticles size ($s_{np} \approx 8$ nm), roughness ($Ra^{MeP1} \sim 7$ nm, $Ra^{MeP2} \approx 13$ nm), and fractal dimension ($Df^{MeP1} \approx 2.48$, $Df^{MeP1} \approx 2.15$). To examine whether the nano-topographical characteristics of the surfaces have the ability to direct cell behavior on the substrate in a controlled way, we put in culture on both Au-MeP_1 and Au-MeP_2 silicon MCF-7 breast cancer cells. We then examined the topological characteristics of the networks that cells formed 24 h from seeding and we correlated them to the topography of the surface. We used nominally flat silicon substrates as a control. Figure 4 shows the spatial layout of cell-nuclei on flat silicon, Au-MeP_1 and Au-MeP_2 silicon imaged 24 h after culture. The initial number of cells deposited in each well for incubation was the same for all the substrates (Section 2). Fluorescence images in Figure 4 show that cells are homogeneously distributed on flat silicon surfaces, showing no preferential points of accumulation. Differently, cells on mesoporous surfaces form complex structures of those cells with a correlation length, cluster size, and topological characteristics that seem to vary from Au-MeP_1 to Au-MeP_2 silicon.

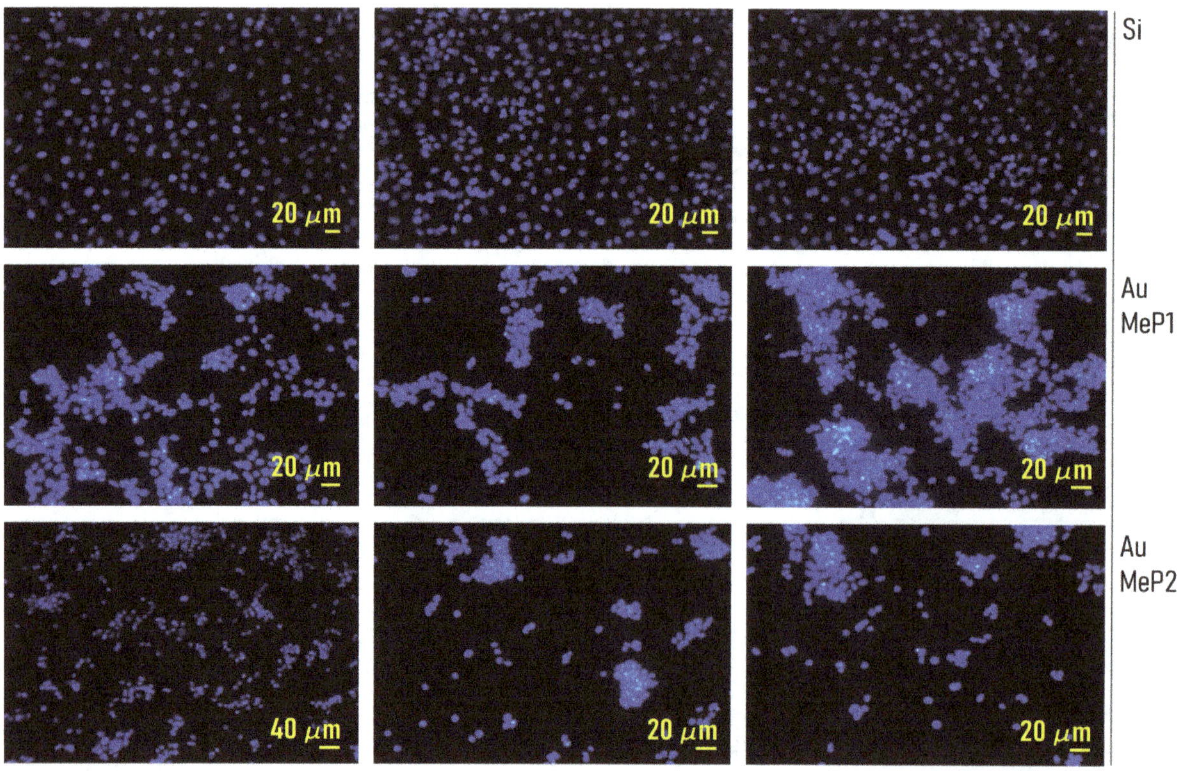

Figure 4. Fluorescence images of MCF-7 cancer cells over MeP_1, MeP_2, and silicon surfaces after 24 h from seeding.

We used image analysis algorithms and the methods of networks analysis, described in [30,40,47,48] and Section 2 of this article, to measure the characteristics of cell-networks quantitatively. Starting from the fluorescence image of a cell configuration, we segmented that image to find the cell-centers. Then, we routed cell-centers using the Waxman algorithm (Figure 5a). The algorithm selected the cell pairs to be connected basing on their distance: cells that were closer than a threshold were connected as described in Section 2. We analyzed more than 30 images per substrate. For each image, we extracted from the resulting network the number of cells in a region of interest (*N*), the clustering coefficient (*Cc*), the characteristic path length (*Cpl*), the small-world-ness (SW). *N* measures the adhesion strength of cells to a substrate [17]. The clustering coefficient, characteristic path length, and small world coefficient are a quantitative measure of the characteristics of the networks that cells form on a surface.

The clustering coefficient is the ratio of active links to the total combinations of connections that cells, around a reference node, can possibly establish, averaged all over the cells of the network [37]. The characteristic path length is the mean shortest distance between nodes of network [37]. The small-world coefficient, found as a combination of the *Cc* and the *Cpl* [42], is a metric that tests whether the distance between nodes grows with the logarithm of the number of nodes in a graph: $Cpl \propto \log(N)$. Typically, small-world-networks are characterized by a few clusters with a high number of elements for a cluster, the identification of small-world networks is of interest because networks with small-world-characteristics communicate more efficiently than equivalent random or ordered graphs of the same size [48,49].

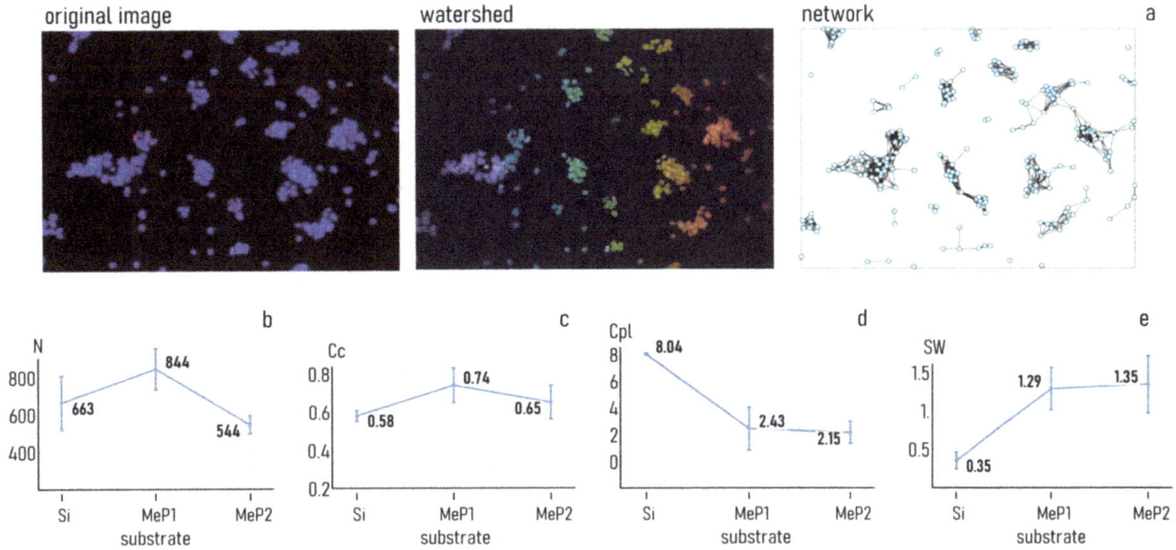

Figure 5. (**a**) Image analysis of fluorescence images: the original images were segmented with a watershed algorithm to identify individual cells, and cell nodes were then connected using the Waxman algorithm to obtain the equivalent graph for each sample. (**b**) Values of adhering cells, (**c**) clustering coefficient, (**d**) characteristic path length, and (**e**) small-world-ness determined for the cultures of MCF-7 cell on MeP_1, MeP_2, and silicon surfaces 24 *h* from seeding.

After network analysis of cell images, we found that the number of adhering cells in a region of interest of 1174 × 882 μm is $N \approx 663$ on flat silicon, $N \approx 884$ for the Au-MeP_1 substrate, $N \approx 544$ for the Au-MeP_2 substrate (Figure 5b). The maximum number of adhering cells is found for the Au-MeP_1 substrate with intermediate values of roughness and higher values of fractal dimension, in line with previous reports [17,29,30,48,49]. Notably, the difference between the number of cells found on Au-MeP_1 and Au-MeP_2 silicon is statistically significant ($p < 0.05$). For the same sets of images, we found that the values of clustering coefficient reach a maximum for the Au-MeP_1 substrate, with $Cc \approx 0.74$, while the clustering coefficient is lower for the Au-MeP_2 substrate ($Cc \approx 0.65$), and significantly lower for simple silicon ($Cc \approx 0.58$) (Figure 5c). At the same time, the values of characteristic path length are nearly identical for the Au-MeP_1 ($Cpl \approx 2.43$) and Au-MeP_2 ($Cpl \approx 2.15$) substrates, and they are statistically different from the values found on flat silicon with $Cpl \approx 8$ (Figure 5d). The resulting small-world-coefficient of cell networks on mesoporous substrates is SW ≈ 1.29 and SW ≈ 1.35 for MeP_1 and MeP_2, respectively, while SW ≈ 0.35 for flat silicon. Thus, cell networks on nanostructured, mesoporous surfaces passed the small-world test, differently from cells on flat silicon that settle on a surface without any appreciable large- or small-scale structure.

3.3. SERS Analysis of Cell Adhesion on Au-Mesoporous Silicon Surfaces

The substrates that we produced induce cell clustering. The increased susceptibility of cells to condensate into compact structures is in turn ascribed to the intermediate values of roughness and large values of fractal dimension of mesoporous silicon compared to flat silicon substrates [17,30]. Since cell clustering and condensation is a side effect of the of the increased adhesive properties of a substrate [48,49], we performed a chemometric analysis of cells cultured on MeP_1 and MeP_2 substrates to examine whether cell adhesion molecules are preferentially expressed from cells on nanostructured surfaces. We mapped the Raman intensity of MCF-7 cells cultivated on MeP_1 and MeP_2 silicon functionalized with gold, compared to the same cells on silicon sputtered with a continuous layer of gold, used as a control (Figure 6a). Raman spectra of cells were acquired following the procedure reported in Section 2 36 h after seeding, that is a sufficiently long time to assure complete adhesion of cells on the substrate. In each point, the Raman maps reported in Figure 6a are proportional to the intensity of the spectra measured at 1569 1/cm, that is typical of integrins as explained in the following of this section. Raman spectra were then subjected to a principal components analysis (PCA), and the principal components resulting from the analysis were in turn clustered into groups using classical k-means algorithms. This allowed to identify in the cell under analysis of five different regions, where points in a region have similar chemometric characteristics (Figure 6b). Moreover, since the principal components are sorted in order of decreasing information content and variance [50], regions in Figure 6b define the portions of the cell that exhibit the more intense and the more vibrantly varying Raman signal.

Integrins are one of four principal cell adhesion molecules families, they play a major role in the process of adhesion of cells to the extracellular matrix (ECM), and especially in tumor cells where they are overexpressed during the process of adhesion [51]. $\alpha5\beta1$ and $\alpha3\beta1$ are integrins specifically expressed by tumour and epithelial cells. In particular, $\alpha3\beta1$ is overexpressed in tumours spreading in ECM with a high content of collagen and laminin, so that an elevated concentration of $\alpha3\beta1$ is a hallmark of cell proliferation and migration [52]. While each of those adhesion molecules have their own distinctive features, nonetheless they exhibit a certain number of peaks that do not vary from spectrum to spectrum representing a fingerprint for those molecules. Those peaks are found at (i) 1126 1/cm related to C-N bond, (ii) 1175 1/cm associated to Tyrosine or Phenylalanine, (iii) 1306 1/cm attributable to amide III, (iv) 1506 1/cm related to Phenylalanine or Hystidine, (v) 1569 1/cm originating from tryptophan, (vi) 1645 1/cm due to the amide I signal [53]. The Raman analysis that we performed on cells on different surfaces was enhanced by the interaction of the electromagnetic (EM) field with gold nanostructures, which amplify the Raman signal by several orders of magnitude in a SERS (surface enhanced Raman spectroscopy) effect [54]. SERS analysis of cells enabled the identification of adhesion markers that are otherwise inaccessible to classical spectroscopy techniques. The Raman intensity profile in Figure 6a for MeP_1 and MeP_2 follows a characteristic and distinguishable spatial distribution. Points in the map with higher values of Raman intensity may be indicative of the expression of integrin cell-adhesion-molecules suggesting that in those spots adhesion is established. The map relative to simple silicon with gold shows less preferential points of adhesion, indicating that smoother unstructured surfaces impair cell adhesion and proliferation. Moreover, SERS maps of cells measured on MeP_1 and MeP_2 substrates show a very high correspondence to the principal components distribution in Figure 6b, and especially to the first two components PC_1 and PC_2. Regions in the maps with greater overlap are at the borders of the cells (Figure 6a,b), with their membrane actively involved in the process of adhesion. The diagram in Figure 6c reports the loading associated to the first principal component measured for the MeP_1, MeP_2, and Si substrates. The loading is a statistical measure of how much different frequencies contribute to a certain principal component. The curves in Figure 6c indicate that the frequency that above all is responsible for the signal is 1569 1/cm for the MeP_1 substrate, while the signal content associated to 1569 1/cm is gradually weaker for the MeP_2 and the simple silicon substrate. Recalling that 1569 1/cm is the distinctive frequency for the integrins, the form of the diagrams of Figure 6c suggests that cell adhesion molecules are preferentially expressed for the foremost on MeP_1 substrates, followed by MeP_2 substrates and by flat silicon. For each substrate we calculated the ratio r between the value of loading intensity measured at 1569 1/cm and the loading averaged over the entire spectral range (Figure 6d). r is a quantitative measure of the relative abundance of integrins at the interface of a cell with a surface. Values of r much larger than one for MeP_1 ($r \approx 4.53$) and MeP_2 ($r \approx 4.34$), compared to the lower value of r measured on silicon ($r \approx 1$), show that the multiscale architecture of mesoporous substrates, with meso-pores functionalized with metal nanoparticles, facilitate cell adhesion compared to flat geometries. The values of r determined for the MeP_1 and MeP_2 substrates are significantly different from that determined for silicon, with $p < 0.05$.

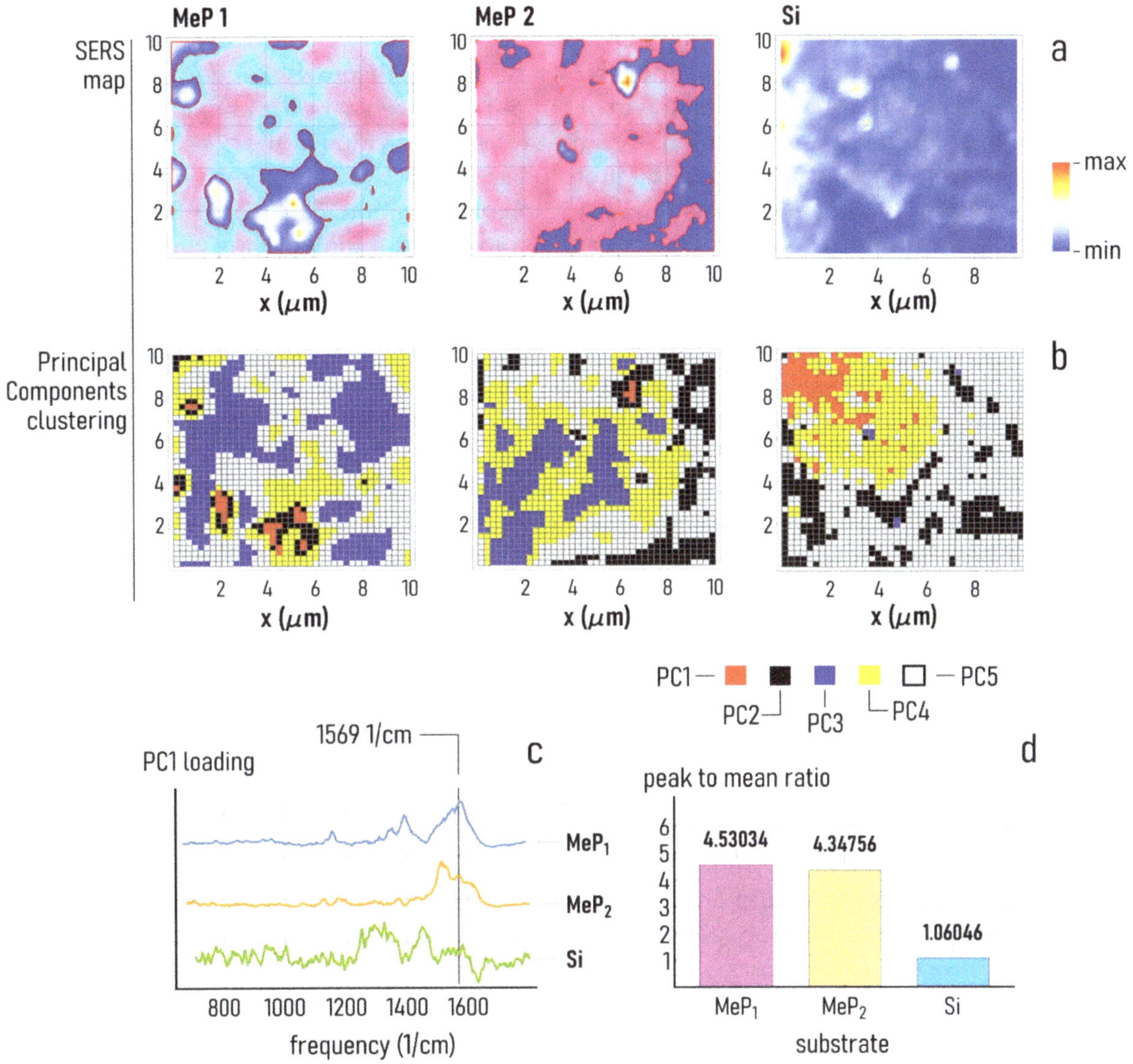

Figure 6. (**a**) Raman maps of MCF-7 cells acquired over a region of interest of 10 × 10 μm for MeP_1, MeP_2, and silicon surfaces, the maps show the Raman intensity measured at 1569 1/cm. (**b**) We show, for each of the considered surfaces (MeP_1, MeP_2, and Si), the first five principal components extracted from the Raman maps, and the spatial distribution of the principal components correlate with the Raman intensity maps previously reported. (**c**) The loading associated to the first principal component measured over MeP_1, MeP_2, and Si surfaces. (**d**) Ratio between the maximum and the mean intensity of the PC1 loading correspondent to MCF-7 cells cultivated over MeP_1, MeP_2, and Si samples.

3.4. Kinetics of Drug Release from the Mesoporous Silicon Matrices

The devices that we produced incorporate networks of nano-pores penetrating deep within their structures. We verified the capability of the device to accumulate and consequently release drug molecules over time using UV spectroscopy techniques as described in Section 2. We incubated MeP_1

and MeP_2 silicon substrates with the antitumor drug PtCl(O,O′-acac)(DMSO) for 60 h. We used two different concentrations of the originating drug during the loading process: $c_1 = 30$ μM and $c_2 = 50$ μM. We then measured the release of the drug in D.I. water up to 10 days from the activation of the process. The diagram in Figure 7a shows the cumulative dose–response curves for different substrates and different initial values of the loading concentration. The dynamics of release from the MeP_2 silicon system is faster compared to MeP_1 silicon, consistently with the fact the pores in MeP_2 silicon are larger (≈21 nm) than those contained in MeP_1 silicon (≈11 nm). Wanting to approximate the curves of release with a function of time of the form $c(t) = c_o + c_s\left(1 - e^{-t/\tau}\right)$, we found after nonlinear fitting of data the following solutions for c_s and τ: (i) $c_s \approx 4.94$ μM and $\tau \approx 46$ h for MeP_1 silicon loaded with an initial concentration equal to c_1, (ii) $c_s \approx 2.81$ μM and $\tau \approx 50$ h for MeP_1 silicon with an initial c_2 concentration, (iii) $c_s \approx 6.7$ μM and $\tau \approx 38$ h for MeP_2 silicon with an initial c_1 concentration, $c_s \approx 7.2$ μM and $\tau \approx 20$ h for MeP_2 silicon with an initial c_2 concentration. c_s is the steady state value of the concentration increment with respect to a zero reference value. τ is the time constant of the drug delivery system, i.e., the time necessary to the system to reach 66% of its final value of concentration. The values that we found for c_s and τ for the different combinations of substrate morphology and initial loading concentration that we used in our study, indicate that the rate of drug release (1/τ) increases moving from MeP_1 to MeP_2 and, for the same substrate, it is higher for an initial higher concentration of the loaded drug. This behavior can be easily described by the first law of Fick, $J = -D\partial c/\partial x$, where the intensity of the flux (J) is proportional to the gradient of concentration from the substrate to the external environment, and the absolute number of molecules transported through the system per unit time depends on the area of the surface actively releasing the drug. In the equation D is the molecular diffusion coefficient [50]. Moreover, the values of c_s and τ and Figure 7a indicate that the total amount of drug released in a system (c_s) is higher for MeP_2 silicon, that has a higher porosity compared to MeP_1, and is higher for an initial higher concentration of the loaded drug. In the neighbor of $t = 0$, the drug release profile can be expanded in a Taylor series yielding, neglecting higher order terms of the expansion, $c(t) \approx c_s/\tau$: this approximate formula enables calculation of the velocity of release (v) at the early stage of the delivery process. Using data from the model fit, we obtained $v \approx 0.06$ μM/h (MeP_1, c_1), $v \approx 0.11$ μM/h (MeP_1, c_2), $v \sim 0.17$ μM/h (MeP_2, c_1), $v \approx 0.37$ μM/h (MeP_2, c_2). Thus, the kinetics of initial release can be varied in the 0.06-0.37 μM/h interval by changing the parameters of the process. Figure 7b displays the drug released from the systems over time, normalized to the initial concentration of the loaded drug. Values in the figure are a measure of the efficiency of the drug delivery system. Data show that the maximum efficiency of release varies between ≈0.12 for MeP_1 silicon with an initial loading concentration c_2, and ≈0.23 for MeP_2 silicon with an initial loading concentration c_1. While the efficiency of delivery is still larger for MeP_2 silicon with higher values of pore size and porosity, it decreases for increasing values of initial loading concentration, possibly because for larger amounts of initial payload the losses associated to the process are also larger. Thus, one of the points of strength of this bio-chip, is that it can artificially increase the half-life of a drug. The half-life ($t\frac{1}{2}$) is the time required to change the amount of a drug in the body by one-half during elimination. Drug clearance from the body is the result of elimination by renal excretion and by non-renal pathways, the latter most often represent clearance by the liver. Remarkably, the characteristic half-life—the duration of action—of anticancer drugs is, on average, small. Clinical studies and reports [55] indicate that the mean half-life of more than 140 small-molecule drugs approved for oncology indications is ≈15 h, with an even smaller value of median of about ≈5 h. The drug delivery system set-up in this study enables the active release of drugs for more than ≈50 h, depending on the configuration. Thus, the chip that we produced can possibly increase the half-life of most anticancer treatments by 300% on average.

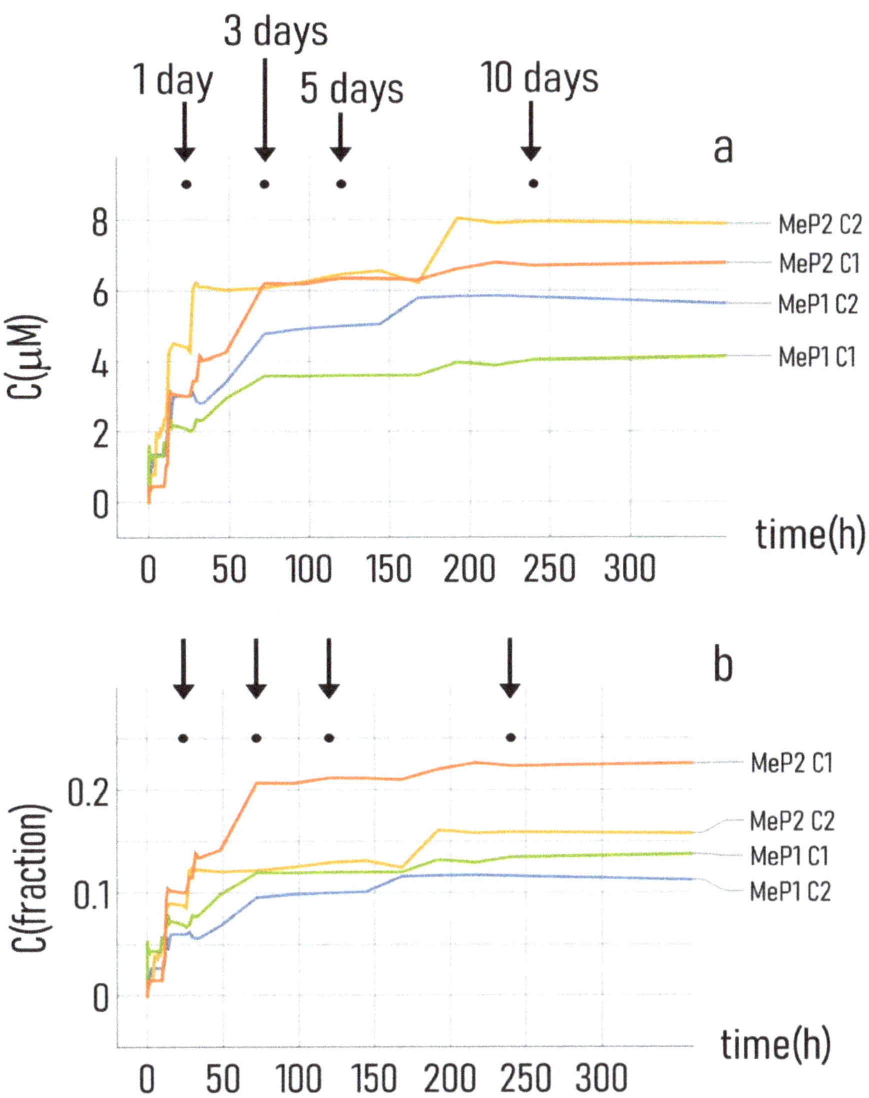

Figure 7. (**a**) Absolute and (**b**) normalized release profile of the anti-tumor drug $PtCl(O, O' - acac)(DMSO)$ measured for MeP_1 and MeP_2 substrates up to 15 days from the beginning of the delivery.

3.5. *Timely Delivery of Drugs Impairs Tumor Cells Adhesion*

The theranostics device presented in the work has the ability to deliver over time the antitumor drug PtCl (O,O′-acac) (DMSO) for several hours from the initial release. We examined the effects of a controlled release of drugs on the adhesion and growth of tumor MCF-7 cells on the mesoporous substrates. MCF-7 cells were cultured on MeP_1 silicon and MeP_2 silicon functionalized with gold nanoparticles and on flat silicon surfaces used as a control. Half of the mesoporous substrates used in this study were loaded with PtCl (O,O′-acac) (DMSO) in a concentration of 50 μM. We then imaged cell-nuclei on different substrates and at different times from incubation. The different number of cells adhering on the substrates is the effect of a combination of factors: (i) the drug released from the system and (ii) the different nano-topographical characteristics of the substrates. Visual examination of samples reveals that already 6 h from culture the number of adhering cells on flat silicon is lower than that observed on MeP_1 with gold, that is in turn different from the number of cells on MeP_1 silicon loaded with drugs (Figure 8). This difference is exacerbated by time. In Figure 9a we report the bar-chart of the number of cells (N) measured on different substrates 36, 48, and 72 h from incubation. N was estimated from more than 20 images per substrate and five technical repeats per sample.

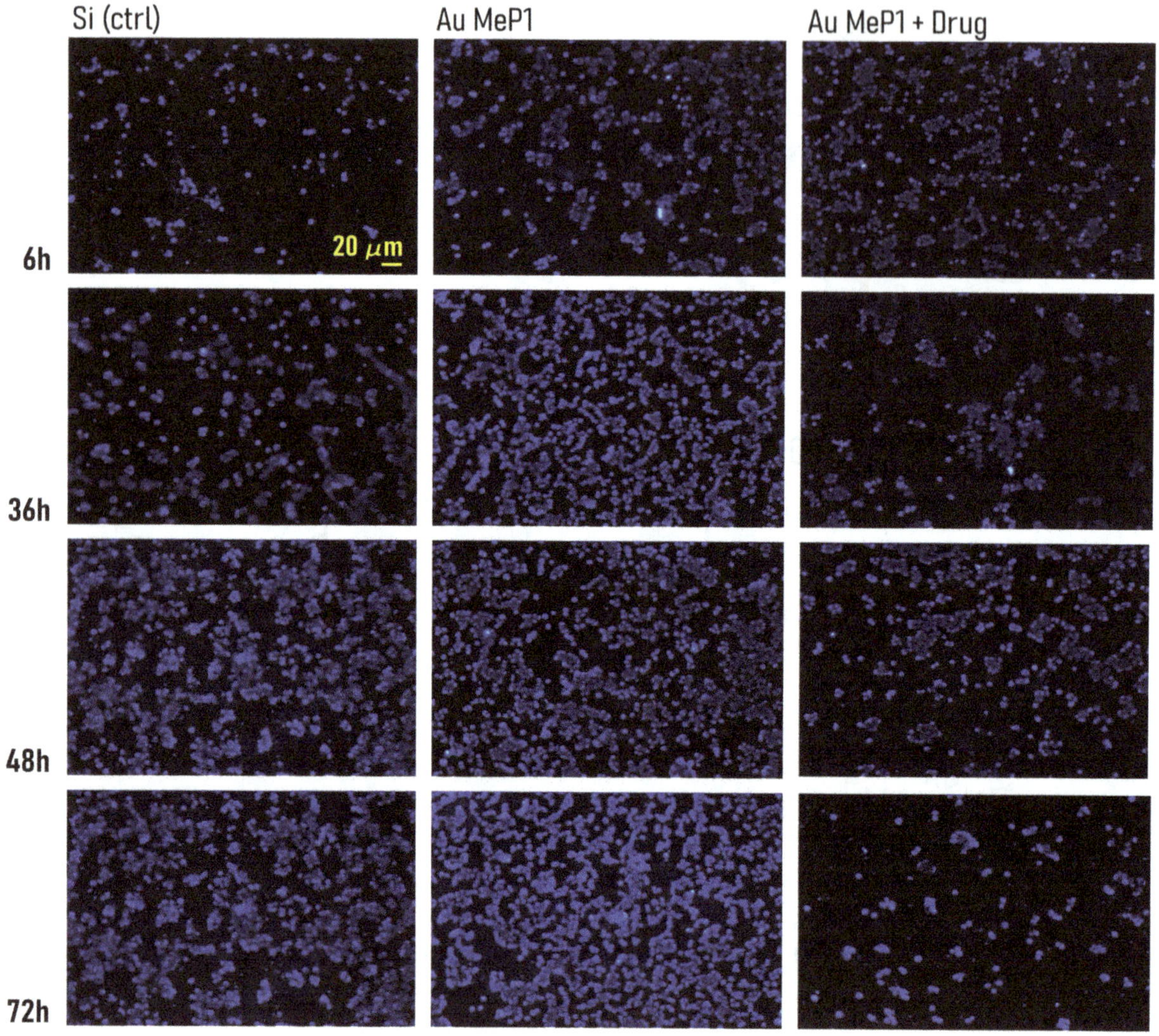

Figure 8. Fluorescence images of MCF-7 cancer cells growing on Au-MeP_1 substrates with and without the delivery of the antitumor agent PtCl(O,O′-acac)(DMSO), at different time frames. In the experiments, unfunctionalized silicon was used as a control.

A total of 36 h after culture, the number of cells on MeP_1 and MeP_2 silicon without drug is not statistically different from that measured on flat silicon, with $N_{MeP1} \approx 1871$, $N_{MeP2} \approx 2100$, and $N_{Si} \approx 1951$. Diversely, N is significantly lower for the mesoporous substrates loaded with drug, being ${N_{MeP1}}^{drug} \approx 675$ and ${N_{MeP2}}^{drug} \approx 424$. A total of 36 h from incubation the effect of topography is negligible compared to the release of drug.

A total of 48 h from incubation, the number of cells on MeP_1 silicon without drug increases to $N_{MeP1} \approx 2928$, significantly larger than the number of cells measured at the same time on simple MeP_2 and flat silicon, with $N_{MeP2} \approx 1983$ and $N_{Si} \approx 2090$. At this time step, the number of cells measured on the mesoporous substrates loaded with drug falls to ${N_{MeP1}}^{drug} \approx 451$ and ${N_{MeP2}}^{drug} \approx 255$, that are significantly different from the values measured for the unloaded substrates. A total of 48 h after cell culture, the improved adhesive characteristics of MeP_1 silicon over simple MeP_2 and simple silicon become apparent, while the delivery of drugs from MeP_2 silicon achieves maximum effects.

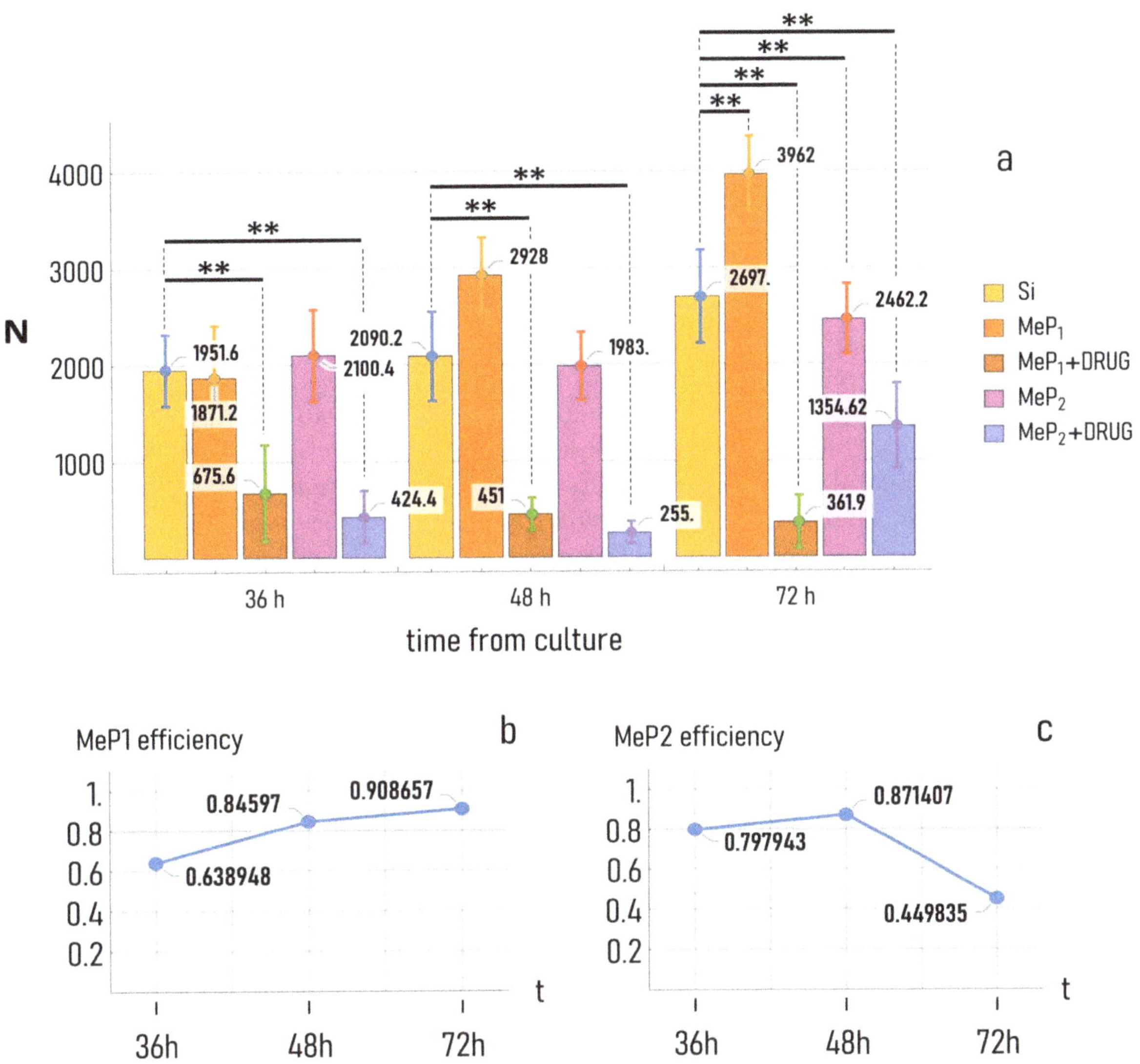

Figure 9. (**a**) Number of adhering cells on Au-MeP_1 and Au-MeP_2 substrates under and without the influence of the antitumor agent PtCl(O,O′-acac)(DMSO), at 36, 48, and 72 h from cell seeding, compared to plain silicon used as a control. All p values less than 0.05 are summarized with two asterisks. Efficacy of the antitumor drug on the cancer cells at different times from the initial release, for the (**b**) Au-MeP_1 (**c**) and Au-MeP_2 substrates.

A total of 72 h from incubation, the number of adhering cells on MeP_1 silicon with drug hits a minimum, $N_{MeP1}{}^{drug} \approx 362$, while N surges to $N_{MeP1} \approx 3962$ for simple MeP_1 silicon without drug. These values are significantly lower and significantly larger than the control: $N_{Si} \approx 2697$. At this time of the analysis, the MeP_2 morphology does not enhance significantly adhesion with respect to the control, with $N_{MeP2} \approx 2462$, while the release of drug from MeP_2 silicon still bears appreciable effects, with $N_{MeP2}{}^{drug} \approx 1355$ significantly lower than the number of cells measured on flat silicon.

Thus, the efficacy of the drug delivery system depends on both of the substrate morphology and the time of the process. For each time, we calculated the efficiency of delivery as the number of adhering cells on the substrate loaded with drug, to the number of cells measured on the same substrate without drug (Figure 9b,c). We observe that the efficiency of the system gradually increases for MeP_1 silicon, varying from ≈0.64 at 36 h, to ≈0.84 at 48 h, to ≈0.90 at 72 h from incubation. For this substrate, more than 90% of cells are killed compared to the same substrate in absence of drug delivery. The curve of efficiency for the MeP_2 silicon is different. For this system, the efficiency of delivery is sufficiently large already 36 h from the initial release (≈0.80), it attains a maximum value at

48 h (≈0.87), to subsequently drop to ≈0.45 at 72 h from incubation. The different efficiency measured for MeP_1 and MeP_2 silicon reflects the different kinetics of release measured for those devices and reported in previous sections of this work.

4. Discussion

The theranostics substrates that we produced are akin to the cell culture glass coverslips used to plate cells for research and analysis—with the notable exception that they enable the targeted delivery of therapeutics to the cells and cell sensing, simultaneously. Moreover, thanks to the fabrication process capability to attain maximum control over surface morphology at the nanoscale, the substrates can be designed to guide cell adhesion, proliferation, and organization. For these characteristics, this bio-device—and its more sophisticated evolutions that will be developed over time—can be integrated into conventional cell culture dishes or multi-wells to test the adhesion and growth of cells against different external factors, including substrate geometry and a controlled delivery of drugs. Researchers can plate cells over several different replica of the device, each of them with its characteristic topography and drug release profile. Then, the researchers will find the combination of surface topography and device payload that guarantees maximum/minimum cell adhesion and proliferation, depending on whether the aim of the research is optimize a structure for tissue engineering or the effects of a drug for personalized medicine. The search for the optimal values of surface topography and kinetics of release should be possibly conducted within the bounds identified by this and other similar works: where the roughness of the surface and the pore size is varied in the 0–30 nm interval, while drugs are released with a maximum initial rate of ≈0.4 μM/h. The output of the experiment—i.e., cell colonies—can be verified at different time steps from seeding using either confocal microscopy or Raman spectroscopy that is, notably, made possible by the distinctive design of the device. While the first technique provides information about cell adhesion, growth, and clustering, Raman analysis of samples describes the conditions of a cell at the level of its adhesion molecules. Thus, the combination of techniques gives a picture of the evolution of a cell over different scales, bridging the divide between the behavior of cells being observed in isolation (individual behavior of cells) or in-group (collective behavior of cells). Consistency between results may indicate that the substrate operates efficiently towards either improving or impairing cell adhesion and organization. Thus, the device can potentially be the basis for a test campaign aimed to optimize the characteristics of biomaterials for tissue engineering, regenerative medicine, or in-vitro-model applications. After identification of the optimal surface characteristics and drug dosage that assure the wanted effect, these values should be copied to the scaffold intended to support cell-growth, or to the implantable device that will release drugs to a disease, for real-life applications. Nonetheless, this implies a process of engineering of the device, aimed to overtake those complications that can possibly emerge when similar devices are used outside of a research context. A list of possible caveats is identified as follows:

(1) Transition from a 2D to 3D geometry. Results of the work and the way the device operates are restricted to 2D geometries. Cells themselves are plated on a surface and cell clusters are described using bi-dimensional variables. Future research that will be conducted over time shall have to clarify whether, and to which extent, cell behavior changes moving from 2D to 3D scaffolds.

(2) Understanding whether the delivery is active. As demonstrated in the work, the delivery of the drugs from the porous matrix does not last indefinitely. Additionally, there could be cases in which, because of unpredictable leakages or occlusions of the pores, the process of release terminates before the expected time. Thus, the substrate should incorporate a sensor sensitive to the released drug, indicating the rate at which release proceeds, warning of possible malfunctions of the device before cells react to the alterations of delivery.

(3) Switching between on-off delivery states of the device. In this configuration, the release of drugs is always active, being driven by the gradients of concentration in the system—and described by the Fick's laws. In a more sophisticated evolution of the device, one should be able to switch between on-off states: i.e., an active (on) state, in which drug molecules are allowed to flow in the

system, and an inactive (off) state, in which release is temporarily paused. This can be possibly accomplished by varying, in a controlled fashion, the levels of pH and temperature of the system, having previously conjugated the drug with a pH-sensitive cleavable linker as described, as for an example, for injectable nanoparticle generators in [56].

(4) Increasing the efficiency of drug loading, either in terms of pore-capacity and total amount of drug loaded in the pores, and in terms of loading time. The time necessary to load the drug into the device (more than 60 h for the present configuration) is unacceptably long for real life/industrial applications of the device.

(5) Integration. While the device offers complementary ways to measure cell performance, using the bio-chip alternatively in a confocal-microscope or in a Raman setup can take time, and slow down the pace of a test campaign, a trial, or a biology/medicine application of the device. The method can take advantage from the integration of the chip in an automatic multi-well plate reader, where different imaging techniques (confocal imaging and Raman spectroscopy) are combined in the same platform.

(6) Optimization. The device can be especially useful in cancer theranostics. While the results obtained in this work are based on an initial cell density of about 10^5 cells per substrate, this value can be optimized: the total number of cells for which the device has some measurable effects may be significantly lower than the 10^5 limit. Miniaturization has as principal consequence the possibility to use the devices in all those cases in which, because of the early stage of a disease, conventional biopsies are ineffective. For the same reason, the device can be used to perform liquid biopsy. Liquid biopsy is based on the detection and isolation of cancer cells directly from the peripheral blood of the patient [57]. The limit of the method is that, often, cancer cells are too few to be detected. Liquid biopsy could realistically benefit from multi-drug array panels based on mesoporous silicon substrates, designed to evaluate the sensitivity of circulating tumor cells to a test drug.

(7) Generality. Further to the end of liquid biopsy: results of the paper suggest that this theranostics device is also effective towards more aggressive cancer cells, such as triple negative breast cancer cells. The integrin expression that we chose to analyze in this work is believed to be a hallmark of more aggressive forms of breast cancer [58]. In particular, the expression of β1 integrins on the cell surface is a predictive marker of triple negative breast cancer. Since the substrates that we produced induce, for certain configurations, an increased production of integrins on the MCF-7 surface, it is legitimate to hypothesize that this theranostics procedure is effective also in the case of triple negative breast cancer cells. Regarding the impact on normal cells, it has been demonstrated in several studies—some of which have been cited throughout the article—that both the porosity and roughness of nanoscale surfaces affect the adhesion, proliferation, and clustering of cells, depending on their degree of differentiation and replication speed. Thus, the method that we developed is general in scope and can be realistically adapted to several different cell types for different applications.

5. Conclusions

Using electrochemical etching, we produced mesoporous silicon substrates functionalized with gold nanoparticles. Due to their porous structures, the substrates behave as a drug delivery system, where drugs or other agents loaded in the matrix are released over time with a first order kinetics and a time constant that can be varied by tuning the characteristics of the pores. Due to its nanostructure, the device can amplify by several orders of magnitude the signal generated by molecules in the cell membrane during the process of adhesion and migration. These nanodevices combine therapy and diagnostics effects in the same device, with the primary advantage of not being limited to therapy or sensing, as they provide coincident diagnostic information plus delivery of therapeutics. For their capabilities to drive cell growth and high capacities of therapeutic loading, these devices can be possibly used in tissue engineering, regenerative medicine, and nanomedicine. In these fields, the ability to assemble cells together has to be associated with the ability of deliver therapeutics accurately to achieve maximum control over cell fate. The ability of the system to measure adhesion at the nanoscale, is an extra feature that makes this theranostics device the ideal candidate for those who want to design substrates for cell growth and proliferation or, vice versa, induce apoptosis in tumor cells with unprecedented control.

In this work, by varying the parameters of the process we obtained substrates with different values of pore size, porosity, and roughness. MeP_1 substrates exhibit smaller values of pore size (PS $\approx$ 11 nm) and roughness (Ra $\approx$ 7 nm), but have a larger fractal dimension (Df $\approx$ 2.48) compared to MeP_2 substrates, with PS $\approx$ 21 nm, $R_a \approx$ 13 nm, and Df $\approx$ 2.15. Adhesion of MCF-7 cells was accelerated on MeP_1 substrates with larger value of fractal dimension compared to MeP_2 substrates and flat silicon used as a control.

When we considered the effect of the release over time of an anti-tumor drug, we observed that the maximum reduction of cell growth is found for MeP_2 substrates 36 and 48 h after seeding, with a decrease in the number of adhering cells up to 87% with respect to the same substrates without drug. A total of 72 h from cell culture, the therapeutics efficacy of MeP_2 substrates falls to 44%, and is overtaken by MeP_1 silicon, with a cell number contraction of 90%, reflecting the different morphological characteristics of surfaces.

Results suggest that the adhesive properties of mesoporous substrates, the kinetics of drug delivery, and the effects that a combination of the two may have on the adhesion and proliferation of cells, can be conveniently modulated by changing the pore size and roughness in the narrow intervals of PS $\approx$ 11–21 nm and Ra $\approx$ 7–13 nm.

Author Contributions: Conceptualization, F.G.; methodology, M.L.C., G.M., M.D.A., S.D.V., A.I. and L.T.; software, V.O.; validation, V.O., M.L.C., G.P., E.D.F., P.C., N.M. and F.G.; formal analysis, M.L.C., V.O., E.D.F., N.M. and F.G.; investigation, M.L.C., N.M. and F.G.; resources, N.M. and F.G.; data curation, M.L.C., V.O., N.M. and F.G.; writing—original draft preparation, F.G.; writing—review and editing, M.L.C., V.O., N.M., F.G.; visualization, M.L.C. and F.G.; supervision, G.P., E.D.F., P.C., N.M., F.G.; project administration, N.M. and F.G.; funding acquisition, N.M. All authors have read and agreed to the published version of the manuscript.

Acknowledgments: We thank the Dresden Center for Nanoanalysis of Technische Universität Dresden for the support provided for the SEM analysis of samples. This publication was supported by the Department of Experimental and Clinical Medicine, University Magna Graecia of Catanzaro.

References

1. Gentile, F. Nanotopographical Control of Cell Assembly into Supracellular Structures. In *Nanomaterials for Advanced Biological Applications*; Rahmandoust, M., Ayatollahi, M., Eds.; Springer: Cham, Switzerland, 2019; Volume 104.
2. Hutmacher, D.W.; Woodfield, T.B.F.; Dalton, P.D. Scaffold Design and Fabrication. In *Tissue Engineering*; Van Blitterswijk, C.A., De Boer, J., Eds.; Academic Press: Boston, MA, USA, 2014; pp. 311–346.
3. Limongi, T.; Schipani, R.; Di Vito, A.; Giugni, A.; Francardi, M.; Torre, B.; Allione, M.; Miele, E.; Malara, N.; Alrasheed, S.; et al. Photolithography and micromolding techniques for the realization of 3D polycaprolactone scaffolds for tissue engineering applications. *Microelectron. Eng.* **2015**, *141*, 135–139. [CrossRef]
4. Lu, T.; Li, Y.; Chen, T. Techniques for fabrication and construction of three-dimensional scaffolds for tissue engineering. *Int. J. Nanomed.* **2013**, *8*, 337–350. [CrossRef]
5. Perozziello, G.; Simone, G.; Candeloro, P.; Gentile, F.; Malara, N.; Larocca, R.; Coluccio, M.L.; Pullano, S.; Tirinato, L.; Geschke, O.; et al. A Fluidic Motherboard for Multiplexed Simultaneous and Modular Detection in Microfluidic Systems for Biological Application. *Micro Nanosyst.* **2010**, *2*, 227–238. [CrossRef]
6. Decuzzi, P.; Ferrari, M. Modulating cellular adhesion through nanotopography. *Biomaterials* **2010**, *31*, 173–179. [CrossRef] [PubMed]
7. Geiger, B.; Bershadsky, A.; Pankov, R.; Yamada, K.M. Transmembrane Extracellular Matrix–Cytoskeleton Crosstalk. *Nat. Rev. Mol. Cell Biol.* **2001**, *2*, 793–805. [CrossRef] [PubMed]
8. Geiger, B.; Spatz, J.P.; Bershadsky, A.D. Environmental sensing through focal adhesions. *Nat. Rev. Mol. Cell Biol.* **2009**, *10*, 21–33. [CrossRef] [PubMed]
9. Kanchanawong, P.; Shtengel, G.; Pasapera, A.M.; Ramko, E.B.; Davidson, M.W.; Hess, H.F.; Waterman, C.M. Nanoscale architecture of integrin-based cell adhesions. *Nature* **2010**, *468*, 580–586. [CrossRef]

10. Perozziello, G.; La Rocca, R.; Cojoc, G.; Liberale, C.; Malara, N.; Simone, G.; Candeloro, P.; Anichini, A.; Tirinato, L.; Gentile, F.; et al. Microfluidic Devices Modulate Tumor Cell Line Susceptibility to NK Cell Recognition. *Small* **2012**, *8*, 2886–2894. [CrossRef]
11. Stevens, M.; George, J. Exploring and engineering the cell surface interface. *Science* **2005**, *310*, 1135–1138. [CrossRef]
12. De Vitis, S.; Coluccio, M.L.; Strumbo, G.; Malara, N.; Fanizzi, F.P.; De Pascali, S.A.; Perozziello, G.; Candeloro, P.; Di Fabrizio, E.M.; Gentile, F. Combined effect of surface nano-topography and delivery of therapeutics on the adhesion of tumor cells on porous silicon substrates. *Microelectron. Eng.* **2016**, *158*, 6–10. [CrossRef]
13. Lane, S.W.; Williams, D.A.; Watt, F.M. Modulating the stem cell niche for tissue regeneration. *Nat. Biotechnol.* **2014**, *32*, 795–803. [CrossRef] [PubMed]
14. Dalby, M.J.; Gadegaard, N.; Oreffo, R.O.C. Harnessing nanotopography and integrin-matrix interactions to influence stem cell fate. *Nat. Mater.* **2014**, *13*, 558–569. [CrossRef]
15. Delcassian, D.; Depoil, D.; Rudnicka, D.; Liu, M.; Davis, D.M.; Dustin, M.L.; Dunlop, I.E. Nanoscale Ligand Spacing Influences Receptor Triggering in T Cells and NK Cells. *Nano Lett.* **2013**, *13*, 5608–5614. [CrossRef]
16. Robinson, J.T.; Jorgolli, M.; Shalek, A.K.; Yoon, M.-H.; Gertner, R.S.; Park, H. Vertical nanowire electrode arrays as a scalable platform for intracellular interfacing to neuronal circuits. *Nat. Nanotechnol.* **2012**, *7*, 180–184. [CrossRef] [PubMed]
17. Gentile, F.; Tirinato, L.; Battista, E.; Causa, F.; Liberale, C.; Di Fabrizio, E.; Decuzzi, P. Cells preferentially grow on rough substrates. *Biomaterials* **2010**, *31*, 7205–7212. [CrossRef] [PubMed]
18. Sorkin, R.; Greenbaum, A.; David-Pur, M.; SaritAnava; Ayali, A.; Ben-Jacob, E.; Hanein, Y. Process entanglement as a neuronal anchorage mechanism to rough surfaces. *Nanotechnology* **2009**, *20*, 015101. [CrossRef] [PubMed]
19. Xie, C.; Hanson, L.; Xie, W.; Lin, Z.; Cui, B.; Cui, Y. Noninvasive Neuron Pinning with Nanopillar Arrays. *Nano Lett.* **2010**, *10*, 4020–4024. [CrossRef]
20. Ankam, S.; Suryana, M.; Chan, L.Y.; Moe, A.A.K.; Teo, B.K.K.; Law, J.B.K.; Sheetz, M.P.; Low, H.Y.; Yim, E.K.F. Substrate topography and size determine the fate of human embryonic stem cells to neuronal or glial lineage. *Acta Biomater.* **2013**, *9*, 4535–4545. [CrossRef]
21. Baranes, K.; Chejanovsky, N.; Alon, N.; Sharoni, A.; Shefi, O. Topographic Cues of Nano-Scale Height Direct Neuronal Growth Pattern. *Biotechnol. Bioeng.* **2012**, *109*, 1791–1797. [CrossRef]
22. Ferrari, A.; Cecchini, M.; Dhawan, A.; Micera, S.; Tonazzini, I.; Stabile, R.; Pisignano, D.; Beltram, F. Nanotopographic Control of Neuronal Polarity. *Nano Lett.* **2011**, *11*, 505–511. [CrossRef]
23. Ligon, S.C.; Liska, R.; Stampfl, J.; Gurr, M.; Mülhaupt, R. Polymers for 3D Printing and Customized Additive Manufacturing. *Chem. Rev.* **2017**, *117*, 10212–10290. [CrossRef] [PubMed]
24. Guvendiren, M.; Molde, J.; Soares, R.M.D.; Kohn, J. Designing Biomaterials for 3D Printing. *ACS Biomater. Sci. Eng.* **2016**, *2*, 1679–1693. [CrossRef]
25. Accardo, A.; Courson, R.; Riesco, R.; Raimbault, V.; Malaquin, L. Direct Laser Fabrication of Meso-Scale 2D and 3D Architectures with Micrometric Feature Resolution. *Addit. Manuf.* **2018**, *22*, 440–446. [CrossRef]
26. Nguyen, A.K.; Narayan, R.J. Two-Photon Polymerization for Biological Applications. *Mater. Today* **2017**, *20*, 314–322. [CrossRef]
27. Fan, D.; Staufer, U.; Accardo, A. Engineered 3D Polymer and Hydrogel Microenvironments for Cell Culture Applications. *Bioengineering* **2019**, *6*, 113. [CrossRef]
28. Accardo, A.; Blatché, M.C.; Courson, R.; Loubinoux, I.; Thibault, C.; Malaquin, L.; Vieu, C. Multiphoton Direct Laser Writing and 3D Imaging of Polymeric Freestanding Architectures for Cell Colonization. *Small* **2017**, *13*, 1700621–1700611. [CrossRef] [PubMed]
29. Gentile, F.; Rocca, R.L.; Marinaro, G.; Nicastri, A.; Toma, A.; Paonessa, F.; Cojoc, G.; Liberale, C.; Benfenati, F.; Di Fabrizio, E.; et al. Differential Cell Adhesion on Mesoporous Silicon Substrates. *ACS Appl. Mater. Interfaces* **2012**, *4*, 2903–2911. [CrossRef]
30. Marinaro, G.; La Rocca, R.; Toma, A.; Barberio, M.; Cancedda, L.; Di Fabrizio, E.; Decuzzi, P.; Gentile, F. Networks of Neuroblastoma Cells on Porous Silicon Substrates Reveal a Small World Topology. *Integr. Biol.* **2015**, *7*, 184–197. [CrossRef]
31. Foll, H.; Christophersen, M.; Carstensen, J.; Hasse, G. Formation and application of porous silicon. *Mater. Sci. Eng.* **2002**, *39*, 93–141. [CrossRef]

32. Gentile, F.; Battista, E.; Accardo, A.; Coluccio, M.; Asande, M.; Perozziello, G.; Das, G.; Liberale, C.; De Angelis, F.; Candeloro, P.; et al. Fractal Structure Can Explain the Increased Hydrophobicity of NanoPorous Silicon Films. *Microelectron. Eng.* **2011**, *88*, 2537–2540. [CrossRef]
33. Coluccio, M.L.; Gentile, F.; Francardi, M.; Perozziello, G.; Malara, N.; Candeloro, P.; Di Fabrizio, E. Electroless Deposition and Nanolithography Can Control the Formation of Materials at the Nano-Scale for Plasmonic Applications. *Sensors* **2014**, *14*, 6056–6083. [CrossRef] [PubMed]
34. Battista, E.; Coluccio, M.-L.; Alabastri, A.; Barberio, M.; Causa, F.; Netti, P.-A.; Di Fabrizio, E.; Gentile, F. Metal enhanced fluorescence on super-hydrophobic clusters of gold nanoparticles. *Microelectron. Eng.* **2017**, *175*, 7–11. [CrossRef]
35. Li, W.; Liu, C.; Zhao, C.; Zhai, L.; Lv, S. Downregulation of β3 integrin by miR-30a-5p modulates cell adhesion and invasion by interrupting Erk/Ets 1 network in triple-negative breast cancer. *Int. J. Oncol.* **2016**, *48*, 1155–1164. [CrossRef] [PubMed]
36. Waxman, B. Routing of multipoint connections. *IEEE J. Sel. Areas Commun.* **1988**, *6*, 1617–1622. [CrossRef]
37. Barabási, A.-L. *Network Science*; Cambridge University Press: Glasgow, UK, 2016; p. 475.
38. Barabási, A.-L.; Albert, R. Emergence of scaling in random networks. *Science* **1999**, *286*, 509–512. [CrossRef]
39. Barabási, A.-L.; Oltvai, Z.N. Network biology: Understanding the cell's functional organization. *Nat. Rev. Genet.* **2004**, *5*, 101–113. [CrossRef]
40. Watts, D.J. *Small Worlds: The Dynamics of Networks between Order and Randomness*; Princeton University Press: Woodstock, UK, 2003.
41. Watts, D.J.; Strogatz, S.H. Collective dynamics of 'small-world' networks. *Nature* **1998**, *393*, 440–442. [CrossRef]
42. Humphries, M.D.; Gurney, K. Network 'Small-World-Ness': A Quantitative Method for Determining Canonical Network Equivalence. *PLoS ONE* **2008**, *3*, e0002051. [CrossRef]
43. Perozziello, G.; Catalano, R.; Francardi, M.; Rondanina, E.; Pardeo, F.; De Angelis, F.; Malara, N.; Candeloro, P.; Morrone, G.; Di Fabrizio, E. A microfluidic device integrating plasmonic nanodevices for Raman spectroscopy analysis on trapped single living cells. *Microelectron. Eng.* **2013**, *111*, 314–319. [CrossRef]
44. Candeloro, P.; Grande, E.; Raimondo, R.; Di Mascolo, D.; Gentile, F.; Coluccio, M.L.; Perozziello, G.; Malara, N.; Francardi, M.; Di Fabrizio, E. Raman database of Amino Acids solutions: A critical study of Extended Multiplicative Signal Correction. *Analyst* **2013**, *138*, 7331–7340. [CrossRef]
45. Muscella, A.; Vetrugno, C.; Migoni, D.; Biagioni, F.; Fanizzi, F.; Fornai, F.; De Pascali, S.; Marsigliante, S. Antitumor activity of [Pt(O,O′-acac)(γ-acac)(DMS)] in mouse xenograft model of breast cancer. *Cell Death Dis.* **2014**, *5*, e1014. [CrossRef] [PubMed]
46. Gentile, F.; Medda, R.; Cheng, L.; Battista, E.; Scopelliti, P.; Milani, P.; Cavalcanti-Adam, E.; Decuzzi, P. Selective modulation of cell response on engineered fractal silicon substrates. *Sci. Rep.* **2013**, *3*, 1461. [CrossRef] [PubMed]
47. Strogatz, S.H. Exploring complex networks. *Nature* **2001**, *410*, 268–276. [CrossRef] [PubMed]
48. Onesto, V.; Cancedda, L.; Coluccio, M.; Nanni, M.; Pesce, M.; Malara, N.; Cesarelli, M.; Fabrizio, E.D.; Amato, F.; Gentile, F. Nano-topography Enhances Communication in Neural Cells Networks. *Sci. Rep.* **2017**, *7*, 1–13. [CrossRef] [PubMed]
49. Onesto, V.; Villani, M.; Narducci, R.; Malara, N.; Imbrogno, A.; Allione, M.; Costa, N.; Coppedè, N.; Zappettini, A.; Cannistraci, C.; et al. Cortical-like mini-columns of neuronal cells on zinc oxide nanowire surfaces. *Sci. Rep.* **2019**, *9*, 4021–4017. [CrossRef]
50. Di Mascolo, D.; Coclite, A.; Gentile, F.; Francardi, M. Quantitative micro-Raman analysis of micro-particles in drug delivery. *Nanoscale Adv.* **2019**, *1*, 1541–1552. [CrossRef]
51. Jin, H.; Varner, J. Integrins: Roles in cancer development and as treatment targets. *Br. J. Cancer* **2004**, *90*, 561–565. [CrossRef]
52. Koistinen, P.; Heino, J. Integrins in Cancer Cell Invasion. In *Madame Curie Bioscience Database [Internet]*; Landes Bioscience: Austin, TX, USA, 2013. Available online: https://www.ncbi.nlm.nih.gov/books/NBK6070/ (accessed on 15 April 2020).
53. Chowdhury, M.H.; Gant, V.A.; Trache, A.; Baldwin, A.M.; Meininger, G.A.; Coté, G.L. Use of surface-enhanced Raman spectroscopy for the detection of human integrins. *J. Biomed. Opt.* **2006**, *11*, 024004. [CrossRef]
54. Gentile, F.; Coluccio, M.L.; Zaccaria, R.P.; Francardi, M.; Cojoc, G.; Perozziello, G.; Raimondo, R.; Candeloroa, P.; Fabrizio, E.D. Selective on site separation and detection of molecules in diluted solutions with superhydrophobic clusters of plasmonic nanoparticles. *Nanoscale* **2014**, *6*, 8208–8225. [CrossRef]

55. Liston, D.R.; Davis, M. Clinically Relevant Concentrations of Anticancer Drugs: A Guide for Nonclinical Studies. *Clin. Cancer Res.* **2017**, *23*, 3489–3498. [CrossRef]
56. Xu, R.; Zhang, G.; Mai, J.; Deng, X.; Segura-Ibarra, V.; Wu, S.; Shen, J.; Liu, H.; Hu, Z.; Chen, L.; et al. An Injectable Nanoparticle Generator Enhances Delivery of Cancer Therapeutics. *Nat. Biotechnol.* **2016**, *34*, 414–418. [CrossRef] [PubMed]
57. Malara, N.; Givigliano, F.; Trunzo, V.; Macrina, L.; Raso, C.; Amodio, N.; Aprigliano, S.; Minniti, A.; Russo, V.; Roveda, L.; et al. In vitro expansion of tumour cells derived from blood and tumour tissue is useful to redefine personalized treatment in non-small cell lung cancer patients. *J. Biol. Regul. Homeost. Agents* **2014**, *28*, 717–731. [PubMed]
58. Yin, H.-L.; Wu, C.-C.; Lin, C.-H.; Chai, C.-Y.; Hou, M.-F.; Chang, S.-J.; Tsai, H.-P.; Hung, W.-C.; Pan, M.-R.; Luo, C.-W. β1 Integrin as a Prognostic and Predictive Marker in Triple-Negative Breast Cancer. *Int. J. Mol. Sci.* **2016**, *17*, 1432. [CrossRef] [PubMed]

5

Sirolimus-Eluting Electrospun-Produced Matrices as Coatings for Vascular Stents: Dependence of Drug Release on Matrix Structure and Composition of the External Environment

Zhanna K. Nazarkina [1,*,†], Boris P. Chelobanov [1,†], Vera S. Chernonosova [1,2], Irina V. Romanova [1], Andrey A. Karpenko [2] and Pavel P. Laktionov [1,2]

1 Institute of Chemical Biology and Fundamental Medicine, Siberian Branch, Russian Academy of Sciences, Novosibirsk 630090, Russia; boris.p.chelobanov@gmail.com (B.P.C.); vera_mal@niboch.nsc.ru (V.S.C.); irin-romanova@yandex.ru (I.V.R.); lakt@niboch.nsc.ru (P.P.L.)

2 Meshalkin National Medical Research Center, Ministry of Health of the Russian Federation, Novosibirsk 630055, Russia; andreikarpenko@rambler.ru

* Correspondence: zha_naz@niboch.nsc.ru

† The first two authors should be regarded as joint first authors.

Abstract: Although a number of drug-eluting coatings for vascular stents (VSs) have been developed and are in commercial use, more efficient stent coatings and drug delivery systems are needed. Sirolimus (SRL) is a clinically important drug with antiproliferative and immunosuppressive activities that is widely used for coating stents. Here, we characterized SRL-enriched matrices, intended for coating vascular stents, that were produced by electrospinning (ES) on a drum collector from a solution of polycaprolactone (PCL) and human serum albumin (HSA), 1,1,1,3,3,3-hexafluoroisopropanol (HFIP), dimethyl sulfoxide (DMSO), and SRL. The release of tritium-labeled SRL (^{3}H-SRL) from matrices in phosphate-buffered saline (PBS) or human blood plasma (BP) was studied. The introduction of DMSO in the ES blend decreased SRL release. The use of BP significantly accelerated SRL release through binding with serum biomolecules. The exchange of PBS or BP after every time point also increased SRL release. The maximum SRL release in BP was observed at 3 days. The matrices produced from the ES solution with DMSO and HSA released no more than 80% SRL after 27 days in BP, even under medium exchange conditions. Therefore, PCL-based matrices containing HSA, SRL, and DMSO can be used for coating VSs with prolonged SRL delivery.

Keywords: sirolimus; electrospinning; drug release; polycaprolactone; 3D matrix; drug-eluting stents

1. Introduction

Stent implantation is one of the most common procedures for the reconstitution of blood flow through atherosclerosis-occluded arteries. The placement of the stent initiates a variety of reactions, including endothelial injury, crushing of the plaque, and stretching and lacerations of the arterial wall, which can lead to stent-induced restenosis [1]. These processes stimulate an inflammatory response—the predominant cause of neointimal proliferation and in-stent restenosis [2] accompanied by the migration and proliferation of smooth muscle cells (SMCs) and fibroblasts from the arterial wall [3]. It was suggested that neointima growth after application of angioplasty drug-eluting stents (DESs) could be prevented by reducing the growth and migration of SMCs and other cell types. Sirolimus (SRL)-eluting stents, which were approved in Europe in 2002 and in the United States in 2003 [4], are the most popular and have been shown to be the most effective among the relevant analogs in reducing coronary restenosis, re-intervention rates, and other adverse cardiac events in patients with coronary artery disease [5,6].

SRL (rapamycin) is a polyketide macrolide compound obtained by a strain of *Streptomyces hygroscopicus* [7]. In mammals, the molecular target of rapamycin, mTOR, is a cell cycle-specific kinase involved in complex intracellular signaling pathways that regulate cell growth and proliferation, immunity, angiogenesis, fibrogenesis, and metabolism [8]. After entering into the cell, SRL interacts with the immunophilin FKBP-12. This complex interacts with mTOR kinase and inhibits its activity [7]. Thus, SRL blocks the activation of p70S6 kinase, which leads to cell cycle arrest at the G1 to S phase.

SRL is a potent inhibitor of the antigen-induced T- and B-cells' proliferation and antibody production [7], as well as the proliferation of a variety of cell types of nonlymphoid origin [9], including the inhibition of human coronary artery SMC proliferation [10]. Complete inhibition of PDGF-induced DNA synthesis in SMCs was achieved at 10 ng/mL SRL, and more than 50% inhibition was observed at an SRL concentration of 0.1 ng/mL. The inhibitory properties of SRL could be observed from a threshold concentration of 0.01 ng/mL. SRL is able to inhibit both quiescent and actively cycling cells [10].

SRL has a broad therapeutic window. Preclinical animal trials have shown that SRL demonstrates biological activity in doses from 18 to 1200 μg, without showing toxicity to the vessel wall [4]. Despite the promising pharmacological activities of SRL, however, its clinical application is complicated by poor aqueous solubility, first-pass metabolism, and nonspecific distribution in off-target sites [8]. SRL has some adverse, dose-dependent effects, including immunosuppression; the inhibition of bone growth; increased cholesterol, triglyceride, and creatinine serum levels; and decreased glomerular filtration rates. Leukopenia, thrombocytopenia, anemia, rash, stomatitis, arthralgia, diarrhea, hypertension, and hypokalemia may also occur [11]. Owing to its lipophilic nature, SRL is widely distributed in lipid membranes, resulting in a large volume of distribution and a relatively long half-life [12,13].

The most commonly used first-generation SRL-eluting stent in clinical practice is Cypher stent (SES; Cordis, Warren, NJ, USA) [14]. This DES consists of a stainless-steel platform with a strut thickness of 140 mm and 140 mg/cm^2 sirolimus with a poly(ethylene-co-vinyl acetate) and poly(n-butyl methacrylate) polymer. A pharmacokinetic study showed that the maximum concentration of SRL in blood is observed between 3 and 4 h after stent implantation, with a peak concentration of 0.57 ng/mL in patients receiving one stent [15]. The average terminal-phase elimination half-life of SRL is 213 h.

It is known that SRL can induce fibrinoid vascular necrosis [16]. A reduction in the SRL dose can reduce this toxic effect in an animal model. A lower SRL dose (25, 40, and 100 μg), released from a nonpolymeric hydroxyapatite-coated stent built by MIV Therapeutics (Atlanta, GA, USA), results in less vascular healing, presenting significantly fewer fibrinoids without increasing neointima formation as compared with Cypher stent (111 μg of SRL) [16]. The REDOX trial showed that lower doses (40% or 70% compared with Cypher stent) of SRL effectively maintain luminal patency for up to at least 12 months, as determined at a follow-up [17].

The stent platform, the antiproliferative drug, and the drug carrier polymer are the three major components that determine stent safety and efficacy [18]. The Cypher stent has not been manufactured since 2011 because the first-generation stents displayed an increased risk for late thrombotic events [19]; this risk was considered to be associated with the permanent presence of the non-erodible polymers poly(ethylene-co-vinyl acetate) and poly(n-butyl methacrylate). Therefore, a second generation of DES was developed using more biocompatible polymer coatings. SRL was also used to develop a new generation of DESs with ultrathin (<70 μm) struts coated with biodegradable polymers, such as Orsiro and BioMime [20]. Another type of SRL-eluting stent is MiStent, which has ultrathin struts composed of crystalline SRL and a biodegradable polymer poly(lactic-co-glycolic acid). Clinical trials have shown the superiority of ultrathin strut biodegradable polymer-coated DESs compared with durable polymer-coated DESs in maintaining a good safety profile [21].

The Tetriflex (Sahajanand Medical Technology, Surat, India) is a new-generation, ultrathin (60 μm), biodegradable SRL-eluting stent with coating composed of a combination of hydrophilic and hydrophobic polymers for controlled and prolonged release of SRL. Clinical studies have demonstrated the safety and effectiveness of the Tetriflex stent [22].

One of the novel DESs is Svelte SRL-eluting stent containing fully bioresorbable polymer and pre-mounted on a single lumen, fixed-wire delivery system [23]. The pharmacokinetics of the Svelte stent mimics the SRL release of the Cypher stent. The Svelte amino-acid based polymer can be enzymatically degraded with complete resorption in 12 months. The OPTMIZE Trial, including 1630 subjects, will estimate the safety and clinical efficacy of the Svelte stent [23].

The DESs used in clinics are manufactured using different techniques for coating metallic vascular stents, including ultrasonic coating [24], dip-coating [25], spray-coating [2], air-brush [26], electrohydrodynamic jetting, plasma-treated coating, electrotreated coating [27], and electrospinning (ES) [28]. Coating techniques have an influence on drug release kinetics and clinical outcomes [27].

ES is based on the generation of polymer fibers from a blend of polymers and drugs in a strong electric field. The advantages of the ES method are the ability to obtain fibers of different diameters and ultrastructures laid in a 3D matrix, as well as its suitability for a broad range of materials, cost effectiveness, and mechanical support from the stented area that covers the inter-strut area (e.g., the InspireMD CGuard stents consisting of a fine mesh that inhibits neointima growth thanks to the prevention of cell migration from the damaged area) [29–31]. Drug release and dissolution of the bioactive substance can be controlled through the structure of polymer fibers, which is determined by the composition of the ES. In recent years, the ES technique and its modifications have been widely used in drug delivery and regenerative medicine. The FDA has approved heart valve prostheses and esophageal stent produced using the ES technique for clinical studies [32].

The materials for coating vascular stents (VSs) must be hemo- and biocompatible, and extensible by at least 2–2.5×. Synthetic materials produced from polycaprolactone (PCL) possess these properties and are widely used in medicine owing to their PCL biocompatibility, mechanical characteristics, and ease of manufacturing. The average degradation time for PCL is about 2–3 years [33]. The PCL matrices produced by ES are convenient for VSs owing to their mechanical properties [29] and good hemo- and biocompatibility [34,35]. The matrices produced from pure PCL possess poor wettability and low cell compatibility, but incorporation of human serum albumin (HSA) into the PCL matrices strongly interferes with its properties, thereby increasing the stiffness and biological properties of such matrices [29]. It is known that HSA reduces platelet adhesion and increases the thromboresistance and hemocompatibility of blood-exposed surfaces [36,37].

In a previous study of paclitaxel release from ES-produced matrices, we showed that drug release depends on the structure of the fibers and the composition of the surrounding medium [29].

In the current study, we investigated SRL release from ES-produced matrices using different solution compositions: 5% PCL/SRL/10% HSA, 5% PCL/SRL/10% HSA/3% dimethyl sulfoxide (DMSO), and 5% PCL/SRL. The physicochemical properties of the materials and the dependence of SRL release on the composition of the surrounding medium were also studied.

2. Materials and Methods

2.1. Production of ^{3}H-Labeled Sirolimus

^{3}H-SRL was synthesized by thermoactivated tritium exchange, as described earlier [38]. ^{3}H-SRL was purified from byproducts using reversed-phase chromatography (RP-HPLC) on a C18 column using a gradient of acetonitrile in water (25–100%). The purity of ^{3}H-SRL was evaluated by autoradiography following thin layer chromatography (TLC) on Kieselgel 60 F254 plates (Merck, Darmstadt, Germany, 25 Alufolien 20 cm × 20 cm) in a chloroform–methanol–water mixture (19:1:0.1, Rf = ~0.7). The radioactivity of the preparation was measured on a Tri-Carb 2800 TR β-counter (PerkinElmer, Waltham, MA, USA) in a "ULTIMA GOLD LTT" scintillator (Perkin Elmer, Waltham, MA, USA). The radioactivity of all samples was evaluated as reported earlier [29], that is, 0.1 mL of the sample was thoroughly mixed with 0.9 mL scintillator, and radioactivity was measured immediately.

2.2. Fabrication of the ES Matrices

The ES solutions were prepared using stock solutions of 9% PCL and 1% HSA (Sigma-Aldrich, St. Louis, MI, USA) in 1,1,1,3,3,3-hexafluoroisopropanol (HFIP, Sigma-Aldrich, USA). The HSA concentration in the matrices was 10% (w/w). SRL (150301, Fujian Kerui Pharmaceutical Co. Ltd., Fujian, China) was dissolved in HFIP or DMSO (Sigma-Aldrich, USA) and added to the ES solutions to a final concentration of 0.9 $\mu g/cm^2$ (0.7 μg per disk). Then, 3% (v/v) DMSO was added to the solution of polymers. ^{3}H-SRL was mixed with unlabeled SRL to reach radioactivity of 27,000 cpm/cm^2 (21,000 per 10 mm diameter disk). To obtain more-uniform fibers, the PCL/SRL ES solution contained 0.1 mm triethylamine (TEA). To obtain the matrices containing ^{3}H-SRL, we used a custom made ES device with an airproof chamber and an exhaust HEPA filter equipped with a Spellman SL 150 (30 kV, Spellman, Brockton, MA, USA) power supply. Matrices of 110–125 μm thickness were prepared using a drum collector (4 cm diameter and 5 cm length). Electrospinning conditions were the same for all matrices: voltage—26.5 kV; feed rate—1 mL/h; nozzle to collector distance—20 cm; collector rotation speed—300 rpm; 23–25 °C; 25–35% humidity. After fabrication, matrices were removed from the collector, dried in vacuum under 10 Pa for 12 h, and stored in sealed ziplock polyethylene containers at 4 °C.

2.3. Characterization of the Matrices

2.3.1. Mechanical Characterization

Strain–stress diagrams were obtained using a universal Zwick/Roell Z100 (Zwick Roell, Ulm, Germany) test bench as described in ISO 7198:1998 [39]. Four 1 × 5 cm rectangular sheets for each matrix were cut and placed between holders at a distance of 2–2.5 cm. Tensile strength testing was performed at a rate of 10 $mm \cdot min^{-1}$ at room temperature (21–23 °C).

2.3.2. Matrix Surface Characterization

The morphology of matrices were studied by scanning electron microscopy (SEM), as described earlier [35]. The size of the pores and the diameter of fibers were estimated from the SEM images according to ISO 7198:1998 [39]. To estimate the stability of the fiber structure, the matrices were incubated in PBS (Sigma-Aldrich, USA) or blood plasma (BP) at 37 °C for 27 days. After incubation, the matrices were rinsed with water, air-dried, and studied by SEM. To evaluate the structure after elongation, the matrices were fixed between clumps of the small device that expands the matrix and fixes it in an SEM camera. Matrices were fixed at conductive colloidal graphite (G303, Agar Scientific Ltd., Cambridge, UK) before gold sputter-coating.

2.3.3. Additional Characterization of the Matrices

The contact angle was measured on a Drop Shape Analyzer–DS A25 (Kruss GmbH, Hamburg, Germany) using water as a solvent (drop volume, 1 μL; shooting speed, 160 frames per second).

The porosity of the matrices was evaluated according to the following formula:

$$\text{Porosity (\%)} = [1 - \text{Da}/\text{Dp}] \times 100$$

where Da = matrix weight/matrix volume and Dp is the PCL density.

2.4. Sirolimus Release Kinetics

To evaluate SRL release, 10 mm diameter disks (~0.785 cm^2) were excised from the matrices by die cutting and placed in wells of a 48-well plate. Then, 400 μL of PBS or EDTA-stabilized BP was added to each well. The investigation was approved by the Local Ethical Committee of Center of Personalized Medicine, Institute of Chemical Biology and Fundamental Medicine of the Siberian Branch of the Russian Academy of Sciences (№1, 15.01.2016). The plate was sealed with a film (Microseal® 'B' PCR Plate Sealing Film, adhesive, Bio-Rad, Hercules, CA, USA) to prevent drying, followed by incubation on a Titramax 1000 shaker (Heidolph, Schwabach, Germany) at 37 °C; platform rotation speed of 200 rpm. Moreover, 0.01% sodium azide was used to prevent bacterial growth. Two series of SRL release kinetics were studied. The matrices were incubated in PBS or BP for 20 min, 60 min, 3 h, 9 h, 27 h, 3 days, 9 days, and 27 days without (Series 1) or with (Series 2) medium replacement. For Series 2, the supernatant was removed at each time point, fresh solution was added, and the matrix was incubated in a fresh solution until the next time point. After incubation, the matrix was washed with H_2O and air-dried at room temperature for SEM analysis. The radioactivity of the supernatants was measured in duplicate, as described above (Section 2.1).

The influence of matrix elongation on SRL release was evaluated as follows. The matrix was fixed in the clamps and then slowly stretched by a screw to double the measured distance. After stretching, the linear sizes of the matrix were measured and the amount of SRL per disk was calculated. The 10 mm diameter discs were then excised from the stretched matrix, and SRL release was estimated as described above. All experiments were performed in duplicate.

2.5. *Statistical Analysis*

The results were processed using Microsoft Excel 2010 and the Statistica 7.0 package (StatSoft Inc., Tulsa, OK, USA).

3. Results and Discussion

3.1. *Preparation and Characterization of the SRL Matrices*

^{3}H-SRL was obtained by thermoactivated tritium exchange. ^{3}H-SRL has the same Rf after RP-HPLC and TLC, suggesting a similar chemical structure of the compound. Purified ^{3}H-SRL preparation with a specific radioactivity of 0.2 mCi/mL (~0.055 Ci/mmol) was thus obtained. The compound was homogenous according to the TLC data, being detected as a single spot on the autoradiograph with the expected Rf corresponding to unlabeled SRL. ^{3}H-SRL was combined with unlabeled SRL to reach a dose of ~1.05 μg/cm^2 SRL and a radioactivity of ~27,000 cpm/cm^2.

ES is a very promising method based on the generation of polymer fibers from a blend of polymers and drugs in a strong electric field. The advantages of the ES method are the ability to obtain fibers with different diameters (from nm to μm) and ultrastructures, broad material suitability, and high cost effectiveness [30,31]. Several parameters have an influence on the structure and morphology of polymer fibers, including voltage, collector to needle distance, solution flow rate, polymer concentration, solvent type, dielectric constant, temperature, pressure, and moisture [31]. The solvent type, polymer concentration, and voltage strongly affect the resulting fiber diameter. Drug release and dissolution of the bioactive substance can be controlled by the structure of the polymer fibers. In this study, we used the same ES conditions to obtain all matrices.

Three different matrices were prepared using ES on a drum collector from solutions containing PCL, HSA, DMSO, SRL, and ^{3}H-SRL. Electrospinning conditions were the same for all matrices: voltage—26.5 kV, feed rate—1 mL/h; nozzle to collector distance—20 cm.

Polymers used for drug-eluting stent coatings need to have mechanical characteristics and biological properties similar to those of natural vessels. The PCL scaffolds exhibit good mechanical properties, flexibility, and nontoxicity [40]. The average degradation time for PCL is about 2–3 years [33]. Earlier, we studied the structure of fibers produced by ES from PCL–HSA solutions [35]; like other authors, we demonstrated that HSA increases the hemocompatibility of blood-exposed surfaces [35–37]. The mechanical properties of PCL/HSA-containing matrices improved compared with pristine PCL, and HSA was tightly bound, with the fiber surface exposed for a long period of time because it is only partially accessible for protease hydrolysis [35]. HSA contains carboxylic and amine groups that promote cell attachment and spreading via integrin-binding sites, and can thus provide endothelization [40]. As such, HSA is the most abundant protein in human blood responsible for fatty acid transport and is the major binding protein for neutral and acidic drugs [41,42].

Its non-immunogenicity, high biocompatibility, and good biodegradability (as well as its binding of drugs) make HSA a prospective compound for DES coatings.

The physical properties of the obtained matrices are shown in Table 1. The tensile strength of the prepared matrices depend on the composition of the ES solution, demonstrating a typical two-phase curve with an extended plastic deformation region, starting from 7–10% to 250–300% and varying from 10.4 to 15 MPa (Table 1). These properties provide elongation without breakage during stent expansion, as well as a low residual load after the stent installation, as previously discussed [29].

Table 1. Physical properties of the matrices. PCL, polycaprolactone; SRL, sirolimus; HSA, human serum albumin: DMSO, dimethyl sulfoxide.

Matrix Type	Thickness (μm)	Strength (MPa)	Mass Per Unit Area (mg/cm²)	Fiber Diameter (μm)	Pore Diameter (μm)	Porosity (%)	Contact Angle (°)
5% PCL/SRL/10% HSA	111	10.45 ± 1.48	2.51	0.27 ± 0.8	1.94 ± 0.33	63.3	117.63 ± 2.72
5% PCL/SRL/10% HSA/3%DMSO	125	12.41 ± 3.11	2.47	0.14 ± 0.05	1.12 ± 0.18	64.7	109.52 ± 2.22
5% PCL/SRL	114	15.04 ± 2.50	2.44	0.36 ± 0.09	2.11 ± 0.34	60.9	127.37 ± 3.41

The structure of the matrices was studied by SEM. All matrices were composed of randomly oriented fibers. The composition of the ES solution influenced the fiber diameter and its variability (Figure 1). The matrices obtained from the blend containing 5% PCL, SRL, and 0.1 mm TEA were more heterogeneous in fiber diameter. The average diameter of the fibers made from the PCL/SRL/HSA and PCL/SRL solution was 0.27 and 0.36 μm, respectively (Table 1, Figure 1). The fiber diameter significantly decreased when DMSO was added (0.14 μm for the PCL/SRL/HSA/DMSO matrix). The SEM at a higher resolution reveals the smooth surface of the PCL fibers. The decrease in the fiber diameter for matrices containing DMSO was previously shown for the PCL-based matrices containing paclitaxel [29].

According to SEM data, incubation in PBS for 27 days did not alter the structure of the PCL/SRL/HSA and PCL/SRL matrices (Figure 1), while fiber fusion and thickening were observed when the PCL/SRL/HSA/DMSO matrix was incubated in PBS or BP for 27 days. A negligible thickening effect was also observed for the PCL/SRL matrix, where the thickness of the PCL/SRL/HSA/DMSO fibers increased almost twofold. There was no significant change in the structure of the PCL/SRL/HSA matrix during incubation. No significant weight change after 27 days of incubation was observed for all matrix types (data not shown). This means that, during the assayed time, there was no substantial matrix degradation. The incorporation of hydrophilic biodegradable components like HSA into the PCL matrices can potentially increase their rate of biodegradation, but we did not observe such an effect for 27 days [40].

The porosity of the matrices was estimated from the matrix weight and polymer density in the range of 60–65% (Table 1). No significant differences were observed for the matrices prepared from different blends. The presence of DMSO in the electrospinning solution resulted in a decrease not only in fiber diameter, but also in pore size. The PCL/SRL/HSA/DMSO matrix containing 3% DMSO had a pore diameter approximately 1.7-fold less than those without DMSO (Table 1, Figure 1). These data correlate with those previously obtained for PCL-based matrices containing paclitaxel [29].

The wettability of the matrices affected the cell distribution in the matrix and cell proliferation [40]. The polar amine and carboxyl groups in HSA might have improved the surface wettability of the matrices. HSA has a high water-binding capacity and can increase the hydrophilicity of materials [40]. Measurement of the contact angle is a commonly used technique to determine wettability. The water contact angles of the matrices are indicated in Table 1. The HSA-containing matrices (PCL/SRL/HSA and PCL/SRL/HSA/DMSO) show a lower contact angle compared with that of PCL/SRL. According to the literature data, hydrophilic matrices are more suitable for implants owing to their lower ability to adsorb proteins and induce inflammation [43,44].

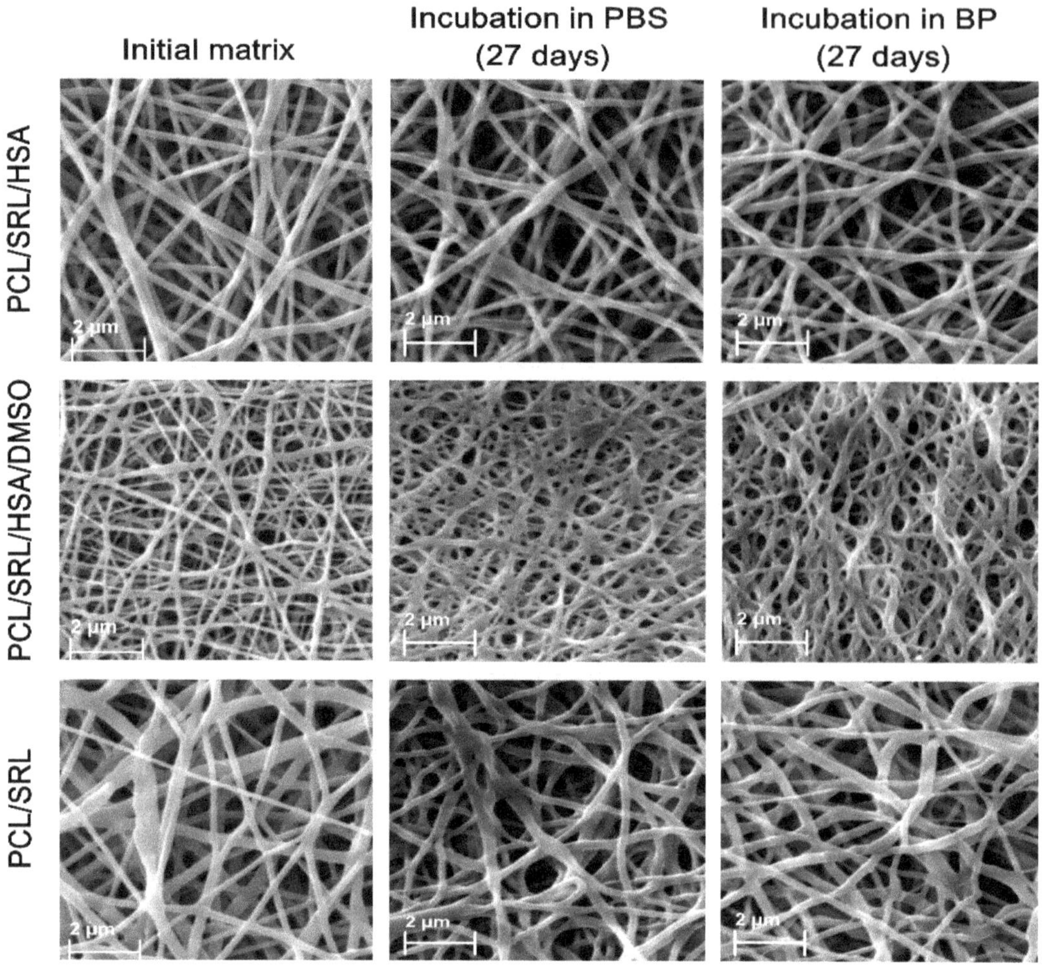

Figure 1. Scanning electron microscopy (SEM) images of the matrices incubated under different conditions. BP, blood plasma; PCL, polycaprolactone; SRL, sirolimus; HSA, human serum albumin: DMSO, dimethyl sulfoxide.

3.2. Study of SRL Release

The SRL release from PCL-based matrices was studied with (2) or without (1) a medium replacement to mimic SRL release in a biological system. The kinetic curves shown for PBS without any medium replacement were similar for all matrices (Supplementary materials, Table S1), although SRL release from the PCL/SRL/HSA/DMSO matrix was slightly slower, with the maximal release of 70% observed at 27 days (Figure 2A). The maximal release observed for the PCL/SRL/HSA and PCL/SRL matrices was 76% and 74%, respectively. When the matrices were incubated with replacement of PBS throughout, the rate of SRL release from the PCL/SRL/HSA/DMSO matrix was significantly slower, with a maximal level of 75% for 27 days (Figure 2B). Meanwhile, the PCL/SRL/HSA and PCL/SRL matrices released 75% SRL during the first three days, and reached maximal levels of 90% and 85%, respectively.

It was shown earlier that paclitaxel is distributed both throughout the volume and on the surface of the fibers in PCL-based matrices [29]. In this work, the SRL distribution seems to be very similar to that of paclitaxel, because we used the same method to obtain matrices. Desorption of SRL from the matrix surface limits the rate of establishing the equilibrium between SRL on the surface and SRL in the solution. This process is the result of the low solubility of SRL in water (2.6 mg/L) [45]. Removing the medium with dissolved SRL led to the additional desorption of SRL from the matrix surface into the solution, thus the amount of dissolved SRL increased. The presence of ions and SRL-binding molecules can also increase the solubility of SRL in PBS and BP.

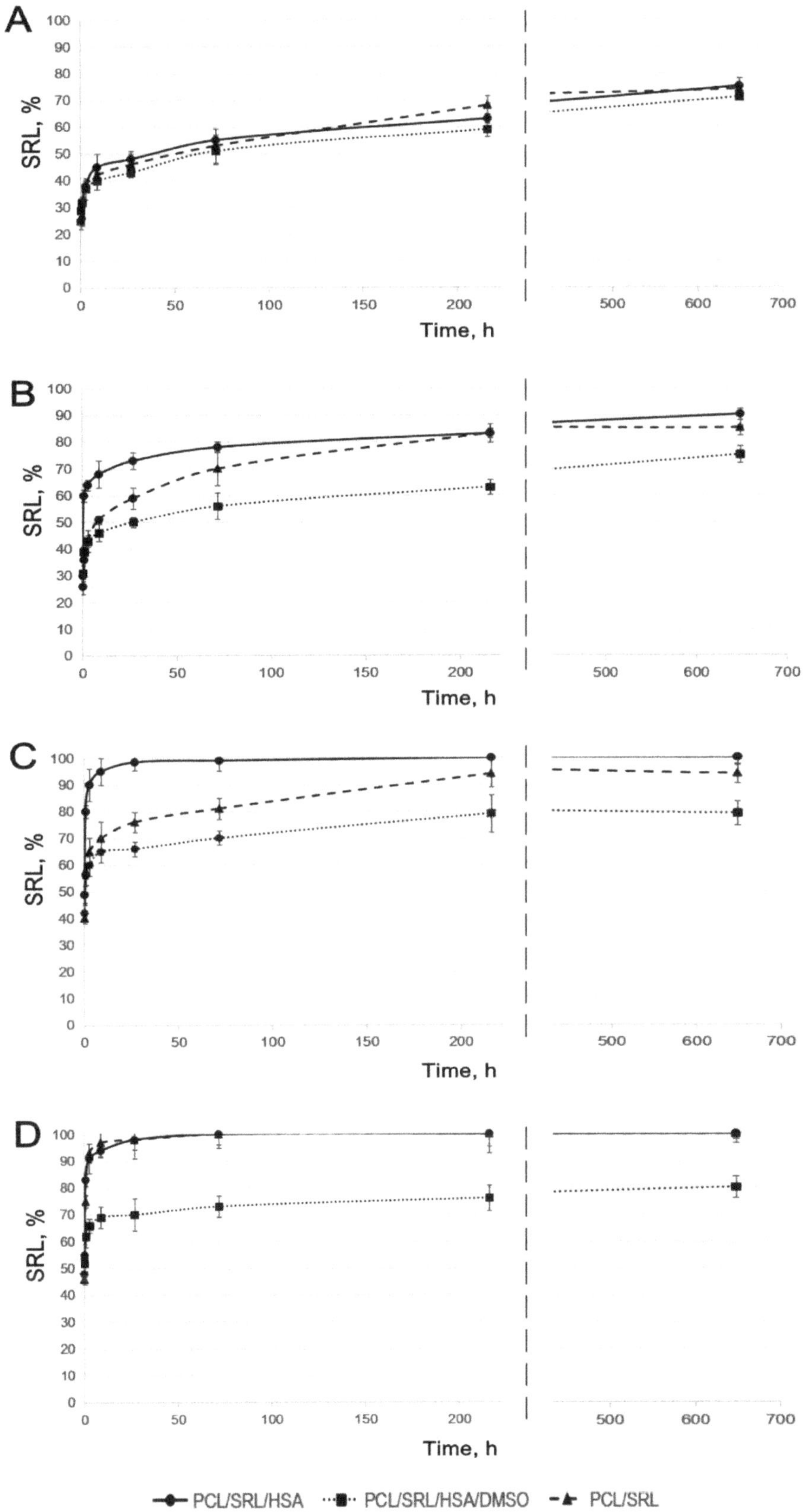

Figure 2. The kinetic curves of SRL release from the matrices. The matrices were incubated (**A**) in PBS without any medium replacement; (**B**) in PBS with medium replacement; (**C**) in BP without any medium replacement; and (**D**) in BP with medium replacement. The data are presented as the means of four independent measurements; the error of the mean did not exceed 7%.

When incubated in BP, SRL was completely released from the PCL/SRL/HSA matrix after 27 h (Figure 2C). The kinetic curve for the PCL/SRL matrix showed a slower SRL release, with saturation achieved over 6–9 days, and a maximal level of 96% was observed at 27 days.

HSA acts as the main transporter of SRL in blood and tissues. HSA has two ligand-specific binding sites for drugs, site I and site II (high-affinity binding and low-affinity binding, respectively) [42,46,47]. SRL binds to albumin at site I more often than at site II. At low BP concentrations, SRL binds to site I. At higher PB concentrations, both sites participate in SRL binding. The affinity association constant for SRL binding to HSA was determined to be 3.99×10^5 M^{-1} [42,46]. Apparently, the SRL resorption on the matrix surface is hindered by the binding of SRL with HSA in BP. It is also possible that other biomolecules in plasma interact with SRL.

Incubation with a BP replacement resulted in an increase in SRL release from the PCL/SRL matrix of up to 100%. According to the SEM data, there were no changes in the fiber structure of PCL/SRL matrices during the 27-day incubation in PBS or BP (Figure 1). This means that long-term SRL release is not associated with matrix structure reorganization or fiber degradation. According to the kinetic study, the PCL/SRL/HSA and PCL/SRL matrices are not capable of prolonged SRL delivery because of rapid SRL release (100% in three days) in BP. The changes in fiber structure and/or SRL distribution inside the fibers are necessary to obtain matrices suitable for prolonged SRL release. Addition of DMSO to the electrospinning blend enabled to obtain porous fibers and retain SRL in the fibers. DMSO is nontoxic, has a boiling point of 189 °C, and dissolves SRL. Moreover, as shown previously, the addition of 3% DMSO to the ES blend significantly reduced paclitaxel release in both PBS and BP [29]. As indicated above, the addition of 3% DMSO to the ES blend resulted in both decreased fiber diameter and pore size. In these matrices, the fiber diameters nearly doubled over the 27 days of incubation owing to the water absorption by HSA. The change in structure of the freshly obtained fibers and those of the fibers after incubation of the PCL/SRL/HSA/DMSO matrices, as well as for the initial and long-term incubation, induced redistribution of SRL in the fibers and obviously affected SRL release. The lowest rate of SRL release in BP (as well as that in PBS) was observed for the matrix containing DMSO. The matrix produced from a 5% PCL/SRL/10% HSA/3% DMSO blend released a maximum of 80% SRL over 27 days, both with and without medium replacement. The data obtained demonstrate the importance of the PCL/SRL/HSA/DMSO matrix as a prospective material for DES coating.

3.3. *Influence of Matrix Elongation on SRL Release*

Considering the twofold elongation of the matrices covering the vascular stents during their installation, the effect of the deformation of the matrices on drug release was studied. To study the influence of twofold elongation on the matrix structures, we used a device that expands the matrix and fixes it in an SEM camera (Figure 3A). This type of deformation differs from the deformation during stent implantation, whereupon uniform deformation of the tube walls occurs, but can simulate the influence of deformation on fiber location and structure. Different areas of the matrices were studied by SEM owing to unequal deformation of the matrices (the maximal deformation was in the center and the minimal deformation was near the clamps) (Figure 3B). In the central area (Figure 3B, 1 and 2; Figure 3C columns 1 and 2), SEM demonstrated that twofold elongation did not lead to a disruption of the fibers, although it was accompanied by the orientation of the fibers along the force vector and compaction of the fiber stack. The structure of the matrix near the clamps with minimal stretching (Figure 3B, 4; Figure 3C column 4) resembles an intact matrix (Figure 1). The intermediate area (Figure 3B, 3; Figure 3C column 3) differs in that fibers are only slightly oriented. After twofold elongation of the matrices and removal of the load, the linear dimensions were reduced by 10–17% (compared with twofold elongation), depending on the type of matrix. According to the SEM data, all obtained matrices are able to withstand elongation during stent installation.

As shown in Figure 4, SRL release from the parent and the twofold expanded matrices were very similar for all matrices under study (Supplementary materials, Table S1). The PCL/SRL/HSA and PCL/SRL matrices present very similar curves of SRL release. SRL was completely released from the

PCL/SRL/HSA and PCL/SRL/TEA matrices, with maximal release in the first 27 h, whereas SRL release from the PCL/SRL/HSA/DMSO matrix was significantly slower, with a maximal level of 80% for 27 days. Data on the SRL release from the matrices with BP replacement demonstrate that twofold elongation barely changes the release kinetics of the matrices (when normalized to the linear/weight/volume characteristics of the matrices). Nevertheless, it is necessary to account for the changes in the areas of the matrices after stent installation when calculating the dose of the drug introduced into the matrix, considering the approximately 1.8-fold increase in the linear size, and thus the decrease in the specific content of the drug in the covered square.

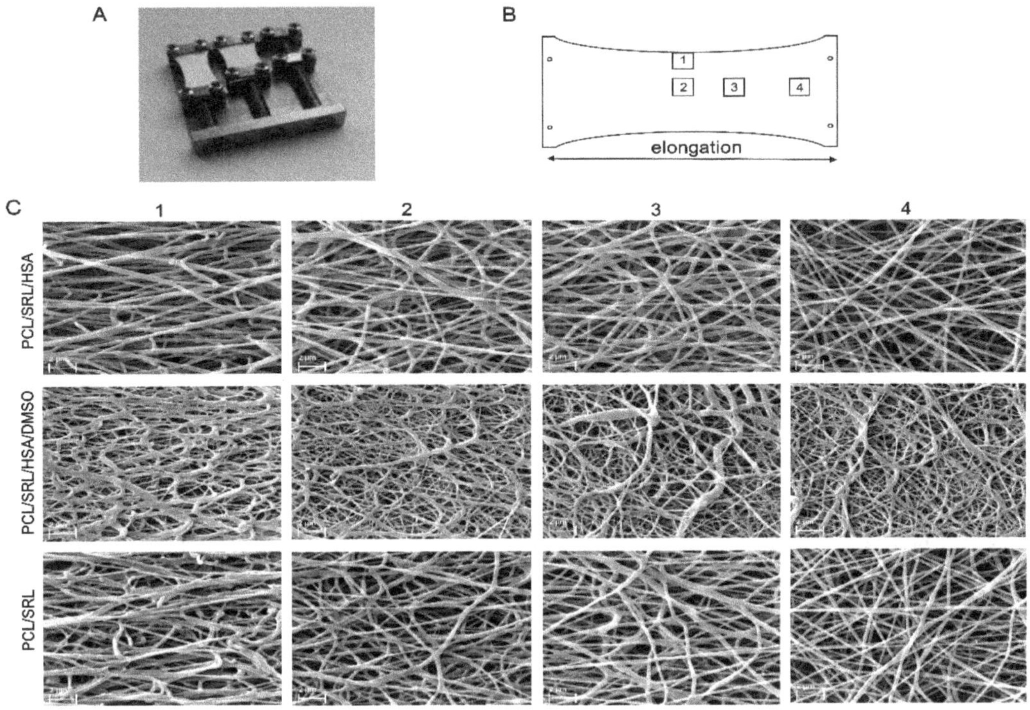

Figure 3. SEM images of the expanded matrices. (**A**) A device allowing one to expand the matrices and fix them in a sputter coater and SEM camera. (**B**) Location of the areas studied by SEM. (**C**) SEM images of different areas of the matrices.

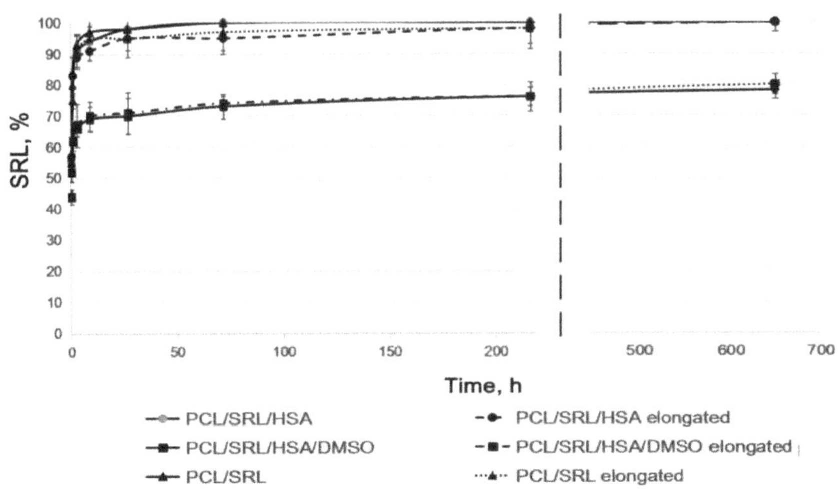

Figure 4. The kinetic curves of SRL release from the expanded matrices. Incubation of the matrices in BP with medium replacement. The data are presented as the means of four independent measurements; error of the mean did not exceed 7%.

4. Conclusions

The structure and physicochemical characteristics of the ES matrices obtained from the solutions of PCL with SRL in HFIP and their blends with HSA, DMSO, and TEA were studied. The matrix produced from 5% PCL/SRL/10% HSA/3% DMSO was shown to be the most suitable for bare-metal stent coating because it is sufficiently strong, exhibited long-term SRL release kinetics, and is thus expected to maintain a concentrations of SRL in the vascular wall that are suitable for antiproliferative activity over a long period. The use of BP increased SRL release. We showed that all matrices can release SRL without fiber degradation. The twofold elongation of the matrices barely changed the SRL release kinetics. Therefore, PCL-based matrices containing HSA, SRL, and DMSO are a promising material for vascular stent coating with prolonged delivery of SRL.

Supplementary Materials:
Table S1: Release curves comparison using Fit factors f1 and f2; Table S2: Release curves comparison using Fit factors f1 and f2. Comparison of kinetic curves of SRL release from the parent and the two-fold expanded matrices. Incubation of the matrices in BP with medium replacement.

Author Contributions: Z.K.N., investigation, matrix characterization and SRL release study, and writing—original draft; B.P.C., investigation, matrix production, and SEM study; V.S.C., investigation and contact angle measurements; I.V.R., investigation and SRL labeling; A.A.K., methodology and resources; P.P.L., supervision, project administration, methodology, funding acquisition, and writing—review & editing. All authors have read and agreed to the published version of the manuscript.

References

1. Costa, M.A.; Simon, D.I. Molecular basis of restenosis and drug-eluting stents. *Circulation* **2005**, *111*, 2257–2273. [CrossRef] [PubMed]
2. Puranik, A.S.; Dawson, E.R.; Peppas, N.A. Recent advances in drug eluting stents. *Int. J. Pharm.* **2013**, *441*, 665–679. [CrossRef] [PubMed]
3. Scott, N.A. Restenosis following implantation of bare metal coronary stents: Pathophysiology and pathways involved in the vascular response to injury. *Adv. Drug Deliv. Rev.* **2006**, *58*, 358–376. [CrossRef] [PubMed]
4. Abizaid, A. Sirolimus-eluting coronary stents: A review. *Vasc. Health. Risk Manag.* **2007**, *3*, 191–201. [CrossRef] [PubMed]
5. Cheng-Lai, A.; Frishman, W.H. Sirolimus-eluting coronary stents: Novel devices for the management of coronary artery disease. *Am. J. Ther.* **2004**, *11*, 218–228. [CrossRef] [PubMed]
6. Piscione, F.; Piccolo, R.; Cassese, S.; Galasso, G.; Chiariello, M. Clinical impact of sirolimus-eluting stent in ST-segment elevation myocardial infarction: A meta-analysis of randomized clinical trials. *Catheter Cardiovasc. Interv.* **2009**, *74*, 323–332. [CrossRef]
7. Sehgal, S.N. Sirolimus: Its discovery, biological properties, and mechanism of action. *Transpl. Proc.* **2003**, *35*, 7S–14S. [CrossRef]
8. Haeri, A.; Osouli, M.; Bayat, F.; Alavi, S.; Dadashzadeh, S. Nanomedicine approaches for sirolimus delivery: A review of pharmaceutical properties and preclinical studies. *Artif. Cells Nanomed. Biotechnol.* **2018**, *46*, 1–14. [CrossRef]
9. Sehgal, S.N.; Camardo, J.S.; Scarola, J.A.; Maida, B.T. Rapamycin (sirolimus, rapamune). *Curr. Opin. Nephrol. Hypertens.* **1995**, *4*, 482–487. [CrossRef]
10. Hafizi, S.; Mordi, V.N.; Andersson, K.M.; Chester, A.H.; Yacoub, M.H. Differential effects of rapamycin, cyclosporine A, and FK506 on human coronary artery smooth muscle cell proliferation and signalling. *Vascul. Pharmacol.* **2005**, *41*, 167–176. [CrossRef]
11. Moes, D.J.; Guchelaar, H.J.; de Fijter, J.W. Sirolimus and everolimus in kidney transplantation. *Drug Discov. Today* **2015**, *20*, 1243–1249. [CrossRef] [PubMed]
12. MacDonald, A.; Scarola, J.; Burke, J.T.; Zimmerman, J.J. Clinical pharmacokinetics and therapeutic drug monitoring of sirolimus. *Clin. Ther.* **2000**, *22*, B101–B121. [CrossRef]
13. Mahalati, K.; Kahan, B.D. Clinical pharmacokinetics of sirolimus. *Clin. Pharmacokinet.* **2001**, *40*, 573–585. [CrossRef] [PubMed]

14. Tada, T.; Byrne, R.A.; Simunovic, I.; King, L.A.; Cassese, S.; Joner, M.; Fusaro, M.; Schneider, S.; Schulz, S.; Ibrahim, T.; et al. Risk of stent thrombosis among bare-metal stents, first-generation drug-eluting stents, and second-generation drug-eluting stents: Results from a registry of 18,334 patients. *JACC Cardiovasc. Interv.* **2013**, *6*, 1267–1274. [CrossRef] [PubMed]
15. Vetrovec, G.W.; Rizik, D.; Williard, C.; Snead, D.; Piotrovski, V.; Kopia, G. Sirolimus PK trial: A pharmacokinetic study of the sirolimus-eluting Bx velocity stent in patients with de novo coronary lesions. *Catheter Cardiovasc. Interv.* **2006**, *67*, 32–37. [CrossRef] [PubMed]
16. Van Der Giessen, W.J.; Sorop, O.; Serruys, P.W.; Peters- Krabbendam, I.; Van Beusekom, H.M.M. Lowering the dose of sirolimus, released from a nonpolymeric hydroxyapatite coated coronary stent, reduces signs of delayed healing. *J. Am. Coll. Cardiol. Intv.* **2009**, *2*, 284–290. [CrossRef]
17. Nakamura, M.; Abizaid, A.; Hirohata, A.; Honda, Y.; Sousa, J.E.; Fitzgerald, P.J. Efficacy of reduced-dose sirolimus-eluting stents in the human coronaryartery: Serial IVUS analysis of neointimal hyperplasia and luminal dimension. *Catheter Cardiovasc. Interv.* **2007**, *70*, 946–951. [CrossRef]
18. Onuma, Y.; Kogame, N.; Serruys, P.W. Unconfirmed very long-term clinical benefit of Xience over Cypher: Should we reset our vision? *JACC Cardiovasc Interv.* **2019**, *12*, 648–650. [CrossRef]
19. Daemen, J.; Wenaweser, P.; Tsuchida, K.; Abrecht, L.; Vaina, S.; Morger, C.; Kukreja, N.; Jüni, P.; Sianos, G.; Hellige, G.; et al. Early and late coronary stent thrombosis of sirolimuseluting and paclitaxel-eluting stents in routine clinical practice: Data from a large two-institutional cohort study. *Lancet* **2007**, *369*, 667–678. [CrossRef]
20. Bangalore, S.; Toklu, B.; Patel, N.; Feit, F.; Stone, G.W. Newer-generation ultrathin strut drug-eluting stents versus older second-generation thicker strut drug-eluting stents for coronary artery disease. *Circulation* **2018**, *138*, 2216–2226. [CrossRef]
21. Tijssen, R.Y.G.; Kraak, R.P.; Lu, H.; Mifek, J.G.; Carlyle, W.C.; Donohoe, D.J.; De Winter, R.J.; Koch, K.T.; Wykrzykowska, J.J. Evaluation of the MiStent sustained sirolimus eluting biodegradable polymer coated stent for the treatment of coronary artery disease: Does uniform sustained abluminal drug release result in earlier strut coverage and better safety profile? *Expert Rev. Med. Devices* **2017**, *14*, 325–334. [CrossRef] [PubMed]
22. Ajmera, P.; Pothineni, R.; Chawla, K.K.; Mantravadi, S.S.; Jariwala, P.V.; Vijan, V.; Vijan, V. Real-world use of ultrathin-strut biodegradable polymer-coated sirolimus-eluting stents in patients with coronary artery disease: 6-month clinical outcomes. *Vasc. Health Risk Manag.* **2019**, *18*, 439–447. [CrossRef] [PubMed]
23. Mauri, L.; Doros, G.; Rao, S.V.; Cohen, D.J.; Yakubov, S.; Lasala, J.; Wong, S.C.; Zidar, J.; Kereiakes, D.J. The OPTIMIZE randomized trial to assess safety and efficacy of the Svelte IDS and RX Sirolimus-eluting coronary stent Systems for the Treatment of atherosclerotic lesions: Trial design and rationale. *Am. Heart J.* **2019**, *216*, 82–90. [CrossRef] [PubMed]
24. Bae, I.H.; Lim, K.S.; Park, D.S.; Shim, J.W.; Lee, S.Y.; Jang, E.J.; Park, J.K.; Kim, J.H.; Jeong, M.H. Sirolimus coating on heparinized stents prevents restenosis and thrombosis. *J. Biomater. Appl.* **2017**, *31*, 1337–1345. [CrossRef] [PubMed]
25. Jelonek, K.; Jaworska, J.; Pastusiak, M.; Sobota, M.; Włodarczyk, J.; Karpeta-Jarzabek, P.; Kaczmarczyk, B.; Kasperczyk, J.; Dobrzyński, P. Effect of vascular scaffold composition on release of sirolimus. *Eur. J. Pharm. Biopharm.* **2018**, *132*, 41–49. [CrossRef] [PubMed]
26. Raval, A.; Parikh, J.; Engineer, C. Mechanism and in vitro release kinetic study of sirolimus from a biodegradable polymeric matrix coated cardiovascular stent. *Ind. Eng. Chem. Res.* **2011**, *50*, 9539–9549. [CrossRef]
27. Livingston, M.; Tan, A. Coating techniques and release kinetics of drug-eluting stents. *J Med. Device.* **2019**, *10*, 1. [CrossRef]
28. Zhang, Y.; Wang, J.; Xiao, J.; Fang, T.; Hu, N.; Li, M.; Deng, L.; Cheng, Y.; Zhu, Y.; Cui, W. An electrospun fiber-covered stent with programmable dual drug release for endothelialization acceleration and lumen stenosis prevention. *Acta Biomater.* **2019**, *94*, 295–305. [CrossRef]
29. Kuznetsov, K.A.; Stepanova, A.O.; Kvon, R.I.; Douglas, T.E.L.; Kuznetsov, N.A.; Chernonosova, V.S.; Zaporozhchenko, I.A.; Kharkova, M.V.; Romanova, I.V.; Karpenko, A.A.; et al. Electrospun produced 3D matrices for covering of vascular stents: Paclitaxel release depending on fiber structure and composition of the external environment. *Materials* **2018**, *11*, 2176. [CrossRef]

30. Rychter, M.; Baranowska-Korczyc, A.; Luleka, J. Progress and perspectives in bioactive agent delivery via electrospun vascular grafts. *RSC Adv.* **2017**, *7*, 32164. [CrossRef]
31. Mirbagheri, M.S.; Mohebbi-Kalhori, D.; Jirofti, N. Evaluation of mechanical properties and medical applications of polycaprolactone small diameter artificial blood vessels. *Int. J. Basic Sci. Med.* **2017**, *2*, 58–70. [CrossRef]
32. Rychter, M.; Milanowski, B.; Grzeskowiak, B.F.; Jarek, M.; Kempinski, M.; Coy, E.L.; Borysiak, S.; Baranowska-Korczyc, A.; Lulek, J. Cilostazol-loaded electrospun three-dimensional systems for potential cardiovascular application: Effect of fibers hydrophilization on drug release, and cytocompatibility. *J. Colloid Interface Sci.* **2019**, *15*, 310–327. [CrossRef] [PubMed]
33. Nair, L.S.; Laurencin, C.T. Biodegradable polymers as biomaterials. *Prog. Polym. Sci.* **2007**, *32*, 762–798. [CrossRef]
34. Michel, S.A.; Knetsch, M.L.; Koole, L.H. Adsorption of albumin on flax fibers increases endothelial cell adhesion and blood compatibility in vitro. *J. Biomater Sci. Polym. Ed.* **2014**, *25*, 698–712. [CrossRef] [PubMed]
35. Chernonosova, V.S.; Kvon, R.I.; Stepanova, A.O.; Larichev, Y.V.; Karpenko, A.A.; Chelobanov, B.P.; Kiseleva, E.V.; Laktionov, P.P. Human serum albumin in electrospun PCL fibers: Structure, release, and exposure on fibersurface. *Polym. Adv. Technol.* **2017**, *28*, 819–827. [CrossRef]
36. Shen, M.; Martinson, L.; Wagner, M.S.; Castner, D.G.; Ratner, B.D.; Horbett, T.A. PEO-like plasma polymerized tetraglyme surface interactions with leukocytes and proteins: In vitro and in vivo studies. *J. Biomater. Sci. Polym. Ed.* **2002**, *13*, 367–390. [CrossRef] [PubMed]
37. Denizli, F.K.; Guven, O. Competitive adsorption of blood proteins on gamma-irradiated-polycarbonate fifilms. *J. Biomater. Sci. Polym. Ed.* **2002**, *13*, 127–139. [CrossRef]
38. Sidorov, V.N.; Polak, Y.V.; Laktionov, P.P.; Roshcke, V.V.; Kist, A.G. Method of production of tritium labeled organic compounds and the device for its implementation. SU Patent 1823961 A3, 18 January 1991.
39. Cardiovascular Implants-Tubular Vacuum Prostheses. International Patent Application No. ISO/FDIS 7198:1998, July 1998.
40. Tiwari, A.P.; Joshi, M.K.; Park, C.H.; Kim, C.S. Nano-nets covered composite nanofibers with enhanced biocompatibility and mechanical properties for bone tissue engineering. *J. Nanosci. Nanotechnol.* **2018**, *18*, 529–537. [CrossRef]
41. Carter, D.C.; He, X.M.; Munson, S.H.; Twigg, P.D.; Gernert, K.M.; Broom, M.B. Three-dimensional structure of human serum albumin. *Science* **1989**, *244*, 1195–1198. [CrossRef]
42. Jr, T.P. Ligand binding by albumin. In *All about Albumin*; Academic Press: San Diego, CA, USA, 1995.
43. Chernonosova, V.S.; Gostev, A.A.; Gao, Y.; Chesalov, Y.A.; Shutov, A.V.; Pokushalov, E.A.; Karpenko, A.A.; Laktionov, P.P. Mechanical properties and biological behavior of 3D matrices produced by electrospinning from protein-enriched polyurethane. *BioMed Res. Int.* **2018**, *2018*, 1380606. [CrossRef]
44. Yasukawa, T.; Ogura, Y.; Sakurai, E.; Tabata, Y.; Kimura, H. Intraocular sustained drug delivery using implantable polymeric devices. *Adv. Drug Deliv. Rev.* **2005**, *57*, 2033–2046. [CrossRef] [PubMed]
45. Kim, M.-S.; Kim, J.-S.; Park, H.J.; Cho, W.K.; Cha, K.-H.; Hwan, S.-J. Enhanced bioavailability of sirolimus via preparation of solid dispersion nanoparticles using a supercritical antisolvent process. *Int. J. Nanomed.* **2011**, *6*, 2997–3009.
46. Rahman, M.; Prianka, F.; Shohel, M.; Mazid, M.A. Interaction of palmitic acid with metoprolol succinate at the binding sites of bovine serum albumin. *Adv. Pharm. Bull.* **2014**, *4*, 379–383. [PubMed]
47. Khodaei, A.; Bolandnazar, S.; Valizadeh, H.; Hasani, L.; Zakeri-Milani, P. Interactions between sirolimus and anti-inflammatory drugs: Competitive binding for human serum albumin. *Adv. Pharm. Bull.* **2016**, *6*, 227–233. [CrossRef] [PubMed]

6

Mesoporous Silica Nanoparticles as Carriers for Therapeutic Biomolecules

Rafael R. Castillo [1,2,3,†], Daniel Lozano [1,2,3,†] and María Vallet-Regí [1,2,3,*]

1 Departamento de Química en Ciencias Farmacéuticas, Facultad de Farmacia, Universidad Complutense de Madrid, Plaza Ramón y Cajal s/n, 28040 Madrid, Spain; rafcas01@ucm.es (R.R.C.); danlozan@ucm.es (D.L.)
2 Centro de Investigación Biomédica en Red—CIBER, 28029 Madrid, Spain
3 Instituto de Investigación Sanitaria Hospital 12 de Octubre—imas12, 28041 Madrid, Spain
* Correspondence: vallet@ucm.es
† These authors contributed equally to this work.

Abstract: The enormous versatility of mesoporous silica nanoparticles permits the creation of a large number of nanotherapeutic systems for the treatment of cancer and many other pathologies. In addition to the controlled release of small drugs, these materials allow a broad number of molecules of a very different nature and sizes. In this review, we focus on biogenic species with therapeutic abilities (proteins, peptides, nucleic acids, and glycans), as well as how nanotechnology, in particular silica-based materials, can help in establishing new and more efficient routes for their administration. Indeed, since the applicability of those combinations of mesoporous silica with bio(macro)molecules goes beyond cancer treatment, we address a classification based on the type of therapeutic action. Likewise, as illustrative content, we highlight the most typical issues and problems found in the preparation of those hybrid nanotherapeutic materials.

Keywords: mesoporous silica; therapeutic biomolecules; proteins; peptides; nucleic acids; glycans

1. Introduction

Since the very first example reported on nanometric mesoporous silica as a drug delivery material [1], many examples were subsequently reported including a broad number of chemical species. One of them includes biomacromolecules, which play a capital role in living beings, as they are responsible for biorecognition [2], signal transduction [3], and replication routes; hence, they are responsible for the adequate development of tissues and organs. Such is the importance of these species that even the immune system and hormone signaling are based on specific affinity interactions between biomacromolecules (BMs). From a therapeutic point of view, hijacking such ligands and receptors may be useful to regulate unbalanced systems, as well as develop new-generation therapeutic nanodevices in oncology [4,5] cancer immunotherapy [6–8], and gene therapy [9–11], among many others.

Unfortunately, most bioactive macromolecules are highly labile in vivo, as a self-regulation mechanism to avoid massive damages. Therefore, to use them, it is necessary to implement chemical modifications or to design vehicles capable of ensuring an adequate preservation and, hence, a long-lasting effect. Among known carriers, viruses have the best performance, although at the expense of having a great associated risk in handling and containment. Additionally, they are only suitable for nucleic acids (NAs), being useless for protein and peptide delivery. To overcome these limitations, nanoparticles emerged as promising vectors for nucleotides, as well as peptides and proteins. This is a consequence of two complementary aspects. On one hand, their size permits establishing intimate interactions with cell's membranes and the receptors therein. On the other hand, they exhibit the possibility to establish non-conventional interactions between particles, cargoes, and target cells.

Amongst all known materials, mesoporous silica nanoparticles (MSNs) arose as promising drug delivery platforms because of their outstanding biocompatibility, their degradability, and their great chemical and biological robustness. Moreover, the unique porous structure of MSNs permits establishing host–guest interactions of high interest for drug delivery purposes, as they allow creating protective environments for labile molecules. In addition to those, the current silica-based nanotechnology also permits creating particles with variable diameters [12,13], pore sizes [14], and structures [15], which permit fine-tuning the final application of the nanosystems, especially those intended to deliver big cargoes such as those reviewed herein. Moreover, MSNs and related hybrid particles with SiO_2 coatings also permit easily tuning the resulting outer layers of nanosystems to enhance biochemical stability and, hence, to reduce side effects and potential toxicities [16–18]. Particle diameter is one of the most critical parameters for achieving a successful therapy. Typically, the accepted window of diameters for cancer treatment comprises particles in a range between 50 and 300 nm, in which the enhanced permeation and retention effect operates. However, depending on the final purpose of the nanosystem, such values may be narrowed. For instance, in cases where a superior trafficking is desired, smaller particles would behave better, while, in nanosystems intended as biomolecule reservoirs, the diameter must unavoidably be increased. Regarding nanoparticle-based drug delivery, we recently reviewed how mesoporous silica-based nanosystems are suitable platforms to combine two or more chemical species, outranging the pharmacological profile of free species [19,20]. However, despite the possible therapeutic improvement, their efficiency and long-term stability could be compromised if the BMs are not properly protected or fully exposed to white blood cells and immune systems. The scarce protection provided by most solid nanoparticles highlights once again the importance of MSNs [21] as platforms for the development of non-viral vectors and protein carriers, whose particular porous morphology can provide a protective environment for those labile molecules, although the typical porosity (2–3 nm) of MSNs may be tuned in order to host the biggest molecules [22] (Figure 1).

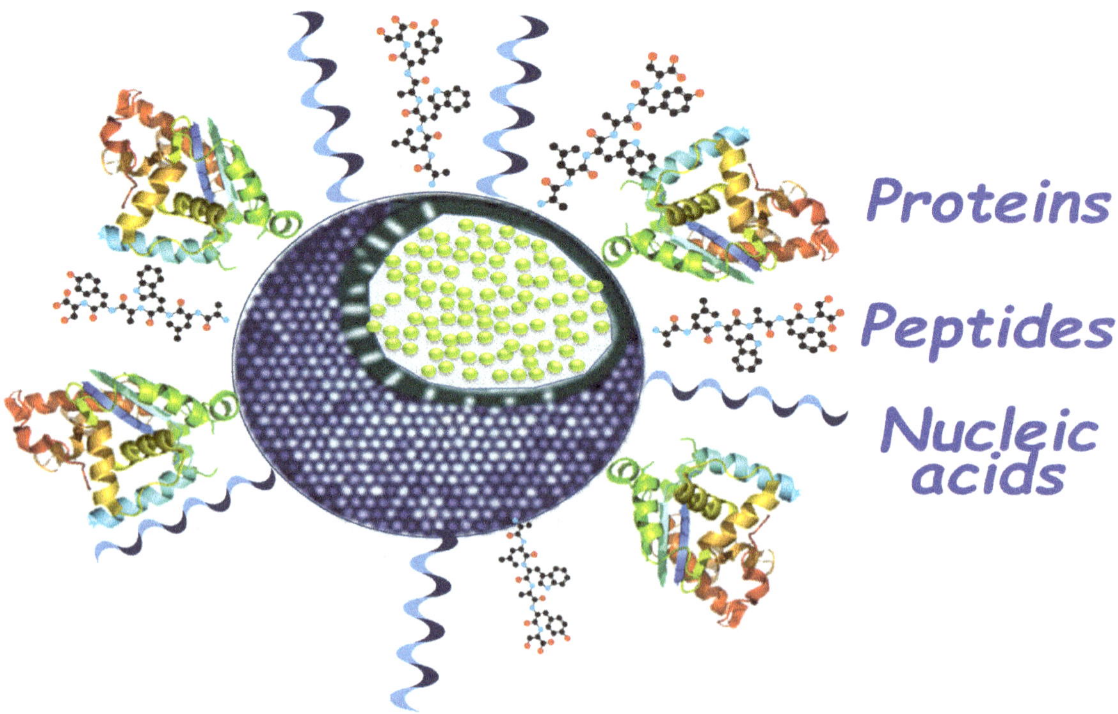

Figure 1. Main groups of therapeutic biomolecules that are possible to deliver using mesoporous nanosilica technology.

As introduced, the use of MSNs in biomedicine has a huge potential impact; in addition to acting as carriers, they also permit creating fancy structures with most functional nanomaterials. However, despite this versatility, the permeation of these materials into clinical trials is still limited [23,24]; this is not caused by poor biocompatibility, but rather by the impossibility of establishing reliable comparisons between different systems, as accounted by Florence [25]. In fact, as can be observed from the growing number of in vivo experiments using MSNs carried out by many groups worldwide, it is logical to assume that they have adequate performance in living systems; thus, MSNs will hopefully soon reach clinical practice.

2. Strategies to Deliver Biomacromolecules with Silica Nanoparticles

Loading effectiveness, cellular internalization, targeting, and cargo delivery are critical issues when developing a nanosystem with maximal therapeutic potential. As we previously mentioned, MSNs are ideal nanocarriers related to the load and delivery of biomolecules due to their unique properties, including shape, size, and surface chemistry [26]. Pore, channel, and cavity sizes can be modified in MSNs to increase the loading of therapeutic molecules [27]. The MSN surface can be functionalized with polyethyleneimine and poly-L-lysine or modified with targeting peptides or antibodies to improve cargo loading, cellular uptake, and endosomal scape rates [26]. The chemical and physical properties of MSNs are critical when designing a nanocarrier with therapeutic efficacy in biomolecule loading and delivery. In the last few years, surface nanoscale topography gained special attention due to the possibility of controlling the interactions between molecules and cells, in the process of molecular loading and cell internalization [28,29].

The chemical functionalization of silica is easily achieved through condensation processes employing functionalized alkoxysilanes. For the functionalization of surfaces, this silanization must be carried out before template removal, while the modification of mesopores could be achieved either via condensation during the template-driven synthesis of MSNs or after surface modification and template removal. In this latter case, it is important to account that pore constriction may occur if the process is not properly controlled. For the preparation of hollow MSNs (HMSNs), the most employed method is the solid template etching of an internal core, typically from solid silica, onto which a mesoporous layer is created. Pore and surface modification can be achieved in a parallel manner as done with conventional MSNs, while, for the functionalization of the internal space, this must be done prior to the formation of the mesoporous layer. Onto this slightly modified MSN, it would be possible to create additional modifications by linking chemical species through conventional chemical reactions. With this strategy, it was possible to create a huge number of functional nanosystems with pore nanogates [30], sensitive bonds [31], recognition elements [5,19], and charged surfaces able to undergo electrostatic interactions.

One common strategy to combine BMs and NPs is surface functionalization; it can be achieved either via a chemical bond or via an electrostatic interaction between charged counterparts. On MSNs, surface grafting is usually accomplished via direct condensation of the remaining Si–OH groups with functional silane reagents; these are typically modified trialkoxysilanes with aliphatic chains bearing an additional functional group. For the bonding of peptides and proteins, the most common functional groups are amino and carboxylate for amide coupling and maleimides for thiol-mediated binding [32]. Additionally, to complement the direct coupling approach, there are also many different bifunctional linkers available which are able to accomplish this task [33]. With regard to this coupling strategy, it is also important to remark the importance of controlling the bonding, which, if produced at the active region of proteins, may lead to inactivation. This is of particular importance when preparing antibody-targeted nanosystems [34,35] and sensors. On this topic, Landry and coworkers studied how the chemical linkage affected the specificity of cluster of differentiation 4 (CD4)-bonded proteins onto MSN against its target, the gp120 glycoprotein [36]. The authors proved that a conventional, unspecific, direct thiol–maleimide linkage behaved worse than a specific linkage placed far away from the active site.

The other approach for surface functionalization is electrostatic deposition. In this case, both nanocarriers and BMs need to establish strong electrostatic interactions through differently charged functional groups. This is of particular importance for NAs, whose permanent negative charge permits strong interactions with positively charged surfaces and polymers such as polyethyleneimine or chitosan among many others. Insights into this strategy are available in References [20,37]. In the most advanced models, a rational deposition of alternating cationic and anionic layers—for instance, polyethyleneimine (PEI)–small interfering RNA (siRNA)–PEI–, also permitted developing multilayered nanosystems in which targeting elements could be added in the outermost layer. This design permits placing NAs in middle layers, obtaining additional protection against nucleases. Moreover, this strategy also enables pH-driven cleavage, which permits disassembling the system in endosomal environments, as a consequence of the proton sponge effect associated with polycationic substances [38]. The main drawback of the surface loading strategy is the absence of protection for BMs, which could be deactivated if exposed to blood (opsonization, enzymatic degradation, macrophage-mediated clearance, etc.) [39] or if not properly handled during processing (non-sterile material, accidental contamination, or physicochemical decomposition).

From a protective point of view, the use of pore-expanded MSNs [40] is the most convenient strategy, but only if the cargo is adequately retained until its final destination. To this end, pore sizes should be tuned to allow cargo hosting and, eventually, pore gates may be required [30]. The typical strategies to prepare enlarged-pore MSNs consist of either using large surfactants such as Pluronic or Brij [14] or employing swelling agents able to increase the diameter of the template cetrimonium micelles during the synthesis [41]. Additionally, the use of non-surfactant species, like tannic acid, was also reported as a pore-forming agent [42]. Regarding NAs, it is also important to remark that raw pores of MSNs need to be chemically modified; otherwise, the negative charges of NAs and silanols would undergo a repulsive interaction that would hinder pore loading. This topic was previously visited by us and other groups in previous contributions [20,37]. In the case of proteins and peptides, this effect is not so relevant, as their isoelectric points are always closer to neutrality. In fact, most peptides behave as small molecules and can be loaded satisfactorily in most raw-pore MSNs.

In summary, the loading strategy must be carefully accounted for depending on the carried biomacromolecule. In this way, short peptides can be easily loaded within pores or grafted onto surfaces, while the delivery of bigger and highly charged molecules may suffer from pore rejection if the mesopores are not properly conditioned [43]. Regarding NAs, their outstanding chemical stability permits creating either fancy layered structures or pore-loaded systems [44–46]. In addition to typical porous particles, the use of hollow mesoporous silica nanoparticles (HMSNs) also receives interest because of their additional enormous internal space. However, to use them as carriers, their mesopores and surfaces must comply with all requirements outlined for in-pore loading, i.e., sufficient diameter, favorable electrostatic environment, and adequate order to permit effective diffusion processes.

In addition to cargo-related modifications, these kinds of nanodevices must also have additional modifications to increase colloidal stability and immune stealth to ensure an adequate trafficking profile (Figure 2). In the case of pore-loaded nanosystems, this can be easily achieved with a common polyethylene glycol (PEG)ylation strategy. On coated nanosystems, it may not be necessary if the particles' coatings are naturally occurring biomolecules, such as those reviewed herein. In this case, although the integrity of supported molecules is not fully ensured, surface deposition is proven to be a synthetic advantage, as it greatly reduces the number of components and synthetic steps.

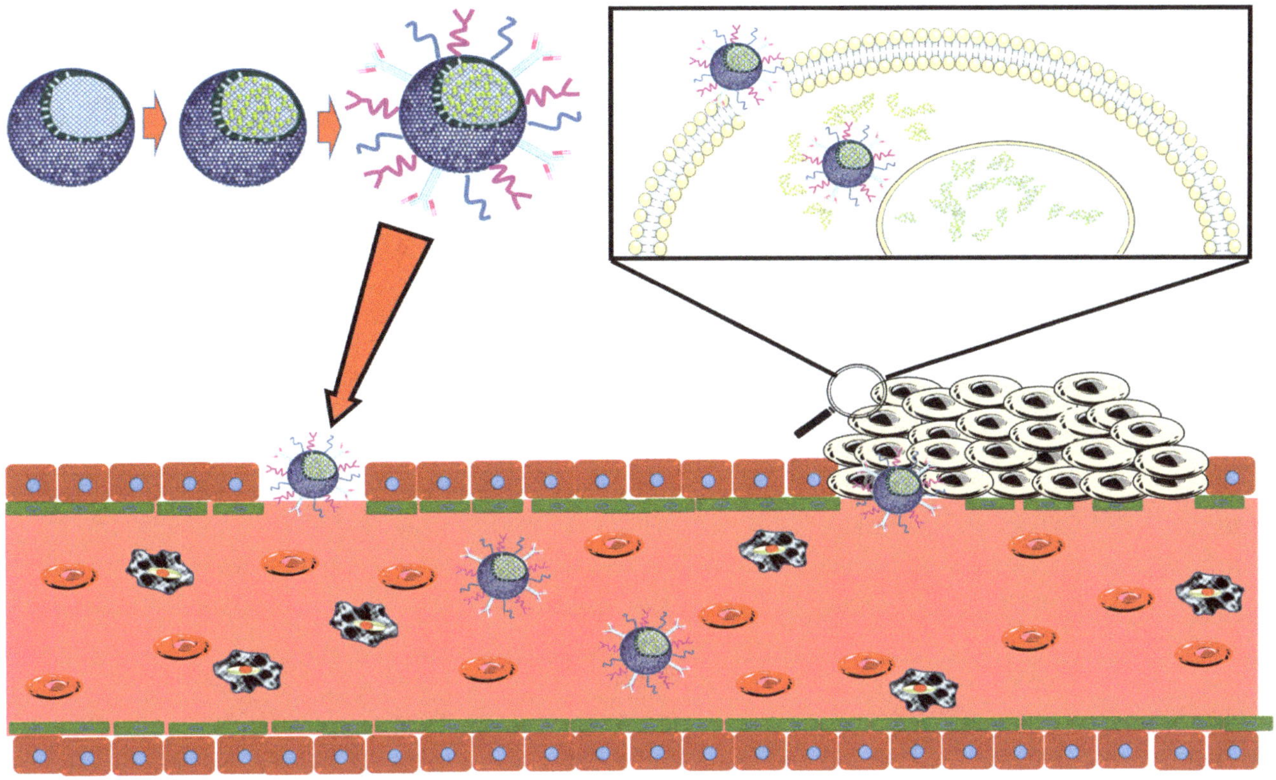

Figure 2. Blood compatibility, colloidal stability, and cell recognition are necessary on therapeutic nanosystems; otherwise, they would not reach their final destination.

3. Delivery of Proteins with Therapeutic Effect

As introduced above, the effect and potency of therapeutic proteins rely on their physiological effect and behavior. For example, cytochrome c (Cyt c) triggers a caspase-mediated apoptosis, while immunoglobulins activate the immune system and induce cell destruction. Additionally, certain enzymes and growth factors may be useful to treat certain genetic diseases based on protein malfunction. Therefore, as there is no common therapeutic effect [47], the different approaches are discussed including pro-apoptotic, immunostimulating, enzymes, growth factors, and antibacterial proteins, according to the classification shown in Table 1 and Figure 3. For the interested reader, previously published outstanding revisions dealt with insights into protein loading and delivery with MSNs [48–51].

Table 1. Examples of therapeutic proteins delivered by silica-based nanocarriers.

Protein	Carrier Type	Protein Location	Loading Strategy	Cell Line(s)	In Vivo	Reference
Anticancer proteins [52,53]						
Cytochrome C	MSNs	Mesopores	Pore filling	HeLa	None	[54,55]
	MSNs	Surface	Adsorption	None	None	[56]
	MSNs	Surface	Grafting	HeLa	None	[57]
	MSNs	Mesopores	Pore filling	SKOV3	None	[58]
Concanavalin A	MSNs	Surface	Grafting	MC3T3-E1, HOS	None	[59]

Table 1. *Cont.*

Protein	Carrier Type	Protein Location	Loading Strategy	Cell Line(s)	In Vivo	Reference
Immunostimulating proteins and vaccines						
IgG	HMSNs	Particle cavity	Cavity loading	HeLa	None	[60]
OVA	HMSNs	Mesopores	Pore filling	NIH3T3	Mice	[61,62]
OVA	DMOHS	Mesopores	Pore filling	None	Mice	[63]
CpG@OVA	MSNs	Mesopores	Pore filling	RAW264.7	Mice	[64]
CpG@OVA GM-CSF	MSNs@ MSRs	Mesopores Mesopores	Pore filling	None	Mice	[65]
Cyt c, IgG, Anti-pAkt	RSNs	Interparticles	In-pocket packing	None	None	[66]
IL-2	HMSNs	Particle cavity	Cavity loading	L929	Mice	[67]
ORF2	HMSNs	Surface	Adsorption	PK15	Mice	[68]
SWAP	MSNs	Surface	Adsorption	None	Mice	[69]
HSP700	MSNs	Surface	Adsorption	None	Mice	[70]
EspA	MSNs	Surface	Adsorption	None	Mice	[71]
rPb27	MSNs	Surface	Adsorption	HEK-293	Mice	[72]
Enzymes						
CA	MSNs	Mesopores	In-pore grafting	HeLa	None	[73]
CA or HPR	MSNs	Mesopores	In-pore grafting	None	None	[74]
β-Galactosidase	MSNs	Mesopores	Adsorption	N2a	None	[75]
SOD	MSNs	Surface	Grafting	HeLa	None	[76]
SOD or GPx	MSNs	Surface	Grafting	HeLa	None	[77]
Proteasomes	MSNs	Surface	Grafting	HEK-293, HeLa	None	[78]
Growth factors						
bFGF	MSNs	Mesopores	Microemulsion	HUVEC	None	[79]
BMP-2	MSNs	Surface	Adsorption	bMSCs	Mice	[80]
	MSN@SPION	Mesopores	Pore filling	bMSCs	None	[81]
Antibacterial proteins						
Lysozyme	MSNs	Surface	Grafting	*Escherichia coli*	Mice	[82]
	MSNs	Pores	Adsorption	*E. coli*	None	[83]
	HMSNs	Surface	Adsorption	*E. coli*	Mice	[84]
	HMSNs	Particle cavity	Cavity loading	*E. coli*	None	[85]
Concanavalin A	MSNs	Surface	Grafting	*E. coli*	None	[86]

Abbreviations: bFGF: basic fibroblast growth factor; BMP-2: bone morphogenetic protein 2; bMSCs: murine bone mesenchymal stem cells; CA: carbonic anhydrase; CpG@OVA: ovalbumin-loaded cytosine–phosphate–guanine (CpG) oligodeoxynucleotide; DMOHS: dendritic mesoporous organosilica hollow spheres; EspA: an immunogenic protein from enterohaemorrhagic *Escherichia Coli*; GM-CSF: murine granulocyte-macrophage colony-stimulating factor; GPx: glutathione peroxidase; HMSNs: hollow mesoporous silica nanoparticles; HRP: horseradish peroxidase; IgG: immunoglobulin G; IL-2: interleukin-2; ORF2: open reading frame from porcine circovirus type 2; OVA: chicken ovalbumin; RSNs: rough (non-porous and core–shell) silica nanoparticles; SOD: superoxide dismutase; SPIONs: superparamagnetic iron oxide nanoparticles.

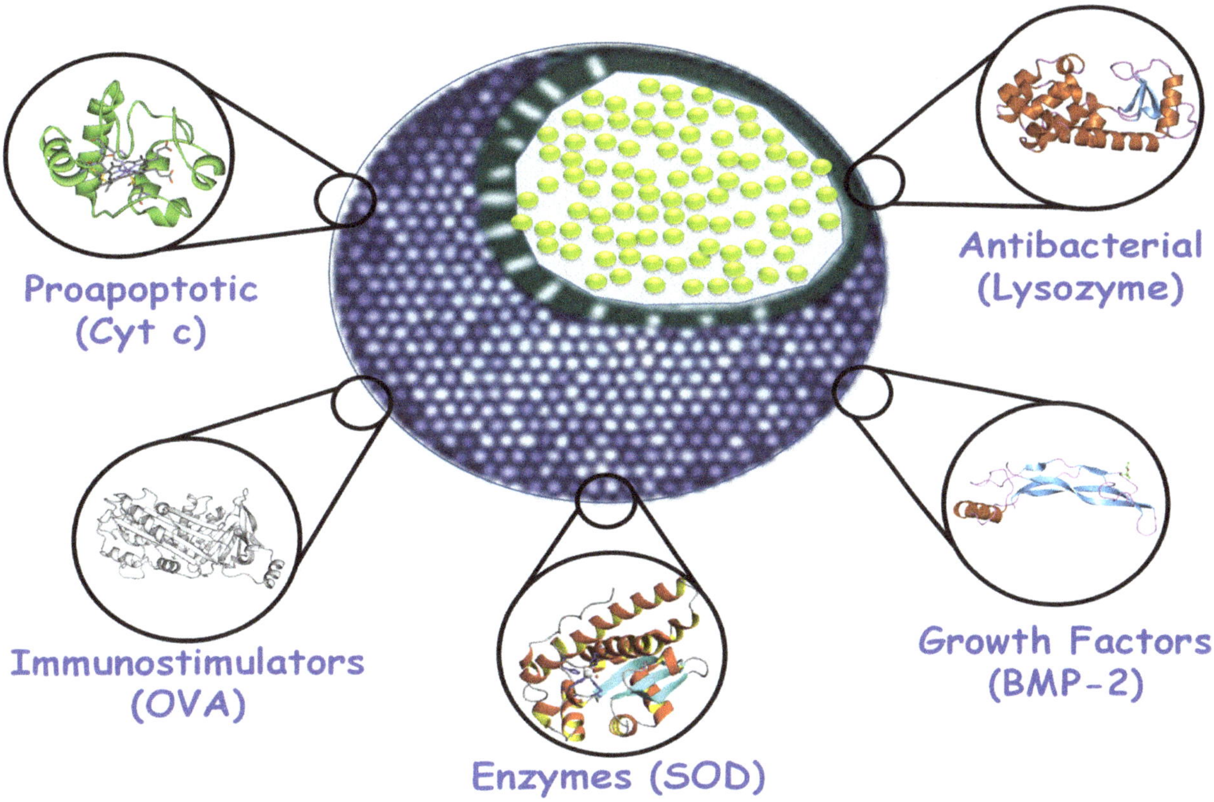

Figure 3. Roles and examples of typical therapeutic proteins delivered with silica-based nanosystems.

3.1. Anticancer Proteins

Historically, Lin's group was the first to describe the potential of MSNs to carry and deliver proteins. To achieve this, they focused on Cyt c, a small protein with a pro-apoptotic effect. In their contribution, they pioneered pore-expanded MSNs to allow protein hosting, highlighting the strategy to follow for the intracellular delivery of membrane-impermeable proteins [54]. Herein, they demonstrated that unmodified MSNs with 5.4-nm mesopores were able to host the globular 3.3-nm-width protein to produce effective intracellular delivery, although with no control. To improve this, Griebenow and coworkers evolved a system including a chemical bond able to retain Cyt c inside the mesopores. Their stimulus-responsive system was based on a redox-sensitive disulfide bond that linked Cyt c to thiol-modified mesopores [55], enabling an intracellular, glutathione-mediated release. Shang et al. also employed Cyt c as a model protein for MSN-based delivery, although, in their system, surface adsorption was preferred [56]. In this contribution, the authors did not evaluate the carrier efficiency or the stability of the protein but studied the loading capacity—protein activity—in relation to nanoparticle size. Their results showed that flatter surfaces—larger diameters—permit adsorbing more proteins and, hence, provide higher activities. Another example employing Cyt c was reported by Davis and coworkers, who studied the best-performing linker to connect the protein onto the particles' surface [57]. In their research, they systematically tested several custom-made linkers against the most critical parameters on optimal delivery for surface-grafted proteins: suitable charging capacity (>40 mV on ξ-potential), cationic character at acidic pH, ability to undergo endosomal escape, and capacity to permanently retain Cyt c immobilized on the surface. They found that MSNs modified with 1 mol.% primary amine were the only material able to satisfactorily accomplish all these tasks, providing a fantastic know-how for subsequent investigations into surface grafting. More recently, Choi et al. explored another possibility to deliver Cyt c, employing eroded MSNs with rougher surfaces and enlarged pores [58]. Herein, these matured MSNs permitted loading the Cyt c instead of obtaining the surface deposition that occurred onto particles bearing conventional (2–3 nm) pores. As a result of the increased in-pore loading, the particles showed an enhanced release compared with both the free Cyt c and the nanosystem with higher surface deposition.

Apart from Cyt c, there were reported numerous anticancer proteins [52,53], albeit few examples in combination with MSNs. A relevant example on the topic was reported with concanavalin A, a lectin with anticancer and antibacterial properties [59,86]. Regarding the anticancer example, the lectin also proved to be an efficient targeting element against human osteosarcoma (HOS) and murine prosteoblast (MC3T3-E1) cells. In our system, MSNs were firstly loaded with the typical chemotherapeutic doxorubicin (DOX) and then coated with a polymeric layer linked to the silica surface through pH-sensitive linkers. To conclude, the concanavalin A (ConA) was grafted onto the surface through amide bonds. The resulting system was able to efficiently deliver the drug intracellularly, but only when the pH dropped enough to cleave the bis-acetal linker. The evaluation of the system demonstrated an enhanced killing effect when both species (ConA and DOX) were co-delivered. This suggested a potent adjuvant effect of the protein, which was able to drop the cell viability from 50% with DOX alone to almost 100%.

3.2. Immunostimulating Proteins

Immunostimulation is one of the most popular strategies for improving cancer treatment, as it promises to recruit the patient's immune system to fight tumors. However, any indiscriminate activation may lead to disastrous results. Therefore, there is interest in developing immunostimulant nanosystems able to induce local immune responses thanks to the enhanced permeability and retention (EPR) effect. MSN-based immunotherapy also has an additional advantage, as these particles were proven to be efficient coadjutants [87–89]. Despite these promising features, the delivery of immune-regulating proteins with silica-based carriers is still in its infancy.

Regarding already reported examples, proteins and MSNs can be combined via either surface deposition—grafted or not—or loading into enlarged pores, although those are not the only options. One such exception was the contribution by Lim et al. who delivered immunoglobulin (IgG) to HeLa cells employing a very special silica particle [60]. These were called unconventional perforated HMSNs. Those particles were able to efficiently deliver large membrane-impermeable cargoes, although without any study on immune response. However, their contribution established the basis for local immunostimulation, opening the way to new therapeutic strategies. In more recent examples, several research groups studied immune inductions in mice using nanoparticles. Along this line, Wang, Ito, Tsuji, and coworkers reported a series of articles which firstly studied the immunostimulating behavior of HMSNs [87–89] in murine models, and then studied how the surface modification of such HMSNs with the T cell-dependent antigen, chicken ovalbumin (OVA), stimulated the overall response [61]. The authors paid special attention to which markers were upregulated when treating the animals with these devices [62]. They found a four-action pathway: an anticancer effect through the use of HMSNs themselves, an effector memory on the $CD4^+$ and $CD8^+$ T-cell population, an overexpression on T helper 1 (Th1) and Th2 cytokines, and an enhanced secretion of immunoglobulin antibodies [62]. Employing another silica nanostructure, a multi-shelled dendritic mesoporous organosilica hollow sphere (DMOHS), Yang et al. also obtained similar stimulation patterns when they employed OVA-loaded particles [63]. Herein, a parallel upregulation on $CD4^+$, $CD8^+$, and Th1 immunoproteins was also reported, characterized by the secretion of interleukin-12 (IL-12), interferon-γ (IFN-γ), and tumor necrosis factor-α (TNF-α). More recently, Cha et al. evolved this system by adding an additional immunostimulating entity. In their model, large-pore MSNs (20–30 nm) were sequentially loaded with OVA plus an additional "danger signal", an agonist for Toll-like receptor 9 (TLR9) [64]. As a result, an increased immunostimulation was obtained, which again suggests the importance of combined therapies for the development of more effective cancer treatments and vaccines. More recently, these authors implemented their immunostimulant nanosystem by designing a combination of these MSNs embedded in large chemokine-loaded mesoporous nanorods suitable for injection [65]. With this system, the authors overcame the limitations of the intravenous dosage of their previous nanosystem, as, with this approach, they could effectively recruit and mature the dendritic cells in order to achieve a more efficient cancer vaccination. Their final formulation demonstrated a significant tumor progression reduction together with great survival rates.

In addition to the typical strategies to link proteins onto nanoparticles, Niu et al. reported another possible approach for protein delivery. They designed different porous systems with variable cavities by controlling a core–shell assembly between solid silica nanoparticles. In their designs, core particles had a preset size, while encircling particles had smaller but variable diameters. The resulting disposition created different interparticle voids able to host different sized proteins [66]. The resulting nanostructures showed variable roughness (14, 21, and 38 nm, respectively) that permitted satisfactorily loading a wide variety of proteins, such as Cyt c, monoclonal rabbit antibodies (IgG), and even antibody fragments (horseradish peroxidase (HRP)-linked anti-rabbit IgG antibody), preserving in all cases their activities, as demonstrated by surface plasmon resonance. From a therapeutic point of view, the most interesting model was the 38-nm hydrophobically modified rough (non-porous and core-shell) silica nanoparticles (RSNs), which were able to deliver the anti-pAkt antibody into MCF-7 breast cancer cells. In this case, the therapeutic effect occurred because the antibody created a significant reduction of cell proliferation, together with a downregulated expression of the anti-apoptotic B-cell lymphoma 2 (Bcl-2) protein.

In addition to immunogenic proteins, another interesting therapeutic possibility enabled by nanotechnology is non-viral-based vaccination [90,91]. Therefore, this could be achieved if antigens are delivered to immune cells, thereby avoiding a general immune response. One of the first examples of vaccination employing silica nanoparticles was reported by Guo et al., who employed HMSNs to deliver the open reading frame of the porcine circovirus type 2 (ORF2) protein using a murine model [68]. In this case, the nanovaccine was prepared via direct adsorption of the protein onto raw nanoparticles. In mice, the MSN-based delivery of ORF2 induced overexpression of the typical markers: IFN-γ, Th1, CD4, and CD8, suggesting an immune activation. This strategy was also successfully employed to create other specific MSN-based non-viral vaccines for mice: (1) against *Schistosoma mansoni* employing homogenates from the parasite [69]; (2) against porcine enzootic pneumonia by using a recombinant heat-shock protein 70 (HSP70) antigen fragment ($HSP70_{212-600}$) from *Mycoplasma hyopneumoniae* [70]; (3) against enterohaemorrhagic *Escherichia coli* by using a recombinant fragment of filamentous immunogenic protein from enterohaemorrhagic *E. coli* (EspA) protein [71]; (4) against the pathogenic fungus *Paracoccidioides brasiliensis* employing the antigenic protein rPb27 [72]. In light of these results, it is noteworthy to highlight that these nanoparticle-based vaccinations permit immunizing against different types of pathogens, such as parasites, fungi, or bacteria, with a better profile than the free antigen or other known pharmacological formulations in which the delivery toward macrophages is not so efficient.

3.3. *Enzymes*

The deregulation of normal enzymatic levels has a fundamental role in many diseases. For example, toxic or metabolic syndromes are a direct consequence of this protein malfunction. In cancer, the deregulation of homeostasis is also a consequence of an abnormal expression of proteins and enzymes. However, the use of enzymes in therapy clearly goes beyond cancer treatment based on the delivery of cell-damaging proteins. Unfortunately, like all proteins, enzymes usually do not nicely tolerate systemic administration unless properly modified [92]. Such is the case of the p53 anticancer protein capsule designed by Zhao et al. [93] or the collagenase capsule reported by Villegas et al. [94], which performed best only when they had a degradable protective shell. With regard to the enzymes delivered by MSNs, it is important to remark that most examples are located at the surface; otherwise, the diffusion of both substrates and products may be difficult. One of the most studied examples is carbonic anhydrase (CA), which, despite not having a significant therapeutic effect, was widely employed as a model for in-pore loading approaches [73,74]. The advantage of CA as a model is a direct consequence of the facile determination of its remaining activity, as both substrate (CO_2)

and final product (HCO_3^-) are small enough to diffuse through the pores with freedom and can be easily determined.

Regarding therapeutic models, the mitigation of toxic syndromes caused by genetic disorders is one of the most promising research fields. One interesting example was reported by Xu et al. [75], who employed MSNs to deliver β-galactosidase (β-Gal) to treat Morquio B syndrome. This disease appears when the enzyme is not able to properly cleave the glycoside bond on oligosaccharides, thus producing the accumulation of substrates. In this case, contrary to other models in which the enzyme was located on the surface, the authors decided to load it into the mesopores to obtain additional protection and long-term stability. In this case, the significant size (119 kDa) of β-Gal made it mandatory to prepare ultra-large-pore MSNs. For this, the authors created core–cone structured MSNs with dahlia-like mesopores that were able to host, preserve, and deliver catalytically active β-Gal to N2a cells. In this case, the large size of mesopores, together with the small sizes of both enzymatic substrates and products, permitted supporting the enzyme within the pores; however, in other cases, in which the substrates have diffusion barriers because of the size or nature, this approach may not be so convenient.

With regard to supported proteins, Mou and coworkers reported the use of two antioxidant enzymes, superoxide dismutase (SOD) and glutathione peroxidase (GPx), to intracellularly deplete reactive oxygen species (ROS). In this case, the different nature of possible substrates demanded an adequate exposure of proteins on the nanosystem; otherwise, they would not be able to prevent oxidative stress. In their first example, the authors developed a mesoporous silica-based multifunctional nanocarrier for SOD [76]. This device employed an Ni^{+2}-chelated nitrilotriacetic acid (Ni-NTA)-modified silane, which was able to connect through a histidine moiety to a TAT-containing peptide sequence bound to the enzyme. At this point, the authors denatured the enzyme with urea in order to have only intracellular refolding and to avoid extracellular ROS depletion. The resulting system was able to internalize into HeLa cells and, therein, refold the enzyme into its active form and reduce the oxidative stress induced by paraquat, a well-known superoxide anion generator. More recently, the authors implemented the antioxidant performance of this model by employing two differently loaded nanodevices: one with SOD and the other with GPx [77]. With this combination, the authors found a complementary synergic effect in which the co-delivery of both antioxidant proteins improved the effect of single treatments.

Another interesting example, reported by Han et al., focused on the delivery of human proteasomes to delay tau aggregation associated with Alzheimer's disease [78]. In this model, the authors employed the same building strategy reported by Mou's group: Ni-NTA able to bind histidine moieties from active human 26S proteasomes isolated from a HEK293-derived cell line. Again, the system proved to deliver proteasomes without a significant proteotoxic effect associated with its enzymatic activity. At this point, the authors claimed that their system was not intended to permeate the blood-brain barrier, although it could be implemented onto permeable systems, opening the way to novel strategies to prevent and treat Alzheimer's.

3.4. *Growth Factors*

Growth factors are biomacromolecules responsible for inducing cellular growth, proliferation, and differentiation; they also play important roles in wound healing, bone formation, and vascularization. The most known growth factor is somatotropin, the human growth factor, which is widely employed to promote impaired growth in healthy individuals. The main drawback of this therapy is the need to accomplish a continuous—intramuscular or subcutaneous—dosage in order to achieve a sustained effect. Because of this, it is a treatment with very low adherence and, therefore, it needs improvement. Among the new strategies developed, the most promising are those that permit reaching long-lasting formulations with noninvasive administration routes [95,96]. With regard to the remaining growth factors, mostly cytokines and steroid hormones, it is typical to have compounds with very little aqueous solubility. As a result, they also require form delivery agents to perform their action properly.

This need could be a niche for non-biogenic carriers, especially those of high loading capacity such as silica-based platforms.

Regarding the examples available in the literature, ten years ago, Zhang et al. already reported the potential of MSNs as carriers for growth factors [79]. In this contribution, a water-in-oil microemulsion strategy was employed to create ad hoc MSNs for the 18-kDa basic fibroblast growth factor (bFGF) protein. The resulting system was able to release the protein for over 20 days, and it could be satisfactorily taken up by HUVEC cells. Moreover, the cytotoxicity assay showed low toxicity even when administered at high concentrations (50 μg/mL). Despite this promising result, the remaining examples with therapeutic growth factors are limited to two contributions by Gan et al., who employed two complementary approaches for the delivery of the bone morphogenetic protein 2 (BMP-2). In their first contribution, they prepared chitosan-coated MSNs to deposit proteins onto the particles' surfaces [80], while, in their second work, SBA-15 microparticles with iron oxide nanocaps were employed to load the protein within the 6.2-nm mesopores [81]. In the first example, the authors included dexamethasone, a corticoid, into the mesopores to increment bone growth due to co-delivery of two osteogenic species. Unfortunately, although a significant osteogenesis was achieved, it was completely uncontrolled, and significant ectopic bone formation occurred. To prevent this, the authors changed the model to deliver only the growth factor. To do so, they employed large-pore silica microparticles to carry the BMP-2 and Fe_3O_4 nanocaps to prevent a premature release. The resulting pH-driven carrier was able to deliver the protein while exhibiting excellent biocompatibility, but only in vitro, where the huge size of the chosen silica particles did not affect the guest survival.

3.5. Antibacterial Proteins

In addition to the previous examples, it is also possible to transport proteins bearing antimicrobial effects. On the delivery of antibacterial proteins with MSNs, most contributions were made with lysozyme, a 14.4-kDa enzyme known to damage bacterial cells by hydrolyzing the major component of Gram-positive bacterial walls, i.e., the β-1,4 bonds between *N*-acetylmuramic acid and *N*-acetyl-D-glucosamine. The first example, reported by Lin et al., employed negatively charged MCM-41 MSNs to bind lysozyme units through electrostatic interactions to provide a stable corona [82]. This model permitted having an antibacterial effect even on Gram-negative bacteria such as *E. coli*. Such an effect was a consequence of the high concentration of lysozyme released in bacterial surroundings. Although forthcoming models improved the antibacterial performance of this device, in this work, the authors set two important advances: the possibility of treating bacterial infections with nanotechnology, and the finding that even Gram-negative bacteria could be highly damaged by these glycoside hydrolase enzymes.

In light of these previous results, Yu's group attempted to improve the antibacterial capacity by using higher-loading carriers. In one contribution, they differently evaluated dendritic pore MSNs, finding that a bigger pore led to a faster release and, thus, higher antibacterial effects [83]. In the second contribution, they developed silica nanopollens, which are engineered non-porous hollow nanoparticles coated with nanosized silica spikes to provide a rough surface [84]. Similarly, to the former model, they evaluated different roughnesses, finding that a rougher surface led to a better loading and the associated antibacterial effect. A comparison between models seemed to indicate that, in the case of large-pore MSNs, the antibacterial effect of lysozyme was a consequence of a faster release, while, in the case of nanopollens, it was a combination of a more sustained release together with an unknown nanoparticle-induced effect. Unfortunately, these models were only tested on planktonic bacteria. To address a more complex situation in which the bacteria form a biofilm, Ye and coworkers studied hollow MSNs as high-capacity nanocarriers (up to 350 mg per gram in the case of their enlarged pore HMSNs) [85]. In this work, the authors reported a threshold for free lysozyme activity (400 μg/mL), over which there was no therapeutic improvement. However, the use of MSN-based delivery raised that maximal effect, as they showed a more sustained release pattern able to induce a long-lasting effect.

Apart from lysozyme, antibacterial effects with other proteins were also reported such as ConA (in this case, in combination with levofloxacin) [86]. In this example, carboxylate-modified MCM-41 MSNs were functionalized with ConA upon drug loading. Herein, the combined action of both species permitted achieving complete biofilm destruction even at minimal concentrations (10 μg MSNs per mL), improving the precedent models due to combination therapy. In addition to these reported models, there are many more proteins that lead to successful combinations [97]. Such is the case of lactoferrin, known for having antibacterial properties [98], which was extensively employed in the preparation of glioblastoma-targeted nanodevices [99,100].

4. Delivery of Peptides with Therapeutic Effect

Many of known bioactive peptides are simplified amino-acid sequences that replicate the active sites of proteins and enzymes. The success of these peptides is a consequence of two complementary aspects: (1) the ability to retain features from their parent proteins, and (2) an outstanding chemical profile that arises from their facile synthesis, significantly low cost, and chemical robustness. Those aspects permitted discovering a large number of peptides of different nature and specificity. For example, regarding targeting, those sequences are selected for their affinity toward eukaryotic [101,102] or prokaryotic [103,104] cell receptors. However, applications of peptides go beyond targeting [105], as they are able to accomplish different tasks in regulating metabolic cycles and signaling. In this section, we focus on the potential of MSN-carried peptides for the development of new therapeutic devices. As shown in Table 2 and Figure 4, their applications range from cancer treatment [106–108] to antibacterial effects [107,109], cell regulation processes [110], and immunostimulation.

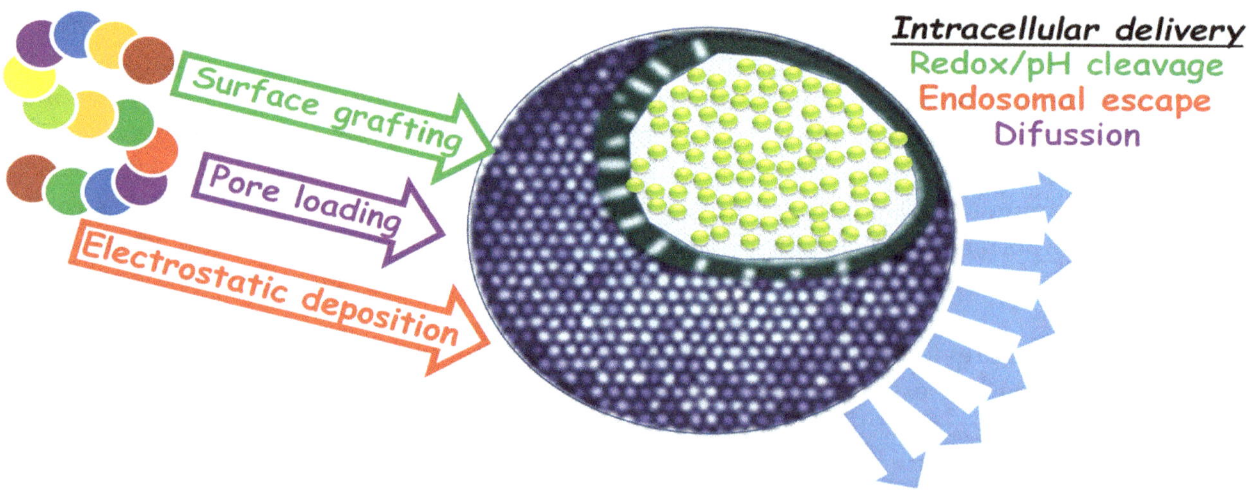

Figure 4. Strategies for delivery of therapeutic peptides employing silica-based carriers.

Table 2. Examples of different types of therapeutic peptides delivered by mesoporous silica-based nanocarriers.

Peptide	Carrier	Pore Cargo	Release Mechanism	Cell Line(s)	In Vivo	Reference
Anticancer Peptides						
K_8-Citraconate $K_8(RGD)_2$	MSNs	Doxorubicin	Electrostatic	COS7, U87 MG	None	[111]
TPP-K-$(KLAKLAK)_2$-	MSNs	Topotecan	Electrostatic/Redox cleavage	KB	None	[112]
C-$GRK_2R_2QR_3P_2Q$-RGDS C-GKGG-D$(KLAKLAK)_2$	MSNs	Doxorubicin	Redox cleavage	HeLa, COS7	None	[113]
$(RGDWWW)_2KC$	MSNs	Doxorubicin	Redox cleavage	COS7, U87 MG	Mice	[114]
$(KLAKLAK)_2$	MSNs	Doxorubicin	Enzymatic degradation Redox cleavage	HeLa	None	[115]
ε-poly-L-lysine C9h	MSNs	C9h	Enzymatic degradation Pore release	HeLa	None	[116]
RDG-Hylin a1	MSNs	RDG-Hylin a1	Pore release	HeLa Hep2	Mice	[117]
Pepstatin A	HMSNs	Pepstatin A	Release from cavity	MCF-7	None	[118]
NuBCP9	MSNs	NuBCP9	Pore release	HeLa, HEK293	Zebrafish	[119]
NuBCP9	PAMAM@MSNs	NuBCP9	Pore release upon PAMAM detachment	HepG2,H292, MCF-7,HeLa	Mice	[120]
Immunostimulating Peptides						
HGP100 TRP2	HMSNs	HGP100 TRP2	Lipid layer disassembly Release from cavity	BMDCs	None	[121]
Antibacterial Peptides						
LL37	SiO_2/MSNs	None/LL37	Surface adsorption vs. pore release	*E. coli*	None	[122]
NZX	MSNs	NZX	Pore release	*Mycobacterium tuberculosis*	Mice	[123]
Melittin	MSNs@ MagMSNs	Melittin Ofloxacin	Pore release upon hyperthermia triggering	*Pseudomonas aeruginosa*	Mice	[124]

Table 2. *Cont.*

Peptide	Carrier	Pore Cargo	Release Mechanism	Cell Line(s)	In Vivo	Reference
Hormones and Growth Factors						
Insulin	MSNs	cAMP	Glucose-mediated displacement	RIN-5F	None	[125]
	MSNs	Insulin	Glucose-sensitive polymer shell	None	None	[126]
	MSNs	Insulin	Pore release	Caco-2	None	[127]
Osteostatin	MSNs	Osteostatin	Pore release	MC3T3-E1	Rabbit	[128–130]
OGP	MSNs MS-HANs	OGP	Pore release	None	None	[131]
BMP-2	MSNs	Surface	None	BMSCs	Rat	[132]

For an illustrative revision of the coupling protocols employed for linking peptides onto nanocarriers, please check Reference [133]. Abbreviations: BMDCs: murine bone-marrow-derived dendritic cells; BMP-2: bone morphogenetic protein 2; BMSCs: rat bone mesenchymal stem cells; cAMP: cyclic adenosine monophosphate; MagMSNs: SPION@MSNs core–shell nanoparticles; MS-HANs: mesoporous silica–hydroxyapatite nanoparticles; OGP: osteogenic growth peptide; PAMAM: polyamidoamine dendrimer.

4.1. Anticancer Peptides

Typically, anticancer effects of peptides occur through two possible mechanisms. One of these arises when the peptide is able to disrupt the normal function of the membrane, while the other occurs when it triggers pro-apoptotic pathways. The membrane-disrupting mechanism operates when the peptides are enriched with cationic amino acids: lysine (Lys, K; amine), arginine (Arg, R; guanidine), and histidine (Hys, H; imidazole). Although this mechanism is not fully clear, these peptides demonstrated a certain membrane-lytic effect similar to other cationic species [134]. The first evidence on the topic was observed with TAT-targeted nanosystems [135], as well with other cell-membrane-penetrating peptides [136].

Regarding the use of cationic peptides as therapeutic agents, it is highly desirable to hide their cationic character to prevent premature damages such as hemolysis and embolisms during trafficking. Apart from pore loading, which preserves cargoes from undesired interactions, another interesting possibility arises from the use of additional negative components to balance the resulting surface charge. One elegant strategy, reported by Zhang and coworkers, employed citraconic anhydride to transform an octa-lysine into a negatively charged peptide able to balance the cationic $K_8(RGD)_2$ functionalized MSNs [111]. The resulting outermost layer was able to accomplish three tasks: target integrin receptors through the RDG moiety, show a highly biocompatible neutral charge, and carry a detachable but toxic K_8 sequence. Unfortunately, the reported studies mainly focused on assessing the effect of carried DOX than on studying the effect of the peptide release, overlooking any potential anticancer effect. In a later contribution by these authors, their system was evolved by including a triphenyl phosphonium group into the KLA peptide sequence (KLAKLAKKLAKLAK) in order to target the mitochondrion. Mitochondria appeared as a key target in cancer treatment because of their roles in regulating cell apoptosis and metabolism [137]. The delivery of antitumoral therapeutic molecules to mitochondria may improve their therapeutic efficacy while avoiding resistance pathways. Furthermore, stimulation of apoptosis mediated by mitochondria could also improve the efficacy of cancer therapy. The resulting organelle-targeted compound was bound to MSNs through disulfide bonds, known to be broken intracellularly by glutathione. Finally, to prevent undesired damages, the authors created a PEGylated anionic polymer shell aimed at increasing biocompatibility and reducing the leakage of topotecan [112]. In this system, the non-loaded model was able to exert a significant pro-apoptotic even at low concentrations, proving the potential of peptides in anticancer therapies; however, as expected, the highest antiproliferative effect occurred when topotecan was loaded within the mesopores.

Encouraged by these results, this group also addressed the synthesis of a multiple pro-apoptotic nanosystem: delivery of DOX, in combination with the delivery of two therapeutic peptides with glutathione-mediated cleavage [113]. In this model, the employed peptides contained different membrane-disrupting sequences, together with two different targeting elements: one of them specific to mitochondrion (C-GKGG-DKLAKLAKKLAKLAK) and the other specific to membranes (C-GRKKRRQRRRPPQ-RGDS). Additionally, to increase the potential cellular damage, the mesopores were loaded with DOX while the peptides were bonded to particles through disulfide bonds, in order to induce oxidative stress upon glutathione depletion. As result, the complete system showed high efficiency against HeLa and COS7 cells, although this effect decreased significantly in the absence of the drug, which highlights the limited effect of membrane-lytic peptides. More recently, this group also employed the glutathione-mediated disulfide cleavage to prepare a drug delivery system for DOX and a membrane-targeted therapeutic peptide rich in tryptophan ($(RGDWWW)_2KC$) [114]. In this case, this peptide was designed to have a DNA-intercalant effect due to the high concentration of indoles. This postulate seems to be justified based on the toxicity obtained for such a nanosystem; however, as expected, the best effect was obtained when DOX was co-delivered. More recently, Feng's group also employed this coating approach to co-deliver DOX and the anticancer peptide KLA. In this model, the final capping was done with a bovine serum albumin (BSA) corona [115], which permitted achieving a double effect: creating a diffusion barrier for both therapeutic agents, and enabling a protease/glutathione-mediated intracellular release. An interesting aspect of the system is that BSA was employed in its wild-type form, which might trigger an additional cellular response when in combination with the remaining multi-apoptotic effects.

Regarding the delivery of peptides that trigger pro-apoptotic routes, the reported examples focused on threading such peptides into the mesopores. For example, Martínez-Máñez's group reported the use of ε-polylysine as a coating layer to prevent the leakage of the pro-apoptotic C9h (YVETLDDIFEQWAHSEDLK) peptide [116]. In this model, the polylysine coating had multiple roles, as it favored cellular uptake due to its cationic character, while maintaining the C9h peptide within the mesopores until proteases cleaved this protective layer. The in vitro testing of this model proved that the encapsulated peptide showed a better therapeutic profile that its free form. However, this effect reached a maximum plateau over which higher dosages did not augment apoptosis. This points out once again the limited anticancer effect of peptides, which demand additional chemotherapeutic agents to obtain satisfactory results. In another similar example employing pore modifications, Cao et al. reported the delivery of a different proapoptotic peptide. In this model, they employed large-pore MSNs to deliver a bifunctional RGD-containing Hylin a1 peptide (IFGAILPLALGALKNLIK) able to target and kill cancerous cells [117]. To accommodate the peptide, the authors functionalized the internal facets of mesopores to favor threading and enable a pH-dependent release. In vitro studies of this system showed that encapsulation drastically reduced the hemolytic rate shown by the free peptide without affecting the potent cytotoxic effect against HeLa and Hep2 cells in vitro. Published in vivo studies with this system showed a clear tumor growth arrest in murine models, although, unfortunately, complete tumor remission could not be achieved.

As previously outlined, the anticancer effect of peptides and proteins is relatively low; thus, their use is generally limited to therapeutic adjuvants of more active species. However, the overall therapeutic effect may be increased if higher doses can be delivered; in this case, high-loading carriers gain interest. Among silica-based carriers, HMSNs are the most suitable candidates, since they theoretically allow loading in larger quantities than their porous analogues. The diverging aspects of MSNs vs. HMSNs in peptide delivery were studied by Rahmani et al., who focused on pepstatin A, a cathepsin D inhibitor peptide [118]. Surprisingly, the authors found two unexpected behaviors: HMSNs loaded less peptide than typical large-pore MSNs, but their effect was higher. Therein, the authors justified such behavior based on the release patterns observed from HMSNs, which provided a more sustained release (longer therapeutic effect), in comparison to regular pore-expended MSNs, which showed a burst-like release.

Another promising anticancer peptide is NuBCP9 (FSRSLHSLL), which is able to bind the Bcl-2 protein, highly overexpressed in cancer cells, turning a cell protector into an apoptosis inductor [138]. Along this line, Wu et al. reported folate-targeted, large-pore MSNs able to deliver this NuBCP9 peptide into HeLa tumors in zebrafish [119]. The resulting ca. 35-nm-width MSNs with pores in the range of 20 nm showed effective internalization into folate-positive HeLa cells, reaching up to 70% reduction of viability when loaded with the peptide. On the other hand, these nanoparticles showed fantastic biocompatibility, as they permitted obtaining fish survival above 80% in concentrations up to 200 μg/mL. In addition to this targeted example, this peptide was also employed in combination with a typical chemotherapeutic. In this contribution, the authors employed ca. 30-nm MSNs with large pores to load the peptide and an outer coating of a fifth-generation polyamidoamine (PAMAM) dendrimer able to load DOX within the structure [120]. As a result, the nanosystem was able to co-deliver both pro-apoptotic species to several cancer cell lines, achieving almost complete cell destruction in concentrations up to 1 μg/mL. To validate the potential of such a combination, the authors tested the efficiency of their nanosystem against resistant cell lines, obtaining outstanding results except for the case of the DOX-resistant MCF-7 line. Nevertheless, these results must be carefully accounted for, as the outermost PAMAM cationic coating may produce a decrease in overall biocompatibility.

4.2. Immunostimulating Peptides

Although most examples of immunostimulation were reported with fully functional proteins, the use of peptides is also possible. Along this line, Xie et al. reported the use of hollow mesoporous silica-based nanocarriers to deliver two melanoma-derived antigen peptides: the hydrophobic H2-K^b peptide $TRP2_{180–188}$ (SVYDFFVWL) and the hydrophilic H2-D^b peptide $HGP100_{25–33}$ (KVPRNQWL) [121]. In order to achieve the desired double loading, the authors modified their HMSNs with amino groups at the internal space and the mesopores with carboxylates in order to create two different preferential locations for peptides within the HMSNs. Then, to provide adequate retention and colloidal stability, the system was further coated with a lipid bilayer. Furthermore, on this lipid layer, another therapeutic species was included to increase the overall effect: monophosphoryl lipid A (MPLA), a Toll-like receptor 4 (TLR4) agonist. The resulting hollow protocells showed time-dependent uptake by murine bone marrow-derived dendritic cells and, according to data shown, induced cell maturation as seen by the overexpression of CD86, TNF-α, IFN-γ, IL-12, and IL-4 proteins. When the system was tested against melanoma lung metastasis in murine models, the vaccinated animals showed less tumor growth and creation of metastatic lymph nodes, demonstrating that the system was able to induce an effective anticancer response in mice.

4.3. Antibacterial Peptides

Although antimicrobial peptides are one of the most promising research lines to fight multi-resistant bacteria, their incorporation into nanocarriers was poorly studied [139]. Among the few systems reported, the contributions made by Braun et al. can be highlighted, who studied the best loading strategy and silica composition for the cationic antibacterial peptide LL37 (LLGDFFRKSKEKIGKEFKRIVQRIKDFLRNLVPRTES). In their first contribution, these authors focused on the membrane interactions between *E. coli* and several silica-based (non-porous, calcined mesoporous, and amino-capped mesoporous) nanoparticles loaded with the LL37 peptide [122]. As expected, the best loading profiles were obtained for the porous calcined—most negatively charged—nanoparticles. In addition, as expected, MSNs provided an adequate protective environment for the peptide and, hence, reduced the associated hemo- and proteolysis. At this point, it is also interesting to remark that these authors also studied how the porous structure affected the delivery, in this case, by comparing regular sized-MSNs with large-pore HMSNs [140]. They found that ca. 2.5-nm-pore MSNs produced a burst release, while the HMSNs showed a more sustained release, in concordance with data obtained by Rahmani et al. [118], suggesting that HMSNs behave better for peptide delivery.

Apart from the activation of immune cells and vaccination, the treatment of infected cells is another big issue that could be solved by applying nanotechnology. One inspiring example was recently reported by Tenland et al., who employed MSNs to deliver an anti-tuberculosis peptide to infected macrophages [123]. In their work, the NZX (GFGCNGPWSEDDIQCHNHCKSIKGYKGG YCARGGFVCKCY) peptide with a proven anti-tuberculosis effect was employed [141]. In this case, the system was assembled by threading the peptide into the mesopores, employing previously optimized nanoparticles [140]. The system demonstrated effective internalization into macrophages and produced peptide release once internalized. As a result, the infecting mycobacterium could the killed without significantly affecting host macrophages; moreover, the MSN-carried peptide showed a longer therapeutic effect than its free form. This effect, seen in other reviewed examples, was justified by the accumulation of nanocarriers within intracellular vacuoles, which created therapeutic reservoirs by maintaining peptide integrity.

Apart from the delivery of antibacterial peptides, combination therapies were also recently reported. Along this line, Zink and coworkers reported the simultaneous delivery of the melittin (MEL, GIGAVLKVLTTGLPALISWIKRKRQQ) peptide and the antibiotic ofloxacin (OFL) with a mesoporous silica-based assembled nanosystem [124]. In this system, the authors employed a very elegant strategy to co-deliver the medium-size peptide together with the small antibiotic. To do so, they prepared large-pore MSNs which were loaded with MEL and capped with a β-cyclodextrin-modified polyethyleneimine and ofloxacin-loaded, adamantane-modified SPION@MSNs capped by cucurbit[6]uril units. The resulting nanoparticles were able to self-assemble and create nanogates able to maintain both drugs within the closed pores. The system was proven to disassemble under magnetothermal induction, thereby releasing both species, which demonstrated efficient destruction of planktonic bacteria and biofilms. Indeed, this system demonstrated its efficiency even when embedded into implants, which were able to prevent bacterial infection in mice.

4.4. Growth Factors

As in many other cases, peptides could also have anabolic properties. These features make them interesting candidates for their use as cargoes in new-generation therapeutic devices aimed at tissue growth induction or hormone therapy. The first example in this field, reported by Lin's group, employed MSNs to intracellularly deliver cyclic adenosine monophosphate (cAMP). To obtain chemical responsiveness, the authors modified the MSNs with a boronic acid $-B(OH)_2$ moiety able to coordinate glucuronic acid moieties. The mesopores were then loaded with cAMP and closed through glucuronate-modified insulin nanocaps [125]. The resulting system was sensitive to glucose, as it could be disassembled by chemical displacement. As a result, this system permitted regulating hyperglycemic levels through a dual release mechanism: Insulin to trigger glucose assimilation by liver, and cAMP delivery to induce glycolysis. Unfortunately, this proof of concept was not further evaluated in vivo.

More recently, Sun et al. revisited insulin delivery with MSNs. To do so, they developed a glucose-sensitive nanodevice employing rod-like MSNs and a polymer shell able to change its conformation upon the presence of glucose [126]. In their investigations, the authors optimized the composition of this polymeric shell by using three different monomers: *N*-isopropylaminomethacrylate (NIPAM) to provide the needed morphological shift, 3-acrylamidophenylboronic acid as a glucose-sensitive fragment, and dextran maleate as an optional hydrophilic component. The resulting system could be loaded with insulin at low temperatures (4 °C), in which the polymer adopted an expanded conformation and closed upon heating (37 °C). Both reported compositions showed effective insulin release when glucose was present; however, when pH was below 7, the polymer was not able to shift morphology, avoiding insulin release. Although only in vitro tests were reported, the possibilities of this model are considerable, as the incorporation of dextran may favor colloidal stability and enhance biocompatibility, as suggested by the high cell viability values obtained. Insulin delivery was also investigated by Zakeri-Siavashani et al., who employed SBA-15 mesoporous microparticles [127]; however, therein, the authors profited from the bigger pore size provided by these particles to achieve higher loading and more sustained release. Although their system showed a nice insulin release profile, the typical bigger sizes of SBA-15 particles (generally above 300 nm) limit their application in intravenous formulations, although they may be used to create biocompatible reservoirs.

The facile aggregation of SBA-15 particles caused by their size, which makes their trafficking through alveoli and capillaries extremely difficult, makes these materials ideal candidates for non-systemic therapies, for example, bone replacement and tissue regeneration. In our first contribution to the topic, we found that the osteostatin peptide, derived from parathyroid hormone-related protein ($PTHrP_{107-111}$), could be efficiently delivered using this kind of material [128]. A clear regenerative effect was observed, which permitted recovering bone mass in peri-implant bone regeneration in cavitary defects [129], as well as in osteoporotic subjects [130]. More recently, our investigations focused on the combination of this peptide with osteogenic elements embedded in bioactive glasses [142,143], finding an enhanced bone formation consequence of the exerted combination therapy.

In addition to these examples, other research groups also focused on the combination of osteoinductive peptides with bone-forming agents. Such is the case of the model reported by Mendes et al., which combined an osteogenic growth peptide (OGP, ALKRQGRTLYGFGG) with hydroxyapatite in an SBA-15-based formulation [131]. Therein, the authors found a substantial behavior difference when hydroxyapatite was present, while deeper studies on the possibilities of such a combination were not addressed. Another interesting combination for remineralizing bone was reported by He and coworkers, who employed MCM-41 to prepare a nanosystem able to deliver a BMP-2-derived peptide (KIPKASSVPTELSAISTLYL) together with dexamethasone, a potent synthetic glucocorticoid [132]. Although, in this case, the peptide was not intended to be released, experimental results showed that its presence exerted a clear osteogenic induction. Moreover, the system was able to promote osteogenic differentiation on mesenchymal stem cells in vitro, as indicated by the upregulation of alkaline phosphatase (ALP) and other bone-forming proteins. Additionally, an increased calcium deposition was observed, demonstrating that mesoporous silica nanoparticles are adequate materials for bone engineering.

5. Delivery of Nucleic Acids: Gene Modulation and Silencing

Gene modulation and silencing are promising strategies to efficiently treat cancer, as well as cardiovascular or inflammatory-related diseases [20]. NAs are rapidly degraded by endonucleases and barely internalized by cells. Therefore, the biggest challenge today is to develop an effective gene delivery vector to transport and introduce NAs into the gene therapy target cells. These carriers must be easy to manipulate and show non-toxic properties in vitro and in vivo.

There are two main carriers for gene delivery therapy: viral and non-viral vector platforms [144]. For non-pathogenic viruses (retro and adenovirus), the most used platforms are viral vectors, but they present some limitations such as high cost and manipulation, immune response, or inadequate accessibility of genetic cargo internalized by cells [144]. Currently, research groups are focusing their efforts on the improvement of cheaper and easier preparation of non-viral platforms as cation polymers, liposomes, or inorganic porous nanoparticles such as MSNs [145]. In this respect, PEI is a widely used polycation in gene delivery systems due to its amino protonation improving gene delivery [20,144,145]. Liposomes are also commonly applied to enhance the cell internalization of NAs. Both polycations and liposomes present some limitations for therapeutic applications related to their molecular weight or disadvantageous gene escape and physicochemical instability, respectively [20,144,145]. Nevertheless, MSNs showed optimal properties for intracellular delivery of NAs due to their easy manipulation, high loading capacity into the mesopores, surface functionalization, and non-toxicity characteristics [20]. In addition, MSNs can be combined with polycations and other therapeutic drugs for personalized treatment related to cancer and other diseases.

In this regard, plasmid DNAs (pDNAs) are the most widely used gene therapy material to treat different diseases [20,144,145], although there is increasing interest in small interfering RNAs (siRNAs) and microRNAs (miRNAs) for therapeutic application. In this section, we focus on NA-loaded (DNA, siRNA, and miRNA) MSN-based drug delivery systems, as shown in Table 3 and Figure 5.

Table 3. Examples of different therapeutic nucleic acids delivered by silica-based nanocarriers.

Nucleic Acid	Carrier Type	NA Location	Loading Strategy	Cell Line(s)	In Vivo	Application	Reference
DNA							
pDNA	MSNs	Surface	Adsorption	Neuro-2A	None	Cancer	[146]
pDNA	MSNs	Surface	Adsorption	HEPA-1	None	Cancer	[147]
dsDNA	MSNs	Surface	Adsorption	HeLa	None	Cancer	[148]
dsDNA	MSNs	Surface	Adsorption	HL-60	None	Cancer	[149]
pDNA	IDMSMs	Surface	Adsorption	QGY-7703	Mice	Cancer	[150]
ssDNA	MSNs	Surface	Disulfide bond Maleimide	MCF-7	None	Cancer	[151]
dsDNA	HMSNs	Surface	Adsorption	MCF-7, A549, HepG2	None	Cancer	[152]
ssDNA	MSNs	Surface	Adsorption	MDA-MB-231	Mice	Cancer	[153]
ssDNA	MSNs	Surface	Adsorption	MCF-7, K-562, U2OS	Mice	Cancer	[154]
pDNA	MSNs	Surface	Adsorption	293T, RAW264.7	Mice	Hepatitis B	[155]
siRNA							
PKM2	MSNs	Surface	Adsorption	MDA-MB-231	Mice	Cancer	[156]
Cell-killing	MSNs	Mesopores	Adsorption	MDA-MB-231	None	Cancer	[157]
HER2	MSNs	Surface	Adsorption	BT474	None	Cancer	[158]
TGFβR-1	MSNs	Surface	Adsorption	RT3	Mice	Cancer	[159]
MDR1	MSNs	Surface	Adsorption	CAL27	None	Cancer	[160]
MDR1	MSNs	Surface	Adsorption	KBV	Mice	Cancer	[161]
Bcl-2	MSNs	Surface	Adsorption	SKOV-3, MCF-7	None	Cancer	[162]
Bcl-2	MSNs	Surface	Adsorption	SKOV-3	Mice	Cancer	[163]

Table 3. *Cont.*

Nucleic Acid	Carrier Type	NA Location	Loading Strategy	Cell Line(s)	In Vivo	Application	Reference
siRNA							
TWIST	MSNs	Surface	Adsorption	F2, Ovcar8	Mice	Cancer	[164]
VEGF	MSNs	Surface	Adsorption	HeLa, HepG2	None	Cancer	[165]
VEGF	MSNs	Surface	Adsorption	HepG2, Huh7	None	Cancer	[166]
HSP47	MSNs	Surface	Adsorption	PMDF	Mice	Fibrosis	[167]
TnC	MSNs	Surface	Adsorption	rHSCs, mHSCs	None	Fibrosis	[168]
COLL1A1	MSNs	Surface	Adsorption	HDFs	Rat	Tissue regeneration	[169]
SOST	MSNs	Surface	Adsorption	MEF, HeLa	Mice	Osteoporosis	[170]
miRNA							
miR-155	MSNs	Mesopores	Adsorption	SW480	Mice	Cancer	[171]
miR-328	MSNs	Mesopores	Adsorption	SW480, SW620, HT-29, Lovo, Caco-2	Mice	Cancer	[172]
miR-34a miR-10b	MSNs	Mesopores	Adsorption	MDA-MB-231, MDA-MB-468	Mice	Cancer	[173]
miR-26a	MSNs	Mesopores	Adsorption	rBMSCs	None	Tissue regeneration	[174]
miR-200c siPlk1	MSNs	Mesopores	Adsorption	MDA-MB-231	Mice	Cancer	[175]

Abbreviations: IDMSN: imidazole dendritic mesoporous silica nanoparticles; PKM2: glycolytic enzyme pyruvate kinase; HER2: human epidermal growth factor receptor 2; TGFβR-1: transforming growth factor, beta receptor I; MDR1: multidrug resistance protein 1; Bcl-2: B-cell lymphoma 2; VEGF: vascular endothelial growth factor; HSP47: heat-shock protein 47; TnC: tenascin-C; COLL1A1: collagen type I; PMDFs: primary mouse dermal fibroblasts; HSCs: human stem cells; HDFs: human dermal fibroblasts; MEF: mouse embryonic fibroblastic cells; rBMSCs: rat bone marrow stromal cells.

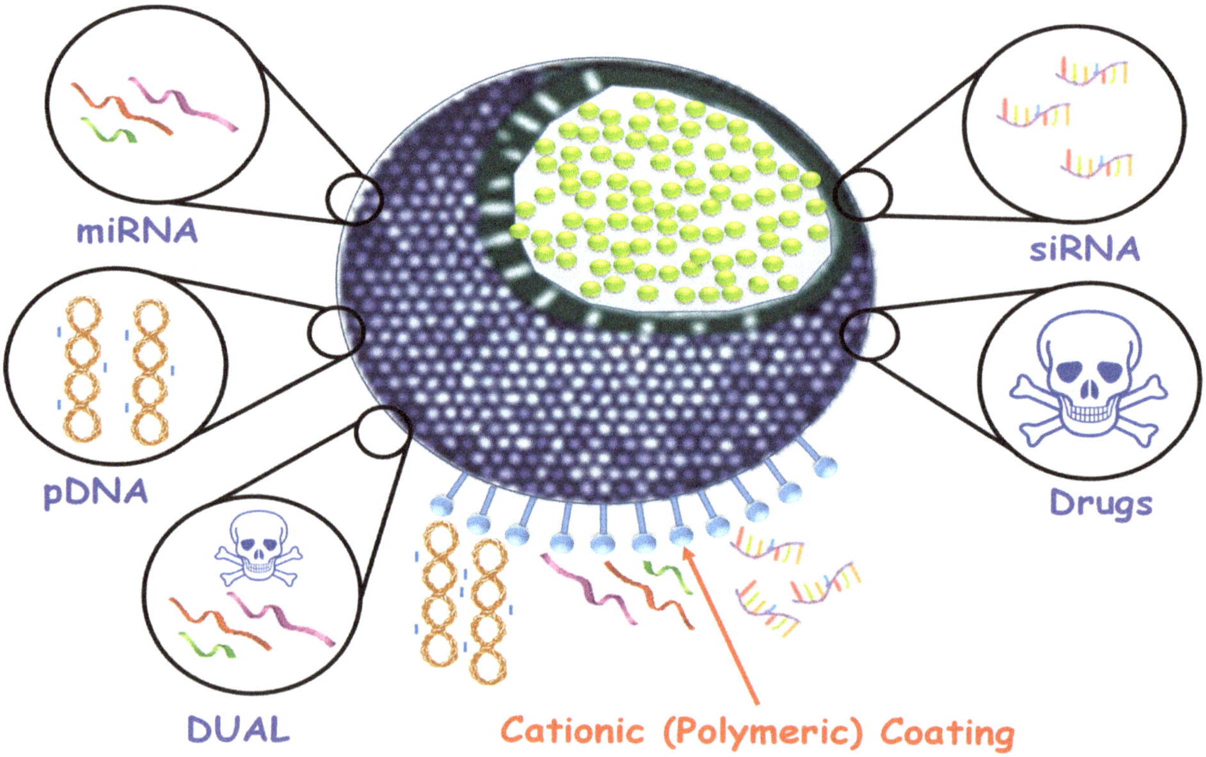

Figure 5. Types of nucleic acids and the possible loading strategies into MSNs for tuning gene expression on cells.

5.1. DNA

As we previously mentioned, MSNs can be functionalized with PEIs for better DNA molecule adsorption and, thus, for a more effective intracellular delivery, protecting NAs from endonuclease degradation due to their positive charge. These positive charges interact with negatively charged cell membranes, inducing higher cell internalization rates and cell death. For example, Zarei et al. [146] developed a functionalized nanosystem based on phosphonate MSNs-PEI loaded with a lysosomotropic factor, chloroquine (CQ), complexed with plasmid DNA. The resulting cell internalization and viability of this pDNA-MSN-PEI was analyzed with the fluorescent protein plasmid (pGFP (green fluorescent protein)), showing a significant increase in transfection of pGFP into the mouse neuroblastoma cell line Neuro-2A. In this respect, Xia et al. [147] proposed the use of a cationic MSN-PEI nanocarrier with a potential therapeutic application. The resulting cationic surface of MSNs facilitated the DNA attachment in order to balance the cationic 10-kDa PEI and, hence, achieve nontoxic effects and higher cellular uptake rates. This nanosystem was loaded with a plasmid DNA (pEGFP) and siRNA construct that was capable of knocking down GFP expression in hepatocellular carcinoma mouse (HEPA-1) cells, with a fluorescent GFP expression of 70% in these cells. In addition, the authors loaded the cationic MSN-PEI nanocarrier with paclitaxel, a hydrophobic anti-tumoral drug used in pancreatic tumor treatment, increasing the cell internalization and delivery of this drug in HEPA-1 cells. On the other hand, Song et al. [29] demonstrated that controlling the nanotopography of MSNs as pDNA vectors had an influence on the transfection efficacy. For example, ambutan-like MSNs-PEI with spiky surfaces showed pDNA-binding capability and a transfection efficacy of 88% in HEK-293T cells, which was a higher rate compared with other MSNs systems. In addition, the authors demonstrated that these types of surface spikes of MSNs induced a continuous open space with two objectives: binding DNA chains through multivalent interactions and protecting the gene cargo covered in the spiky layer against enzymatic degradation, without negative effects on transfection rates. These results indicated that this nanosystem is an interesting approach as a non-viral vector for effective gene delivery.

In a study by Wang et al. [148], an MSN based nanoplatform functionalized with a DNA gate was evaluated in vitro. In this report, the authors developed a fluorometric method for adenosine triphosphate (ATP) recognition using rolling circle amplification (RCA) consisting of proximity ligation-mediated amplification. In addition, the nanosystem was functionalized with graphene oxide modified with folic acid (FA) as a DNA vehicle and loaded with DOX, to evaluate the control release efficacy in HeLa tumoral cells. Following the RCA process, long DNA chains that contained a complementary strand to the DNA at the gate permitted dehybridizing such a nanogate and producing DOX release into tumoral cells. This nanoplatform was effectively internalized by the FA receptor, upregulated in those tumoral cells, while the DOX release induced increased cell toxicity compared with control systems, improving the targeted cancer therapeutics on these HeLa cells. In another study by Wang et al. [149], a DNA-capped MSN nanocarrier loaded with DOX for tumor marker-triggered on-demand drug release was developed and evaluated in vitro. As a first step, a DNA biomolecular gate adsorbed on the MSN–NH_2 was developed at neutral pH via electrostatic adsorption. In the absence of a stimulus, the pores were locked, and it was not possible to release the drug. However, when the nanosystem recognized the internal stimulus (survivin messenger RNA (mRNA) or miR-21, overexpressed biomarkers in cancer), the DNA caps were removed from the MSNs, allowing DOX release. This stimulus-responsive behavior was confirmed by different microscopy techniques in cell-acute myeloblastic leukemia (HL-60) cells. This nanocarrier was effectively internalized by these cells, releasing DOX cargo into the cytoplasm and inducing significant cell death. Therefore, this nanoplatform is a very useful novel system for both imaging diagnosis and therapeutic controlled drug delivery applications. In this regard, Li et al. [150] designed and evaluated another anti-tumoral and gene drug co-delivery nanosystem with on-demand release properties in vitro and in vivo. For this purpose, the authors developed dendritic MSNs modified with imidazole groups employing a Schiff-base imine linkage, which permitted loading DOX within the pores and electrostatically depositing the survivin short hairpin RNA (shRNA)-expressing plasmid (iSur-pDNA). The imidazole functionalization triggered efficient endosomal escape, improving the accumulation of iSur-pDNA and gene knockdown efficacy. Such nanosystems were successfully internalized by QGY-7703 hepatoma cells and decreased tumoral cell viability in vitro, due to the pH-sensitive co-delivery of DOX and iSur-pDNA. In addition, this nanoplatform induced tumor growth reduction in H-22 tumor-bearing mice, indicating that it could be a promising nanocarrier for co-delivery cancer treatment.

On the other hand, aptamers are short single-stranded oligonucleotides with high affinity and specificity to several molecule targets, and they exhibit potential properties as therapeutic and diagnostic factors in different diseases [176]. In this regard, Sun et al. [151] developed an MSN-based nanocarrier with different DNA molecules on the surface for self-assembly. For the controlled delivery of anti-tumoral drug cargo (DOX), the authors used an aptamer oligonucleotide as a gatekeeper and other oligonucleotides on the MSN surface to allow DNA-guided immobilization bearing single-stranded capture oligonucleotides. This nanovalve induced an increase in cell adhesion rates in MCF-7 adenocarcinoma cells, with an efficient triggered release of DOX drug in these cells. The DNA-directed self-assembly aptamer-based nanosystem is efficient in surface-bound monolayers and can be used as a delivery system for different applications and treatments, allowing site-specific delivery of anti-tumoral drugs. In the same way, Li et al. [152] developed a dual multi-locked DNA valve HMSN-based nanosystem to intracellular cancer-related mRNAs for controlled DOX drug release. The upregulated endogenous targeted mRNAs (K1 and GalNAc-T mRNAs) were able to dehybridize the multi-locked DNA valves and open the pores to release DOX. As a result, a synergic effect was obtained, caused by the intratumoral delivery of the drug together with the depletion of TK1 mRNA, implicated in cell division as a tumor growth factor, and GalNAc-T, upregulated in several tumoral cells. The nanocarrier was evaluated in vitro in different cancer cells, inducing higher rates of cytotoxicity compared to non-tumoral cells. In an in vivo study, Pascual et al. [153] designed another novel non-viral drug delivery and diagnostic nanocarrier based on a capped MSN-NH_2 hybrid platform, which was loaded with DOX and gated with Mucin 1 (MUC1) aptamer (S-apMUC1). MUC1 is a protein present in the cell surface and upregulated in breast cancer cells. The S-apMUC1-MSNs nanosystem was efficiently and specifically internalized only by tumoral MDA-MB-231 cells related to MUC1 receptor overexpression of these cells. After S-apMUC1-MSNs internalization by tumoral cells, the DOX cargo was released into the cytoplasm of tumoral cells, inducing a decrease in cell viability. This nanoplatform exhibited reduced cargo release when DNAse I was not present. In vivo, S-apMUC1-MSNs were radionuclide-labeled with ^{99}Tc for a radio-imaging study in MDA-MB-231 tumor-bearing Balb/c mice. S1-apMUC1-Tc displayed significant tumor signaling and accumulation in these mice. These results suggest that MSN nanosystems capped with aptamers showing radiopharmaceutical properties are promising hybrid nanomaterials in the clinical context.

Of particular interest is a study by Srivastava et al. [154], where the authors proposed a novel telomerase-responsive delivery of DOX loaded in an MSN nanosystem against telomerase-positive tumoral cells. DOX loading was performed using a telomeric repeat complementary sequence and a telomerase substrate primer sequence, allowing controlled release in MCF-7 cancer cells. This functionalized nanocarrier was efficiently internalized, and it significantly reduced the tumoral cell viability, with an inhibition of function when a specific telomerase inhibitor was present. This oligo-wrapped nanoprobe specific for telomerase was used in a telomerase-positive Dalton's lymphoma mice model. The nanosystem induced a significant inhibition of tumors, enhanced survival, and re-established histopathological parameters, including neo-angiogenesis.

Furthermore, DNA vaccination was proven to provide an immune response to viruses or infectious diseases [177]. In this regard, Wang et al. [155] developed a layered double hydroxide (LDH) MSN nanocarrier as a vaccine delivery platform and immune stimulant, using a GFP expression plasmid as model DNA. The pDNA-MSN-LDH nanosystem showed high internalization rates in monocyte-derived dendritic cells (MDDCs) and stimulated macrophage activation via nuclear factor kappa B (NF-κB) signaling pathway, increasing IFN-γ, IL-6, CD86, and major histocompatibility complex class I (MHC-I). In vivo, the nanocarrier immunized BALB/c mice, indicating that the DNA vaccine-MSN-LDH system increased the serum antibody response and promoted T-cell proliferation, skewing T helper to Th1 polarization. Taken together, these results indicated that MSN-LDH nanosystems could operate as a potential non-viral gene delivery platform.

5.2. siRNAs

Small interfering RNA (siRNA) are highly potent, short, double-stranded RNA molecules (20–25 bp) used in gene-based therapy of different diseases that can be delivered in a sustained manner [178]. Moreover, siRNAs are anti-cancer targets because they can modify the expression of pro-apoptotic oncogenes and cell-cycle key regulators. However, siRNAs have a very short half-life and poor cell internalization capability [178]. In this regard, MSNs attracted pronounced consideration for the intracellular delivery of NAs due to their high loading capacity into the mesopores and surfaces. Polycations such as PEI combined onto the surface of MSNs permit a more stable encapsulation, loading, controlled release, and intracellular internalization of potential siRNA cargoes [178]. In addition, positively charged amine-rich nanosystems are required for a better result in siRNA/MSN cellular uptake rates [178]. Future in vivo efforts are necessary to validate the tissue-specific siRNA therapeutic efficacy using imaging techniques to analyze MSN biodistribution at the whole-body level. On the other hand, it is mandatory to find nanosystems able to efficiently deliver those therapeutic siRNAs in vivo with enough efficiency, as well as with protective features against nucleases, able to enhance their gene-silencing capabilities at the target tissues.

In this respect, Shen et al. [156] developed a universal siRNA multi-component system carrier based on MSNs functionalized with cyclodextrin-grafted polyethyleneimine (CP). CP offers a positive charge to improve the siRNA loading on MSNs through electrostatic interaction, allowing endosomal escape. To analyze the effectiveness of the proposed delivery system, an siRNA of the M2 isoform of the glycolytic enzyme pyruvate kinase (PKM2) was used, due to it being overexpressed in several cancer types. Firstly, siRNA-loaded CP-MSNs were positively evaluated in vitro in MDA-MB-231 human breast cancer cells with higher rates of cellular internalization and gene silencing capability. The nanosystem showed specific tumor accumulation and gene silencing in an orthotopic mouse model of MDA-MB-231 cells, inhibiting tumor cell growth, invasion, and migration. Prabhakar et al. [157] designed a new nanosystem based on MSNs with expanded mesopores and pore–surface-hyperbranched PEI tethered with redox-cleavable organic linkers that could carry high concentrations of siRNAs. This stimulus-responsive nanosystem was highly internalized by MDA-MB-231 cells, releasing the cell-killing siRNA as cargo into the cytoplasm, followed by endosomal escape triggered by the intracellular redox situation, with high efficiency in long-term gene knockdown for several days. In addition, long-term stability of therapeutic nanosystems is mandatory to provide personalized medicine. In this respect, lyophilization or freeze-drying are useful and common methods to ensure this aim. Ngamcherdtrakul et al. [158] successfully reported a lyophilized nanosystem consisting of MSNs modified with cationic polymers (PEI), PEG, and antibody (trastuzumab), which was loaded with a human epidermal growth factor receptor 2 (HER2) siRNA upon reconstitution. This nanosystem was successfully internalized by $HER2^+$ human breast cancer cells, BT474, decreasing their viability; it maintained a cake-like structure and retained hydrodynamic size, charge, siRNA loading ability, and silencing efficacy. With the tested method, the lyophilized nanocarrier can be stored stably for eight weeks at 4 °C and at least six months at −20 °C.

Oral cancer is the seventh most frequent cancer and the ninth most frequent cause of death in the world [179]. About 90% of oral cancer is of squamous cell carcinoma type (SCC) [179]. Currently, surgery and radiation, combined or not with chemotherapy, are the main treatments, but this approach presents several limitations due to multidrug resistance; thus, new therapeutic drugs must be evaluated. Lio et al. [159] developed a topical formulation for the transdermal delivery of siRNA built on MSNs for the treatment of skin disorders. In this regard, transforming growth factor beta receptor I (TGFβR-1) is overexpressed in patients with skin SCC, and the anti-tumor effects of TGFβR-1 inhibitors were proven in several types of cancer. The nanosystem was built by loading TGFβR-1 siRNA into the pores of MSNs and further coating the resulting particle with a layer of poly-L-lysine (PLL) to improve transdermal delivery. The tested platform demonstrated positive cellular uptake rates and detection of specific gene biomarkers in human SCC cells in vitro. This system induced a topical delivery of TGFβR-1 siRNA targeting the SCC in a mouse xenograft model, decreasing the TGFβR-1 siRNA levels and reducing tumor volume. These results indicated that this platform is a promising non-invasive transdermal drug delivery system. Moreover, multidrug resistance plays an important role in the failure of oral cancer chemotherapy. In this sense, in a study by Wang et al. [160], a novel MSN loaded with both multidrug resistance protein 1 (MDR1) siRNA and DOX was evaluated in vitro and in vivo to directly kill tumor cells without the effect of multidrug resistance. MSNP-PEI@siRNA loaded with DOX was efficiently transfected into human oral squamous carcinoma DOX-resistant (KBV) cells, decreasing the gene expression of MDR1 and increasing the apoptosis of these cells. This nanocarrier significantly reduced the tumor size and decelerated tumor growth rate in vivo, showing a huge potential therapeutic application for multidrug-resistant cancer. On the other hand, Shi et al. [161] developed hyaluronic acid (HA)-assembled MSNs nanosystems loaded with MDR1 siRNA and protein MutT homolog 1 (MTH1) inhibitor TH287. Downregulation of MTH1 protein expression increased oxidative stress levels and significantly decreased tumor survival and proliferation. TH287 is a potent small molecule that inhibits the MTH1 protein, and it could act as a potential chemotherapeutic drug. The HA-MSNs nanosystem was successfully internalized by CAL27 cancer cells, inducing a high rate of cell apoptosis when TH287 and MDR1 siRNA were present. In vivo, this nanocarrier reduced the tumor growth compared with untreated control and free TH287 in male Balb/c mice. These results suggest that HA-MSN-based nanosystems are a promising vehicle to control the delivery of MDR1 siRNA and TH287, with a possible combination with other therapeutic agents for oral cancer treatment.

Regarding multidrug resistance as a persistent limitation for cancer treatment, Pan et al. [162] proposed a novel pH-responsive delivery nanosystem based on carboxylated MSNs (MSN-COOH) with a zeolitic imidazole framework-8 (ZIF-8) film synthesized for pore blocking and efficient loading of anti-apoptotic B-cell lymphoma 2 (Bcl-2) siRNA. The nanosystem developed was efficiently internalized by MCF-7/ADR and SKOV-3/ADR tumoral cells. The ZIF-8 film can be degraded in the acidic endo-lysosome and trigger the intracellular release of both siRNAs and potential antitumor drugs, decreasing cancer cell proliferation. In this regard, Choi et al. [163] developed a new biodegradable and biocompatible amine-free, neutral MSN-based nanocarrier for siRNA delivery. In this study, Bcl-2 siRNA was loaded via a calcium ion (Ca^{2+})-mediated interconnection between phosphates of siRNA and surface silicates of MSNs, reducing the risk of amine-related cytotoxicity and immunogenicity. This nanosystem showed positive results in internalization rates in tumoral SKOV-3 cells, inducing a significant decrease in cell viability when the siRNA was released, compared with MSNs or siRNA alone. This reduction in tumoral cell proliferation was dramatically enhanced when the nanocarrier was loaded with DOX. The therapeutic potential of the co-delivery system was also analyzed in SKOV3 xenografts in nude mice. The authors found that co-delivery of Bcl-2-siRNA and DOX MSNs-Ca^{2+} reduced tumor volume with an inhibition rate of 72%, higher than MSNs-Ca^{2+} loaded with DOX and MSNs-Ca^{2+} with siRNA. The results indicated that Ca^{2+}-bound MSNs can act as an siRNA nanocarrier with a less toxic, more effective, and safer siRNA potential clinical application. On the other hand, patients with epithelial ovarian cancer (EOC) metastases relapse after initial effective chemotherapy treatment due to multiple drug resistance. In order to resolve this problem, Shahin et al. [164] proposed a novel nanoparticle delivery platform to reverse chemoresistance based on HA-MSNs loaded with TWIST siRNA. Hyaluronic acid (HA) is a ligand for CD44, which is overexpressed and correlates with worse prognosis in EOC. TWIST is a key protein implicated in epithelial–mesenchymal transition, cancer metastasis, angiogenesis, and drug resistance. The developed nanocarrier was successfully internalized in vitro by F2 and Ovcar8 cell lines, inducing a sustained TWIST gene knockdown. MSN-HA@siRNA showed safety and specific tumor targeting in an EOC mouse model. Mice treated with the complete nanosystem induced significant tumor reduction, and, when the authors combined this nanocarrier with cisplatin, the reduction of tumor growth was greater compared with the corresponding control groups.

For the metastatic spread of cancer, growth of the vascular network is a critical event [29]. Vascular endothelial growth factor (VEGF) is a glycoprotein and key mediator of angiogenesis in tumoral cells [180]. Keeping this in mind, Zheng et al. [165] proposed a new nanocarrier based on MSNs functionalized with FA-targeted tumoral cells and co-loading of VEGF siRNA and ursolic acid (UA), a pentacyclic triterpenoid with anticancer efficacy. HeLa (FA receptor-overexpressed) and HepG2 tumoral cell lines were used to analyze the MSN-FA-UA@siRNA nanosystems in vitro. The MSN-FA nanocarrier enhanced transfection efficiency and siVEGF stability, improving the targeted antitumoral efficacy of siVEGF and UA, with a significant decrease in cancer-related VEGF protein levels in HeLa cells. In this sense, the same authors [166] developed an alternative MSN nanosystem consisting of an asialoglycoprotein receptor (ASGPR)-targeting drug delivery system for co-delivery of siVEGF and sorafenib (SO), a multi-kinase inhibitor that can target VEGF for the inhibition of tumor growth and neo-angiogenesis in hepatocellular carcinoma (HCC). Lactobionic acid (LA) is derived from lactose oxidation, and it was able to effectively target human HCC. In addition, ASGPR is overexpressed in several types of cancer cells, facilitating hepatic infection, and it is specifically recognized by glycoproteins which bind with it. The MSN-LA-SO@siVEGF nanocarrier induced synthesis (S) phase cell-cycle arrest, increasing the anti-cancer efficacy (cell apoptosis) of SO and siVEGF through the active targeting of LA in ASGPR-overexpressing Huh7 tumoral cells. Furthermore, this nanosystem enhanced the siVEGF transfection efficiency and inhibited the expression of angiogenesis-related VEGF proteins in these tumoral cells. Taking both studies together, these types of functionalized MSN-based nanosystems could be potential nanocarriers for targeted delivery of anti-tumoral drugs and VEGF siRNAs to improve anti-tumor capability.

On the other hand, fibrotic diseases are related to augmented oxidative stress and upregulation of pro-fibrotic genes [181]. Oxygen species (ROS), nicotinamide adenine dinucleotide phosphate

(NADPH) oxidase 4 (NOX4) and heat-shock protein 47 (HSP47) are implicated in this disease [181], producing disproportionate collagen synthesis. Morry et al. [167] proposed an MSN platform with PEI and PEG coating that effectively delivered HSP47 siRNA in vitro and in vivo. This nanocarrier induced a knockdown of the HSP47 gene and a decrease in ROS and NOX4 levels in an in vitro model of fibrosis based on TGF-β-stimulated fibroblasts. Intradermal administration of MSNs@siHSP47 successfully decreased HSP47 protein levels in a bleomycin-induced scleroderma mouse model in vivo, reducing ROS production and different pro-fibrotic markers. These nanocarriers could be a very interesting platform to treat both fibrotic and inflammation diseases. On the other hand, it is necessary to develop anti-fibrotic drugs for chronic liver fibrotic diseases. Hepatic stellate cell (HSC) activation is present in the progression of liver fibrosis, secreting extracellular matrix proteins as tenascin-C (TnC). Vivero-Escoto et al. [168] proposed an MSN@siTnC based nanosystem as a favorable alternative to evaluate the siRNA therapy of chronic liver disease in preclinical trials. This novel nanocarrier was successfully internalized by human stem cells in vitro and produced a downregulation in TnC mRNA and protein levels, inducing a decrease in inflammatory cytokine expression by macrophages and hepatoma migration. These promising results must be tested in a liver fibrosis in vivo model.

As demonstrated in this section, siRNA-MSN based nanosystems were widely studied and showed a high efficiency in silencing genes and reducing tumoral growth related to cancer processes in vivo. Nevertheless, in tissue engineering applications, scaffold-mediated delivery is desired to achieve local and sustained release of drugs. In this respect, Pinese et al. [169] developed an MSN-PEI@siRNA nanocarrier delivered from electrospun scaffolds via surface adsorption and nanofiber encapsulation. These nanosystems were either combined with the surfaces of nanofiber substrates or directly encapsulated. MSN-PEI@siRNA coated scaffolds offered sustained availability of siRNA for at least 30 days and five months in the case of MSN-PEI@siRNA-encapsulated scaffolds within the electrospun fibers in human dermal fibroblasts cells in vitro. The scaffolds showed excellent bifunctionality in vitro and in vivo by targeting collagen type I (COLL1A1) as a target gene to reduce fibrous capsule formation. These platforms were subcutaneously implanted in a rat model in vivo and COLL1A1 siRNA/MSN-PEI induced a reduction of 45.8% in fibrous capsule formation after four weeks compared to negative siRNA treatment. This method improved siRNA internalization rates and sustained targeted protein silencing in vitro and in vivo. The nanoplatform proposed by these authors can be used to release and internalize siRNA/miRNA combined with other specific low-molecular-weight drugs in long-term tissue engineering applications and cancer. In addition, the current pharmacological therapy of bone diseases such as osteoporosis presents several limitations related to bioavailability and toxicity. In this sense, gene knockdown through siRNA delivery received great attention as a promising treatment in osteoporosis [182]. In a recent study by Mora-Raimundo et al. [170], a nanosystem based on MSN-PEI, which can effectively deliver SOST siRNA and osteostatin inside cells, was evaluated in vitro and in vivo. The SOST gene inhibits the Wnt signaling pathway, decreasing osteoblast differentiation, whereas osteostatin is a pentapeptide with osteogenic and anti-osteoclastic properties [183]. SOST siRNA/MSN-PEI loaded with osteostatin induced a dramatic suppression of SOST gene expression in mouse embryonic fibroblastic cells with the consequent upregulation of several osteogenic markers with a synergistic effect. In vivo, the complete nanosystem was injected in the femoral bone marrow of ovariectomized mice, and the results were in concordance with in vitro studies, knocking down SOST and upregulating the osteogenic marker levels in a synergistic manner. The nanoplatform proposed by these authors was able to transport, co-deliver, and internalize SOST siRNA and osteostatin in cells, preserving its activity and achieving an effective silencing effect.

5.3. *miRNAs*

MiRNAs are small endogenous noncoding RNA molecules (17–25 nucleotides) that act as regulators of gene expression and downregulate target proteins via miRNA degradation or translational inhibition [184]. The aberrant expression of miRNAs in several cancers is associated with several mechanisms such as cellular differentiation, proliferation, survival, and apoptosis [184,185]. MiRNAs can accomplish a gene knockdown effect by regulating multiple miRNAs compared to siRNA, which is very useful when treating complex multifactorial diseases such as cancer [184,185]. Several drugs based on miRNAs were used in clinical trials in cancer [186]; however, the effective and safe delivery of anti-miRNAs or miRNA mimics is a key challenge for clinical applications.

Regarding these objectives, Li et al. [171] proposed a novel nanosystem based on MSN functionalized with polymerized dopamine (PDA) and AS1411 aptamer loaded with microRNA-155 (anti-miRNA-loaded MSN@PDA-Apt) for the specific treatment of colorectal cancer (CRC). Upregulation of miR-155 (oncogenic microRNA) was found in several cancer-related pathways, including in CRC. Firstly, the authors demonstrated that nuclear factor kappa B (NF-κB), an important transcription factor with a crucial role in the process of tumor growth, has a positive feedback loop with miR-155 in vitro and in CRC tissues. MSNs-anti-miR-155@PDA-Apt decreased miR-155 expression in SW480 cells and successfully targeted the CRC tumor, leading to gene knockdown and tumor growth reduction, thanks to both active targeting of AS1411 aptamer and passive targeting of the EPR effect. In addition, the same authors [172] explored the miR-328 pathway and developed a new pH-responsive nanoplatform consisting of MSNs-miRNA-328 decorated with PDA, a cell adhesion molecule aptamer, and bevacizumab (MSNs-miR-328@PDA-PEG-Apt-Bev) for the dual-targeting treatment of CRC. MiR-328 is a tumor suppressor downregulated in several human cancers, including CRC, and it is correlated with drug resistance. The authors demonstrated for the first time that CPTP, a ubiquitously expressed lipid transfer protein associated with inflammation and CRC, is a direct target of miR-328. MSNs-miR-328@PDA-PEG-Apt-Bev increased miR-328 levels and inhibited CPTP expression in SW480 cells, increasing binding ability and showing much higher cytotoxicity in vitro and in vivo. In addition, this nanoplatform showed efficient gene silencing and tumor growth inhibition of the target tumor in a SW480 xenograft mouse tumor model in vivo. Taken together, these results indicate that the MSN-based functionalized nanoplatforms reported herein show promise for miRNA therapy in cancer, specifically CRC. In a recent study by Ahir et al. [173], a nanosystem based on MSN-HA@miRNA with an appended PEG–poly(lactic-*co*-glycolic acid) (PLGA) polymer to target triple-negative breast cancer (TNBC) was evaluated in vitro and in vivo. In this context, miR-34a is downregulated and miR-10b is upregulated in TNBC disease, inducing tumorigenesis and metastatic dissemination. These authors proposed the MSN nanocarrier for co-delivery of miR-34a-mimic and antisense-miR-10b, targeting the CD44 receptor. In vitro, this nanosystem showed positive results in terms of cellular internalization rates, release profile, and a subsequent pro-apoptosis effect in human mammary carcinoma cell lines (MDAMB-231 and MDAMB-468). In vivo studies exhibited a high specificity in TNBC tumor targeting, leading to effective tumor growth reduction and metastasis delay in mice.

As previously mentioned, MSN nanosystems emerged as a promising bone regeneration methodology in bone tissue engineering. In this regard, Yan et al. [174] developed a novel miR-26a delivery nanosystem based on MSNs. MiR-26a was confirmed to regulate several pathways of osteogenic differentiation and promote bone regeneration. The authors demonstrated the protection effectiveness of the vectors to the miRNA and the positive internalization rates in rat bone marrow stromal cells (BMSCs) in vitro, releasing miR-26a into the cytoplasm without cytotoxicity effects. This nanosystem promoted stem-cell osteogenic differentiation, inducing an increase in alkaline phosphatase activity and mineralization, as well as in several genes and proteins implicated in osteogenesis in BMSCs. The nanocarrier proposed by these authors provides new methods and strategies for the delivery of mRNAs in bone tissue engineering, but it is necessary to further validate them in vivo.

On the other hand, a combined siRNA/miRNA therapy would be a very interesting approach, especially for cancer treatment, targeting multiple disease-related pathways and silencing specific genes. Currently, the use of this combination in clinical studies shows several limitations such as the availability of safe and effective systemic delivery nanocarriers with efficient tumor penetration. In this respect, Wang et al. [175] developed multifunctional tumor-penetrating MSNs for co-delivery of siRNA (siPlk1) and miRNA (miR-200c), upregulated in several types of tumor and implicated in cancer development and progression. In addition, the authors functionalized the nanosystem to facilitate endosomal scape using a photosensitizer indocyanine green (ICG) and surface conjugation of the iRGD peptide to allow deep tumor penetration. The complete nanosystem induced an increase in internalization rates in MDA-MB-231 cells and three-dimensional (3D) tumor spheroids in vitro, whereas ROS produced by ICG upon light irradiation induced the endosomal scape of the siRNA/miRNA into the cytoplasm with a deleterious effect on cell viability. In vivo, a significant reduction in tumor growth and metastasis upon short-light irradiation was found when the nanosystem was intravenously administrated in mice with metastatic breast cancer.

6. Delivery of Glycan-Based Biomolecules

Beyond the use of proteins, peptides, and nucleotides, glycan-based structures were also successfully employed in MSN-based delivery. Among them, the most recurrent examples are reported with heparin, chondroitin sulfate (CS), chitosan, and HA. Those compounds, apart from being important components of structural matrices, are known to affect many biochemical processes. For instance, HA is a valuable targeting element for the development of new therapeutic tools, as it is able to interact with CD44 and CD168, which are upregulated in many cancerous cells and are closely related to cell adhesion and migration in metastases [187,188].

Similarly, chitosan [188–190] and chondroitin sulfate [191–193] were employed for the development of high colloidally stable and biocompatible nanosystems with certain targeting capabilities. Moreover, as both substances are important structural components of extracellular matrices on vertebrates and crustaceans, they can act as bioactive components for tissue regeneration. Such was the case in the contributions by Kavya et al. [194] and Porgham Daryasari et al. [195], who employed those elements to induce osteogenesis through two different approaches. In the first approach, Kavya et al. designed a crosslinked chitosan/CS scaffold reinforced with nanometric SiO_2. In this system, the presence of silica permitted improving the mechanical properties and obtaining slower degradation, while the glycans permitted obtaining an adequate moisture swelling for creating a favorable environment for cell proliferation [194]. In the article by Porgham Daryasari et al., the authors employed chitosan-coated, dexamethasone-loaded MSNs as a bioactive component in a poly-L-lactic acid scaffold. The system was proven to induce osteogenic differentiation of human adipose stem cells according to the ALP activity [195]. Although both models offered promising results, the absence of osteoregeneration experiments in vivo makes these materials a mere design exercise, in which the presence of glycans is not completely justified. Apart from its use as a stabilizer, CS was also successfully employed as a functional coating able to interact with blood lipoproteins through a double effect: electrostatic interaction plus saccharide recognition [196]. Although these CS-modified dendritic MSNs permitted selectively binding and isolating low-density lipoproteins (LDL) for analytical purposes, the potential of such a nanosystem as a therapeutic agent is of enormous interest, as it may enable an interesting therapeutic effect against hypercholesterolemia and blood vessel atheromatosis.

Heparin is a highly sulfated, negatively charged glycosaminoglycan with outstanding properties as an anticoagulant. Beyond injectable applications, heparin is employed as an anticoagulant surface in medical devices like test tubes and dialysis machines. Regarding additional uses in combination with mesoporous silica, its capacity as a targeting moiety was also described against human hepatocyte carcinoma HepG2 [197,198] and HUVEC cell lines [198].

Additionally, as a consequence of its anticoagulant effect, some investigations focused on improving its release profile from silica-based carriers as nanodepots. Along this line, the research articles authored by Zhu and coworkers performed two systematic studies on how different types of mesoporous silica, with varying pore sizes and functionalization, affected the loading-release process [199,200]. Based on their results, the authors established that a slight pore enlargement of MCM-41 yielded better adsorption and release. Indeed, they also demonstrated that the presence of amino groups in the mesopores increased the amount of heparin adsorbed, albeit at the expense of slowing down the release [199]. With regard to SBA-15, they found that, apart from pore size and charge, the presence of rough pore surfaces caused by carbonaceous deposits upon calcination boosted both the retention and the release of heparin, improving the performance of such a material and enabling access to better-performing nanodepots.

Apart from its use as a drug delivery agent, there are examples of heparin-loaded silica-based materials used as anticoagulant coatings for medical devices. For example, Wei et al. reported the use of SBA-15 to prepare a heparin-releasing anticoagulant coating [201]. Their system employed amino-modified mesopores to favor heparin loading and delay its release. To incorporate these particles into chosen substrates (silicon wafer, glass, or polyvinylchloride), the authors coated the particles with polydopamine and the substrate with a catechol-modified chitosan polymer. This configuration permitted depositing the negatively charged, heparin loaded MSNs onto chitosan, which was further bound to the catechol–dopamine coating of substrates. Finally, to prevent undesired detachment, this dopamine–catechol bond was oxidized with $NaIO_4$ in order to create a non-degradable polymeric layer. When the authors tested this coating against blood, they found a very low fibrinogen adsorption, as well as platelet adhesion and hemolysis, which is in concordance with a sustained anticoagulant release and good biocompatibility. More recently, Wu et al. reported a similar approach but with an added feature: antibacterial adhesion. To achieving this, the authors loaded the mesopores of MSNs with two glycan-based structures: agarose for an antibacterial effect and heparin as an anticoagulant [202]. The agarose-heparin loaded MCM-41 nanoparticles were electrostatically immobilized onto the prepared device, i.e., an amino-modified silicone film. Therefore, the final coating presented a negative charge and exposed mesopores, which were able to produce effective agarose and heparin release. The system demonstrated a low hemolytic effect comparable with that of the previous model but with an additional antibacterial effect against *E. coli*, gaining additional applicability. However, regarding the design, the possibility of detaching SBA-15 particles within the bloodstream has to be considered as a potential risk and must be accounted for in the further development of such devices.

7. Challenges and Future Perspectives

As reviewed, the number of developing therapeutic hybrid nanosystems employing biomolecules together with mesoporous silica nanoparticles is enormous, as reported over the last few years. In general, and according to the literature here visited, cancer therapy is by far the most active research field and the one that exploits the most up-to-date technological advances such as PEGylation, controlled drug delivery, or the implementation of hybrid nanomaterials, among many others. However, such technology permitted developing alternative therapies to cancer, applied to other not-so-common diseases with a promising prognosis. This fact is largely due to the particular structure of MSNs, with a high capacity to load and release therapeutic molecules within their porous matrix. However, the advancement of knowledge and the need to adapt these nanomaterials to advanced preclinical in vivo models, with new aspects in loading and release systems, must be considered when designing these medical nanosystems. In this context, short therapeutic peptides and small molecules seem to be the ideal target for transfer to preclinical studies because they can be easily designed, developed, functionalized, and coupled. Among these new emerging therapeutic strategies with biomolecules that came to light recently, the most promising for implementation together with mesoporous silica materials seem to be immune therapy, gene modulation, and anti-infective nano-agents, as can be determined from the number and quality of related papers. In any case, there are different issues to be addressed regarding the nanocarriers themselves such as the absence of reliable in vivo pre-clinical studies, methods of clearance of the nanoplatforms, and how different particles properties (shape, size, pore symmetry and connectivity, and chemical composition) affect their application in nanomedicine.

Author Contributions: D.L. and R.R.C. contributed equally to this work, M.V.-R. coordinated the work. All authors have read and agreed to the published version of the manuscript.

Abbreviations

ATP	Adenosine triphosphate
Bcl-2	B-cell lymphoma 2
bFGF	Basic fibroblast growth factor
BM	Biomacromolecule
BMP-2	Bone morphogenetic protein 2
bMSCs	Murine bone mesenchymal stem cells
BSA	Bovine serum albumin
CA	Carbonic anhydrase
cAMP	Cyclic adenosine monophosphate
COLL1A1	Collagen type 1
ConA	Concanavalin A
CS	Chondroitin sulfate
DMOHS	Dendritic mesoporous organosilica hollow spheres
DNA	Deoxyribonucleic acid
Cyt c	Cytochrome c
DOX	Doxorubicin
FA	Folic acid/folate
gG	Immunoglobulin G
GFP	Green fluorescent protein
GM-CSF	Murine granulocyte-macrophage colony-stimulating factor
GPx	Glutathione peroxidase
HMSNs	Hollow mesoporous silica nanoparticles
HA	Hyaluronic acid
HDFs	Human dermal fibroblasts
HOS	Human osteosarcoma
HRP	Horseradish peroxidase
HSCs	Human stem cells
HSP47	Heat-shock protein 47
IDMSN	Imidazole dendritic mesoporous silica nanoparticles
IL-2	Interleukin-2
kDa	Kilodaltons
LA	Lactobionic acid
LDL	Low-density lipoprotein
MCM-41	Mobil composition of matter formulation 41
MDR1	Multidrug resistance protein 1
MEF	Mouse embryonic fibroblastic cells
MPLA	Monophosphoryl lipid A
miRNA	Micro ribonucleic acid
mRNA	messenger ribonucleic acid
MSNs	Mesoporous silica nanoparticles
NA	Nucleic acid
NOX4	NADPH oxidase 4
OGP	Osteogenic growth peptide
OVA	Chicken ovalbumin
PAMAM	Polyamidoamine dendrimer
PDA	Polydopamine
PEG	Polyethylene glycol
PEI	Polyethyleneimine
pGFP	Fluorescent protein plasmid

PKM2	Glycolytic enzyme pyruvate kinase
PMDFs	Primary mouse dermal fibroblast
ROS	Oxygen species
RSNs	Rough (non-porous and core–shell) silica nanoparticles
SBA-15	Santa Barbara amorphous formulation 15
rBMSCs	Rat bone marrow stromal cells
RCA	Rolling circle amplification
shRNA	Short hairpin ribonucleic acid
siRNA	Small interfering ribonucleic acid
SO	Sorafenib
SOD	Superoxide dismutase
SPIONs	Superparamagnetic iron oxide nanoparticles.
TAT	Transactivator of transcription
TnC	Tenascin-C
TGFβR-1	Transforming growth factor beta receptor I
VEGF	Vascular endothelial growth factor

References

1. Vallet-Regi, M.; Rámila, A.; del Real, R.P.; Pérez-Pariente, J. A New Property of MCM-41: Drug Delivery System. *Chem. Mater.* **2001**, *13*, 308–311. [CrossRef]
2. Yang, J.; Li, L.; Kopeček, J. Biorecognition: A key to drug-free macromolecular therapeutics. *Biomaterials* **2019**, *190*, 11–23. [CrossRef]
3. Sever, R.; Brugge, J.S. Signal Transduction in Cancer. *Cold Spring Harb. Perspect. Med.* **2015**, *5*, a006098. [CrossRef]
4. Núñez-Lozano, R.; Cano, M.; Pimentel, B.; de la Cueva-Méndez, G. 'Smartening' anticancer therapeutic nanosystems using biomolecules. *Curr. Opin. Biotechnol.* **2015**, *35*, 135–140. [CrossRef]
5. Castillo, R.R.; Lozano, D.; González, B.; Manzano, M.; Izquierdo-Barba, I.; Vallet-Regí, M. Advances in mesoporous silica nanoparticles for targeted stimuli-responsive drug delivery: An update. *Expert Opin. Drug Deliv.* **2019**, *16*, 415–439. [CrossRef]
6. Dempke, W.C.M.; Fenchel, K.; Uciechowski, P.; Dale, S.P. Second-and third-generation drugs for immuno-oncology treatment—The more the better? *Eur. J. Cancer* **2017**, *74*, 55–72. [CrossRef]
7. Topalian, S.L.; Taube, J.M.; Anders, R.A.; Pardoll, D.M. Mechanism-driven biomarkers to guide immune checkpoint blockade in cancer therapy. *Nat. Rev. Cancer* **2016**, *16*, 275–287. [CrossRef]
8. Ribas, A.; Wolchok, J.D. Cancer immunotherapy using checkpoint blockade. *Science* **2018**, *359*, 1350–1355. [CrossRef]
9. Ahuja, N.; Sharma, A.R.; Baylin, S.B. Epigenetic Therapeutics: A New Weapon in the War Against Cancer. *Annu. Rev. Med.* **2016**, *67*, 73–89. [CrossRef]
10. Das, S.K.; Menezes, M.E.; Bhatia, S.; Wang, X.-Y.; Emdad, L.; Sarkar, D.; Fisher, P.B. Gene Therapies for Cancer: Strategies, Challenges and Successes. *J. Cell. Physiol.* **2015**, *230*, 259–271. [CrossRef]
11. Fukuhara, H.; Ino, Y.; Todo, T. Oncolytic virus therapy: A new era of cancer treatment at dawn. *Cancer Sci.* **2016**, *107*, 1373–1379. [CrossRef]
12. Yamada, H.; Urata, C.; Aoyama, Y.; Osada, S.; Yamauchi, Y.; Kuroda, K. Preparation of colloidal mesoporous silica nanoparticles with different diameters and their unique degradation behavior in static aqueous systems. *Chem. Mater.* **2012**, *24*, 1462–1471. [CrossRef]
13. Yamada, H.; Urata, C.; Ujiie, H.; Yamauchi, Y.; Kuroda, K. Preparation of aqueous colloidal mesostructured and mesoporous silica nanoparticles with controlled particle size in a very wide range from 20 nm to 700 nm. *Nanoscale* **2013**, *5*, 6145–6153. [CrossRef] [PubMed]
14. Knežević, N.Ž.; Durand, J.-O. Large pore mesoporous silica nanomaterials for application in delivery of biomolecules. *Nanoscale* **2015**, *7*, 2199–2209. [CrossRef] [PubMed]
15. Wu, S.H.; Lin, H.P. Synthesis of mesoporous silica nanoparticles. *Chem. Soc. Rev.* **2013**, *42*, 3862–3875. [CrossRef]

16. Lindén, M. Biodistribution and Excretion of Intravenously Injected Mesoporous Silica Nanoparticles: Implications for Drug Delivery Efficiency and Safety. In *The Enzymes*; Elsevier: Amsterdam, The Netherlands, 2018; Volume 43, pp. 155–180.
17. Croissant, J.G.; Fatieiev, Y.; Khashab, N.M. Degradability and Clearance of Silicon, Organosilica, Silsesquioxane, Silica Mixed Oxide, and Mesoporous Silica Nanoparticles. *Adv. Mater.* **2017**, *29*, 1604634. [CrossRef]
18. Castillo, R.R.; Vallet-Regí, M. Functional Mesoporous Silica Nanocomposites: Biomedical applications and Biosafety. *Int. J. Mol. Sci.* **2019**, *20*, 929. [CrossRef]
19. Castillo, R.R.; Colilla, M.; Vallet-Regí, M. Advances in mesoporous silica-based nanocarriers for co-delivery and combination therapy against cancer. *Expert Opin. Drug Deliv.* **2017**, *14*, 229–243. [CrossRef]
20. Castillo, R.R.; Baeza, A.; Vallet-Regí, M. Recent applications of the combination of mesoporous silica nanoparticles with nucleic acids: Development of bioresponsive devices, carriers and sensors. *Biomater. Sci.* **2017**, *5*, 353–377. [CrossRef]
21. Narayan, R.; Nayak, U.; Raichur, A.; Garg, S. Mesoporous Silica Nanoparticles: A Comprehensive Review on Synthesis and Recent Advances. *Pharmaceutics* **2018**, *10*, 118. [CrossRef]
22. Vallet-Regí, M.; Balas, F.; Colilla, M.; Manzano, M. Bone-regenerative bioceramic implants with drug and protein controlled delivery capability. *Prog. Solid State Chem.* **2008**, *36*, 163–191. [CrossRef]
23. Anselmo, A.C.; Mitragotri, S. A Review of Clinical Translation of Inorganic Nanoparticles. *AAPS J.* **2015**, *17*, 1041–1054. [CrossRef] [PubMed]
24. Anselmo, A.C.; Mitragotri, S. Nanoparticles in the clinic: An update. *Bioeng. Transl. Med.* **2019**, *4*, e10143. [CrossRef]
25. Florence, A.T. Nanotechnologies for site specific drug delivery: Changing the narrative. *Int. J. Pharm.* **2018**, *551*, 1–7. [CrossRef]
26. Baeza, A.; Manzano, M.; Colilla, M.; Vallet-Regí, M. Recent advances in mesoporous silica nanoparticles for antitumor therapy: Our contribution. *Biomater. Sci.* **2016**, *4*, 803–813. [CrossRef]
27. Singh, R.K.; Knowles, J.C.; Kim, H.-W. Advances in nanoparticle development for improved therapeutics delivery: Nanoscale topographical aspect. *J. Tissue Eng.* **2019**, *10*, 1–9. [CrossRef]
28. Niu, Y.; Yu, M.; Meka, A.; Liu, Y.; Zhang, J.; Yang, Y.; Yu, C. Understanding the contribution of surface roughness and hydrophobic modification of silica nanoparticles to enhanced therapeutic protein delivery. *J. Mater. Chem. B.* **2016**, *4*, 212–219. [CrossRef]
29. Song, H.; Yu, M.; Lu, Y.; Gu, Z.; Yang, Y.; Zhang, M.; Fu, J.; Yu, C. Plasmid DNA Delivery: Nanotopography Matters. *J. Am. Chem. Soc.* **2017**, *139*, 18247–18254. [CrossRef]
30. Aznar, E.; Oroval, M.; Pascual, L.; Murguía, J.R.; Martínez-Máñez, R.; Sancenón, F. Gated Materials for On-Command Release of Guest Molecules. *Chem. Rev.* **2016**, *116*, 561–718. [CrossRef]
31. Thi, T.T.H.; Nguyen, T.N.Q.; Hoang, D.T.; Nguyen, D.H. Functionalized mesoporous silica nanoparticles and biomedical applications. *Mater. Sci. Eng. C* **2019**, *99*, 631–656. [CrossRef]
32. Hu, J.J.; Xiao, D.; Zhang, X.Z. Advances in Peptide Functionalization on Mesoporous Silica Nanoparticles for Controlled Drug Release. *Small* **2016**, *12*, 3344–3359. [CrossRef] [PubMed]
33. Bruno, B.J.; Miller, G.D.; Lim, C.S. Basics and recent advances in peptide and protein drug delivery. *Ther. Deliv.* **2013**, *4*, 1443–1467. [CrossRef] [PubMed]
34. Baker, M. Reproducibility crisis: Blame it on the antibodies. *Nature* **2015**, *521*, 274–276. [CrossRef] [PubMed]
35. Montenegro, J.-M.; Grazu, V.; Sukhanova, A.; Agarwal, S.; de la Fuente, J.M.; Nabiev, I.; Greiner, A.; Parak, W.J. Controlled antibody/(bio-) conjugation of inorganic nanoparticles for targeted delivery. *Adv. Drug Deliv. Rev.* **2013**, *65*, 677–688. [CrossRef] [PubMed]
36. Cheng, K.; El-Boubbou, K.; Landry, C.C. Binding of HIV-1 gp120 Glycoprotein to Silica Nanoparticles Modified with CD4 Glycoprotein and CD4 Peptide Fragments. *ACS Appl. Mater. Interfaces* **2012**, *4*, 235–243. [CrossRef]
37. Kamegawa, R.; Naito, M.; Miyata, K. Functionalization of silica nanoparticles for nucleic acid delivery. *Nano Res.* **2018**, *11*, 5219–5239. [CrossRef]
38. Benjaminsen, R.V.; Mattebjerg, M.A.; Henriksen, J.R.; Moghimi, S.M.; Andresen, T.L. The Possible "Proton Sponge" Effect of Polyethylenimine (PEI) Does Not Include Change in Lysosomal pH. *Mol. Ther.* **2013**, *21*, 149–157. [CrossRef]

39. Boraschi, D.; Duschl, A. (Eds.) *Nanoparticles and the Immune System*; Academic Press: Cambridge, MA, USA, 2014; ISBN 9780124080850.
40. Tu, J.; Boyle, A.L.; Friedrich, H.; Bomans, P.H.H.; Bussmann, J.; Sommerdijk, N.A.J.M.; Jiskoot, W.; Kros, A. Mesoporous Silica Nanoparticles with Large Pores for the Encapsulation and Release of Proteins. *ACS Appl. Mater. Interfaces* **2016**, *8*, 32211–32219. [CrossRef]
41. Kruk, M. Access to Ultralarge-Pore Ordered Mesoporous Materials through Selection of Surfactant/ Swelling-Agent Micellar Templates. *Acc. Chem. Res.* **2012**, *45*, 1678–1687. [CrossRef]
42. Gao, Z.; Zharov, I. Large Pore Mesoporous Silica Nanoparticles by Templating with a Nonsurfactant Molecule, Tannic Acid. *Chem. Mater.* **2014**, *26*, 2030–2037. [CrossRef]
43. Balas, F.; Manzano, M.; Horcajada, P.; Vallet-Regi, M. Confinement and controlled release of bisphosphonates on ordered mesoporous silica-based materials. *J. Am. Chem. Soc.* **2006**, *128*, 8116–8117. [CrossRef] [PubMed]
44. Wu, M.; Meng, Q.; Chen, Y.; Du, Y.; Zhang, L.; Li, Y.; Zhang, L.; Shi, J. Large-Pore Ultrasmall Mesoporous Organosilica Nanoparticles: Micelle/Precursor Co-templating Assembly and Nuclear-Targeted Gene Delivery. *Adv. Mater.* **2015**, *27*, 215–222. [CrossRef] [PubMed]
45. Na, H.-K.; Kim, M.-H.; Park, K.; Ryoo, S.-R.; Lee, K.E.; Jeon, H.; Ryoo, R.; Hyeon, C.; Min, D.-H. Efficient Functional Delivery of siRNA using Mesoporous Silica Nanoparticles with Ultralarge Pores. *Small* **2012**, *8*, 1752–1761. [CrossRef] [PubMed]
46. Ashley, C.E.; Carnes, E.C.; Epler, K.E.; Padilla, D.P.; Phillips, G.K.; Castillo, R.E.; Wilkinson, D.C.; Wilkinson, B.S.; Burgard, C.A.; Kalinich, R.M.; et al. Delivery of Small Interfering RNA by Peptide-Targeted Mesoporous Silica Nanoparticle-Supported Lipid Bilayers. *ACS Nano* **2012**, *6*, 2174–2188. [CrossRef]
47. Akash, M.S.H.; Rehman, K.; Tariq, M.; Chen, S. Development of therapeutic proteins: Advances and challenges. *Turk. J. Biol.* **2015**, *39*, 343–358. [CrossRef]
48. Liu, H.-J.; Xu, P. Smart Mesoporous Silica Nanoparticles for Protein Delivery. *Nanomaterials* **2019**, *9*, 511. [CrossRef]
49. Xu, C.; Lei, C.; Yu, C. Mesoporous Silica Nanoparticles for Protein Protection and Delivery. *Front. Chem.* **2019**, *7*, 290. [CrossRef]
50. Yu, M.; Gu, Z.; Ottewell, T.; Yu, C. Silica-based nanoparticles for therapeutic protein delivery. *J. Mater. Chem. B* **2017**, *5*, 3241–3252. [CrossRef]
51. Deodhar, G.V.; Adams, M.L.; Trewyn, B.G. Controlled release and intracellular protein delivery from mesoporous silica nanoparticles. *Biotechnol. J.* **2017**, *12*, 1600408. [CrossRef]
52. Karpiński, T.; Adamczak, A. Anticancer Activity of Bacterial Proteins and Peptides. *Pharmaceutics* **2018**, *10*, 54. [CrossRef]
53. Liu, X.; Wu, F.; Ji, Y.; Yin, L. Recent Advances in Anti-cancer Protein/Peptide Delivery. *Bioconjug. Chem.* **2019**, *30*, 305–324. [CrossRef] [PubMed]
54. Slowing, I.I.; Trewyn, B.G.; Lin, V.S.-Y. Mesoporous Silica Nanoparticles for Intracellular Delivery of Membrane-Impermeable Proteins. *J. Am. Chem. Soc.* **2007**, *129*, 8845–8849. [CrossRef] [PubMed]
55. Méndez, J.; Morales Cruz, M.; Delgado, Y.; Figueroa, C.M.; Orellano, E.A.; Morales, M.; Monteagudo, A.; Griebenow, K. Delivery of chemically glycosylated cytochrome c immobilized in mesoporous silica nanoparticles induces apoptosis in HeLa cancer cells. *Mol. Pharm.* **2014**, *11*, 102–111. [CrossRef] [PubMed]
56. Shang, W.; Nuffer, J.H.; Muñiz-Papandrea, V.A.; Colón, W.; Siegel, R.W.; Dordick, J.S. Cytochrome c on silica nanoparticles: Influence of nanoparticle size on protein structure, stability, and activity. *Small* **2009**, *5*, 470–476. [CrossRef]
57. Huang, W.-Y.; Davies, G.-L.; Davis, J.J. Engineering Cytochrome-Modified Silica Nanoparticles To Induce Programmed Cell Death. *Chem. A Eur. J.* **2013**, *19*, 17891–17898. [CrossRef]
58. Choi, E.; Lim, D.-K.; Kim, S. Hydrolytic surface erosion of mesoporous silica nanoparticles for efficient intracellular delivery of cytochrome c. *J. Colloid Interface Sci.* **2020**, *560*, 416–425. [CrossRef]
59. Martínez-Carmona, M.; Lozano, D.; Colilla, M.; Vallet-Regí, M. Lectin-conjugated pH-responsive mesoporous silica nanoparticles for targeted bone cancer treatment. *Acta Biomater.* **2018**, *65*, 393–404. [CrossRef]
60. Lim, J.-S.; Lee, K.; Choi, J.-N.; Hwang, Y.-K.; Yun, M.-Y.; Kim, H.-J.; Won, Y.S.; Kim, S.-J.; Kwon, H.; Huh, S. Intracellular protein delivery by hollow mesoporous silica capsules with a large surface hole. *Nanotechnology* **2012**, *23*, 085101. [CrossRef]

61. Wang, X.; Li, X.; Ito, A.; Yoshiyuki, K.; Sogo, Y.; Watanabe, Y.; Yamazaki, A.; Ohno, T.; Tsuji, N.M. Silica Nanospheres: Hollow Structure Improved Anti-Cancer Immunity of Mesoporous Silica Nanospheres In Vivo. *Small* **2016**, *12*, 3510–3515. [CrossRef]
62. Wang, X.; Li, X.; Yoshiyuki, K.; Watanabe, Y.; Sogo, Y.; Ohno, T.; Tsuji, N.M.; Ito, A. Comprehensive Mechanism Analysis of Mesoporous-Silica-Nanoparticle-Induced Cancer Immunotherapy. *Adv. Healthc. Mater.* **2016**, *5*, 1169–1176. [CrossRef]
63. Yang, Y.; Lu, Y.; Abbaraju, P.L.; Zhang, J.; Zhang, M.; Xiang, G.; Yu, C. Multi-shelled Dendritic Mesoporous Organosilica Hollow Spheres: Roles of Composition and Architecture in Cancer Immunotherapy. *Angew. Chem. Int. Ed.* **2017**, *56*, 8446–8450. [CrossRef] [PubMed]
64. Cha, B.G.; Jeong, J.H.; Kim, J. Extra-Large Pore Mesoporous Silica Nanoparticles Enabling Co-Delivery of High Amounts of Protein Antigen and Toll-like Receptor 9 Agonist for Enhanced Cancer Vaccine Efficacy. *ACS Cent. Sci.* **2018**, *4*, 484–492. [CrossRef] [PubMed]
65. Nguyen, T.L.; Cha, B.G.; Choi, Y.; Im, J.; Kim, J. Injectable dual-scale mesoporous silica cancer vaccine enabling efficient delivery of antigen/adjuvant-loaded nanoparticles to dendritic cells recruited in local macroporous scaffold. *Biomaterials* **2020**, *239*, 119859. [CrossRef] [PubMed]
66. Niu, Y.; Yu, M.; Zhang, J.; Yang, Y.; Xu, C.; Yeh, M.; Taran, E.; Hou, J.J.C.; Gray, P.P.; Yu, C. Synthesis of silica nanoparticles with controllable surface roughness for therapeutic protein delivery. *J. Mater. Chem. B* **2015**, *3*, 8477–8485. [CrossRef] [PubMed]
67. Kong, M.; Tang, J.; Qiao, Q.; Wu, T.; Qi, Y.; Tan, S.; Gao, X.; Zhang, Z. Biodegradable Hollow Mesoporous Silica Nanoparticles for Regulating Tumor Microenvironment and Enhancing Antitumor Efficiency. *Theranostics* **2017**, *7*, 3276–3292. [CrossRef]
68. Guo, H.C.; Feng, X.M.; Sun, S.Q.; Wei, Y.Q.; Sun, D.H.; Liu, X.T.; Liu, Z.X.; Luo, J.X.; Yin, H. Immunization of mice by hollow mesoporous silica nanoparticles as carriers of porcine circovirus type 2 ORF2 protein. *Virol. J.* **2012**, *9*, 1–10. [CrossRef]
69. Oliveira, D.C.d.P.; de Barros, A.L.B.; Belardi, R.M.; de Goes, A.M.; de Oliveira Souza, B.K.; Soares, D.C.F. Mesoporous silica nanoparticles as a potential vaccine adjuvant against Schistosoma mansoni. *J. Drug Deliv. Sci. Technol.* **2016**, *35*, 234–240. [CrossRef]
70. Virginio, V.G.; Bandeira, N.C.; dos Anjos Leal, F.M.; Lancellotti, M.; Zaha, A.; Ferreira, H.B. Assessment of the adjuvant activity of mesoporous silica nanoparticles in recombinant Mycoplasma hyopneumoniae antigen vaccines. *Heliyon* **2017**, *3*, e00225. [CrossRef]
71. Hajizade, A.; Salmanian, A.H.; Amani, J.; Ebrahimi, F.; Arpanaei, A. EspA-loaded mesoporous silica nanoparticles can efficiently protect animal model against enterohaemorrhagic E. coli O157: H7. *Artif. Cells Nanomed. Biotechnol.* **2018**, *46*, S1067–S1075. [CrossRef]
72. Ferreira Soares, D.C.; Soares, L.M.; Miranda de Goes, A.; Melo, E.M.; Branco de Barros, A.L.; Alves Santos Bicalho, T.C.; Leao, N.M.; Tebaldi, M.L. Mesoporous SBA-16 silica nanoparticles as a potential vaccine adjuvant against Paracoccidioides brasiliensis. *Microporous Mesoporous Mater.* **2020**, *291*, 109676. [CrossRef]
73. Méndez, J.; Monteagudo, A.; Griebenow, K. Stimulus-responsive controlled release system by covalent immobilization of an enzyme into mesoporous silica nanoparticles. *Bioconjug. Chem.* **2012**, *23*, 698–704. [CrossRef] [PubMed]
74. Gößl, D.; Singer, H.; Chiu, H.Y.; Schmidt, A.; Lichtnecker, M.; Engelke, H.; Bein, T. Highly active enzymes immobilized in large pore colloidal mesoporous silica nanoparticles. *N. J. Chem.* **2019**, *43*, 1671–1680. [CrossRef]
75. Xu, C.; Yu, M.; Noonan, O.; Zhang, J.; Song, H.; Zhang, H.; Lei, C.; Niu, Y.; Huang, X.; Yang, Y.; et al. Core-Cone Structured Monodispersed Mesoporous Silica Nanoparticles with Ultra-large Cavity for Protein Delivery. *Small* **2015**, *11*, 5949–5955. [CrossRef] [PubMed]
76. Chen, Y.P.; Chen, C.T.; Hung, Y.; Chou, C.M.; Liu, T.P.; Liang, M.R.; Chen, C.T.; Mou, C.Y. A new strategy for intracellular delivery of enzyme using mesoporous silica nanoparticles: Superoxide dismutase. *J. Am. Chem. Soc.* **2013**, *135*, 1516–1523. [CrossRef] [PubMed]
77. Lin, Y.H.; Chen, Y.P.; Liu, T.P.; Chien, F.C.; Chou, C.M.; Chen, C.T.; Mou, C.Y. Approach to Deliver Two Antioxidant Enzymes with Mesoporous Silica Nanoparticles into Cells. *ACS Appl. Mater. Interfaces* **2016**, *8*, 17944–17954. [CrossRef] [PubMed]

78. Han, D.H.; Na, H.-K.; Choi, W.H.; Lee, J.H.; Kim, Y.K.; Won, C.; Lee, S.-H.; Kim, K.P.; Kuret, J.; Min, D.-H.; et al. Direct cellular delivery of human proteasomes to delay tau aggregation. *Nat. Commun.* **2014**, *5*, 5633. [CrossRef]
79. Zhang, J.; Postovit, L.M.; Wang, D.; Gardiner, R.B.; Harris, R.; Abdul, M.M.; Thomas, A.A. In situ loading of basic fibroblast growth factor within porous silica nanoparticles for a prolonged release. *Nanoscale Res. Lett.* **2009**, *4*, 1297–1302. [CrossRef]
80. Gan, Q.; Zhu, J.; Yuan, Y.; Liu, H.; Qian, J.; Li, Y.; Liu, C. A dual-delivery system of pH-responsive chitosan-functionalized mesoporous silica nanoparticles bearing BMP-2 and dexamethasone for enhanced bone regeneration. *J. Mater. Chem. B* **2015**, *3*, 2056–2066. [CrossRef]
81. Gan, Q.; Zhu, J.; Yuan, Y.; Liu, C. pH-Responsive Fe3O4 Nanopartilces-Capped Mesoporous Silica Supports for Protein Delivery. *J. Nanosci. Nanotechnol.* **2016**, *16*, 5470–5479. [CrossRef]
82. Li, L.-L.; Wang, H. Enzyme-coated mesoporous silica nanoparticles as efficient antibacterial agents in vivo. *Adv. Healthc. Mater.* **2013**, *2*, 1351–1360. [CrossRef]
83. Wang, Y.; Nor, Y.A.; Song, H.; Yang, Y.; Xu, C.; Yu, M.; Yu, C. Small-sized and large-pore dendritic mesoporous silica nanoparticles enhance antimicrobial enzyme delivery. *J. Mater. Chem. B* **2016**, *4*, 2646–2653. [CrossRef] [PubMed]
84. Song, H.; Ahmad Nor, Y.; Yu, M.; Yang, Y.; Zhang, J.; Zhang, H.; Xu, C.; Mitter, N.; Yu, C. Silica Nanopollens Enhance Adhesion for Long-Term Bacterial Inhibition. *J. Am. Chem. Soc.* **2016**, *138*, 6455–6462. [CrossRef] [PubMed]
85. Xu, C.; He, Y.; Li, Z.; Ahmad Nor, Y.; Ye, Q. Nanoengineered hollow mesoporous silica nanoparticles for the delivery of antimicrobial proteins into biofilms. *J. Mater. Chem. B* **2018**, *6*, 1899–1902. [CrossRef]
86. Martínez-Carmona, M.; Izquierdo-Barba, I.; Colilla, M.; Vallet-Regí, M. Concanavalin A-targeted mesoporous silica nanoparticles for infection treatment. *Acta Biomater.* **2019**, *96*, 547–556. [CrossRef]
87. Wang, X.; Li, X.; Ito, A.; Sogo, Y.; Ohno, T. Particle-size-dependent toxicity and immunogenic activity of mesoporous silica-based adjuvants for tumor immunotherapy. *Acta Biomater.* **2013**, *9*, 7480–7489. [CrossRef]
88. Li, X.; Wang, X.; Sogo, Y.; Ohno, T.; Onuma, K.; Ito, A. Mesoporous Silica-Calcium Phosphate-Tuberculin Purified Protein Derivative Composites as an Effective Adjuvant for Cancer Immunotherapy. *Adv. Healthc. Mater.* **2013**, *2*, 863–871. [CrossRef]
89. Wang, X.; Li, X.; Ito, A.; Watanabe, Y.; Sogo, Y.; Tsuji, N.M.; Ohno, T. Stimulation of In Vivo Antitumor Immunity with Hollow Mesoporous Silica Nanospheres. *Angew. Chem. Int. Ed.* **2016**, *55*, 1899–1903. [CrossRef]
90. Kim, M.-G.; Park, J.Y.; Shon, Y.; Kim, G.; Shim, G.; Oh, Y.-K. Nanotechnology and vaccine development. *Asian J. Pharm. Sci.* **2014**, *9*, 227–235. [CrossRef]
91. Pati, R.; Shevtsov, M.; Sonawane, A. Nanoparticle Vaccines Against Infectious Diseases. *Front. Immunol.* **2018**, *9*, 2224. [CrossRef]
92. Villegas, M.R.; Baeza, A.; Vallet-Regí, M. Nanotechnological Strategies for Protein Delivery. *Molecules* **2018**, *23*, 1008. [CrossRef]
93. Zhao, M.; Liu, Y.; Hsieh, R.S.; Wang, N.; Tai, W.; Joo, K.-I.; Wang, P.; Gu, Z.; Tang, Y. Clickable Protein Nanocapsules for Targeted Delivery of Recombinant p53 Protein. *J. Am. Chem. Soc.* **2014**, *136*, 15319–15325. [CrossRef] [PubMed]
94. Villegas, M.R.; Baeza, A.; Usategui, A.; Ortiz-Romero, P.L.; Pablos, J.L.; Vallet-Regí, M. Collagenase nanocapsules: An approach to fibrosis treatment. *Acta Biomater.* **2018**, *74*, 430–438. [CrossRef] [PubMed]
95. Mohammed, G.K.; Obaidat, R.M.; Assaf, S.; Khanfar, M.; Al-Taani, B. Formulations and Technologies in Growth Hormone Delivery. *Int. J. Pharm. Pharm. Sci.* **2017**, *9*, 1–12. [CrossRef]
96. Rohrer, T.R.; Horikawa, R.; Kappelgaard, A.-M. Growth hormone delivery devices: Current features and potential for enhanced treatment adherence. *Expert Opin. Drug Deliv.* **2017**, *14*, 1253–1264. [CrossRef] [PubMed]
97. Kuijpers, A.J.; Engbers, G.H.; van Wachem, P.B.; Krijgsveld, J.; Zaat, S.A.; Dankert, J.; Feijen, J. Controlled delivery of antibacterial proteins from biodegradable matrices. *J. Control. Release* **1998**, *53*, 235–247. [CrossRef]
98. Jenssen, H.; Hancock, R.E.W. Antimicrobial properties of lactoferrin. *Biochimie* **2009**, *91*, 19–29. [CrossRef]
99. Zhu, Y.; Feijen, J.; Zhong, Z. Dual-targeted nanomedicines for enhanced tumor treatment. *Nano Today* **2018**, *18*, 65–85. [CrossRef]

100. Song, Y.; Du, D.; Li, L.; Xu, J.; Dutta, P.; Lin, Y. In Vitro Study of Receptor-Mediated Silica Nanoparticles Delivery across Blood–Brain Barrier. *ACS Appl. Mater. Interfaces* **2017**, *9*, 20410–20416. [CrossRef]
101. Kalmouni, M.; Al-Hosani, S.; Magzoub, M. Cancer targeting peptides. *Cell. Mol. Life Sci.* **2019**, *76*, 2171–2183. [CrossRef]
102. Zhao, N.; Qin, Y.; Liu, H.; Cheng, Z. Tumor-Targeting Peptides: Ligands for Molecular Imaging and Therapy. *Anticancer Agents Med. Chem.* **2018**, *18*, 74–86. [CrossRef]
103. Robinson, J.A. Folded Synthetic Peptides and Other Molecules Targeting Outer Membrane Protein Complexes in Gram-Negative Bacteria. *Front. Chem.* **2019**, *7*, 45. [CrossRef] [PubMed]
104. Malanovic, N.; Lohner, K. Antimicrobial Peptides Targeting Gram-Positive Bacteria. *Pharmaceuticals* **2016**, *9*, 59. [CrossRef] [PubMed]
105. Jiang, Z.; Guan, J.; Qian, J.; Zhan, C. Peptide ligand-mediated targeted drug delivery of nanomedicines. *Biomater. Sci.* **2019**, *7*, 461–471. [CrossRef]
106. Marqus, S.; Pirogova, E.; Piva, T.J. Evaluation of the use of therapeutic peptides for cancer treatment. *J. Biomed. Sci.* **2017**, *24*, 21. [CrossRef]
107. Gaspar, D.; Salomé Veiga, A.; Castanho, M.A.R.B. From antimicrobial to anticancer peptides. A review. *Front. Microbiol.* **2013**, *4*, 294. [CrossRef]
108. Kurrikoff, K.; Aphkhazava, D.; Langel, Ü. The future of peptides in cancer treatment. *Curr. Opin. Pharmacol.* **2019**, *47*, 27–32. [CrossRef]
109. Mahlapuu, M.; Håkansson, J.; Ringstad, L.; Björn, C. Antimicrobial Peptides: An Emerging Category of Therapeutic Agents. *Front. Cell Infect. Microbiol.* **2016**, *6*, 194. [CrossRef]
110. Lau, J.L.; Dunn, M.K. Therapeutic peptides: Historical perspectives, current development trends, and future directions. *Bioorg. Med. Chem.* **2018**, *26*, 2700–2707. [CrossRef]
111. Luo, G.-F.; Chen, W.-H.; Liu, Y.; Zhang, J.; Cheng, S.-X.; Zhuo, R.-X.; Zhang, X.-Z. Charge-reversal plug gate nanovalves on peptide-functionalized mesoporous silica nanoparticles for targeted drug delivery. *J. Mater. Chem. B* **2013**, *1*, 5723–5732. [CrossRef]
112. Luo, G.F.; Chen, W.H.; Liu, Y.; Lei, Q.; Zhuo, R.X.; Zhang, X.Z. Multifunctional enveloped mesoporous silica nanoparticles for subcellular co-delivery of drug and therapeutic peptide. *Sci. Rep.* **2014**, *4*, 6064. [CrossRef]
113. Cheng, Y.J.; Zeng, X.; Cheng, D.B.; Xu, X.D.; Zhang, X.Z.; Zhuo, R.X.; He, F. Functional mesoporous silica nanoparticles (MSNs) for highly controllable drug release and synergistic therapy. *Colloids Surfaces B Biointerfaces* **2016**, *145*, 217–225. [CrossRef] [PubMed]
114. Xiao, D.; Hu, J.-J.; Zhu, J.-Y.; Wang, S.-B.; Zhuo, R.-X.; Zhang, X.-Z. A redox-responsive mesoporous silica nanoparticle with a therapeutic peptide shell for tumor targeting synergistic therapy. *Nanoscale* **2016**, *8*, 16702–16709. [CrossRef] [PubMed]
115. Zhang, J.; Shen, B.; Chen, L.; Chen, L.; Meng, Y.; Feng, J. A dual-sensitive mesoporous silica nanoparticle based drug carrier for cancer synergetic therapy. *Colloids Surfaces B Biointerfaces* **2019**, *175*, 65–72. [CrossRef] [PubMed]
116. De la Torre, C.; Domínguez-Berrocal, L.; Murguía, J.R.; Marcos, M.D.; Martínez-Máñez, R.; Bravo, J.; Sancenón, F. ϵ-Polylysine-Capped Mesoporous Silica Nanoparticles as Carrier of the C9h Peptide to Induce Apoptosis in Cancer Cells. *Chem. A Eur. J.* **2018**, *24*, 1890–1897. [CrossRef] [PubMed]
117. Cao, J.; Zhang, Y.; Shan, Y.; Wang, J.; Liu, F.; Liu, H.; Xing, G.; Lei, J.; Zhou, J. A pH-dependent Antibacterial Peptide Release Nano-system Blocks Tumor Growth in vivo without Toxicity. *Sci. Rep.* **2017**, *7*, 1–13. [CrossRef] [PubMed]
118. Rahmani, S.; Budimir, J.; Sejalon, M.; Daurat, M.; Aggad, D.; Vivès, E.; Raehm, L.; Garcia, M.; Lichon, L.; Gary-Bobo, M.; et al. Large pore mesoporous silica and organosilica nanoparticles for pepstatin A delivery in breast cancer cells. *Molecules* **2019**, *24*, 332. [CrossRef]
119. Wu, Y.; Ge, P.; Xu, W.; Li, M.; Kang, Q.; Zhang, X.; Xie, J. Cancer-targeted and intracellular delivery of Bcl-2-converting peptide with functional macroporous silica nanoparticles for biosafe treatment. *Mater. Sci. Eng. C* **2020**, *108*, 110386. [CrossRef]
120. Xie, J.; Xu, W.; Wu, Y.; Niu, B.; Zhang, X. Macroporous organosilicon nanocomposites co-deliver Bcl2-converting peptide and chemotherapeutic agent for synergistic treatment against multidrug resistant cancer. *Cancer Lett.* **2020**, *469*, 340–354. [CrossRef]

121. Xie, J.; Yang, C.; Liu, Q.; Li, J.; Liang, R.; Shen, C.; Zhang, Y.; Wang, K.; Liu, L.; Shezad, K.; et al. Encapsulation of Hydrophilic and Hydrophobic Peptides into Hollow Mesoporous Silica Nanoparticles for Enhancement of Antitumor Immune Response. *Small* **2017**, *13*, 1701741. [CrossRef]
122. Braun, K.; Pochert, A.; Lindén, M.; Davoudi, M.; Schmidtchen, A.; Nordström, R.; Malmsten, M. Membrane interactions of mesoporous silica nanoparticles as carriers of antimicrobial peptides. *J. Colloid Interface Sci.* **2016**, *475*, 161–170. [CrossRef]
123. Tenland, E.; Pochert, A.; Krishnan, N.; Rao, K.U.; Kalsum, S.; Braun, K.; Glegola-Madejska, I.; Lerm, M.; Robertson, B.D.; Lindén, M.; et al. Effective delivery of the anti-mycobacterial peptide NZX in mesoporous silica nanoparticles. *PLoS ONE* **2019**, *14*, e0212858. [CrossRef]
124. Yu, Q.; Deng, T.; Lin, F.-C.; Zhang, B.; Zink, J.I. Supramolecular Assemblies of Heterogeneous Mesoporous Silica Nanoparticles to Co-deliver Antimicrobial Peptides and Antibiotics for Synergistic Eradication of Pathogenic Biofilms. *ACS Nano* **2020**. [CrossRef]
125. Zhao, Y.; Trewyn, B.G.; Slowing, I.I.; Lin, V.S.-Y. Mesoporous Silica Nanoparticle-Based Double Drug Delivery System for Glucose-Responsive Controlled Release of Insulin and Cyclic AMP. *J. Am. Chem. Soc.* **2009**, *131*, 8398–8400. [CrossRef] [PubMed]
126. Sun, L.; Zhang, X.; Zheng, C.; Wu, Z.; Li, C. A pH gated, glucose-sensitive nanoparticle based on worm-like mesoporous silica for controlled insulin release. *J. Phys. Chem. B* **2013**, *117*, 3852–3860. [CrossRef] [PubMed]
127. Zakeri Siavashani, A.; Haghbin Nazarpak, M.; Fayyazbakhsh, F.; Toliyat, T.; McInnes, S.J.P.; Solati-Hashjin, M. Effect of amino-functionalization on insulin delivery and cell viability for two types of silica mesoporous structures. *J. Mater. Sci.* **2016**, *51*, 10897–10909. [CrossRef]
128. Lozano, D.; Manzano, M.; Doadrio, J.C.; Salinas, A.J.; Vallet-Regí, M.; Gómez-Barrena, E.; Esbrit, P. Osteostatin-loaded bioceramics stimulate osteoblastic growth and differentiation. *Acta Biomater.* **2010**, *6*, 797–803. [CrossRef]
129. Trejo, C.G.; Lozano, D.; Manzano, M.; Doadrio, J.C.; Salinas, A.J.; Dapía, S.; Gómez-Barrena, E.; Vallet-Regí, M.; García-Honduvilla, N.; Buján, J.; et al. The osteoinductive properties of mesoporous silicate coated with osteostatin in a rabbit femur cavity defect model. *Biomaterials* **2010**, *31*, 8564–8573. [CrossRef]
130. Lozano, D.; Trejo, C.G.; Gómez-Barrena, E.; Manzano, M.; Doadrio, J.C.; Salinas, A.J.; Vallet-Regí, M.; García-Honduvilla, N.; Esbrit, P.; Buján, J. Osteostatin-loaded onto mesoporous ceramics improves the early phase of bone regeneration in a rabbit osteopenia model. *Acta Biomater.* **2012**, *8*, 2317–2323. [CrossRef]
131. Mendes, L.S.; Saska, S.; Martines, M.A.U.; Marchetto, R. Nanostructured materials based on mesoporous silica and mesoporous silica/apatite as osteogenic growth peptide carriers. *Mater. Sci. Eng. C* **2013**, *33*, 4427–4434. [CrossRef]
132. Zhou, X.; Feng, W.; Qiu, K.; Chen, L.; Wang, W.; Nie, W.; Mo, X.; He, C. BMP-2 Derived Peptide and Dexamethasone Incorporated Mesoporous Silica Nanoparticles for Enhanced Osteogenic Differentiation of Bone Mesenchymal Stem Cells. *ACS Appl. Mater. Interfaces* **2015**, *7*, 15777–15789. [CrossRef]
133. Du, A.W.; Stenzel, M.H. Drug carriers for the delivery of therapeutic peptides. *Biomacromolecules* **2014**, *15*, 1097–1114. [CrossRef] [PubMed]
134. Mader, J.S.; Hoskin, D.W. Cationic antimicrobial peptides as novel cytotoxic agents for cancer treatment. *Expert Opin. Investig. Drugs* **2006**, *15*, 933–946. [CrossRef] [PubMed]
135. Torchilin, V.P. Tat peptide-mediated intracellular delivery of pharmaceutical nanocarriers. *Adv. Drug Deliv. Rev.* **2008**, *60*, 548–558. [CrossRef]
136. Boohaker, R.J.; Lee, M.W.; Vishnubhotla, P.; Perez, J.L.M.; Khaled, A.R. The Use of Therapeutic Peptides to Target and to Kill Cancer Cells. *Curr. Med. Chem.* **2012**, *19*, 3794–3804. [CrossRef]
137. Naz, S.; Wang, M.; Han, Y.; Hu, B.; Teng, L.; Zhou, J.; Zhang, H.; Chen, J. Enzyme-responsive mesoporous silica nanoparticles for tumor cells and mitochondria multistage-targeted drug delivery. *Int. J. Nanomed.* **2019**, *14*, 2533–2542. [CrossRef]
138. Kolluri, S.K.; Zhu, X.; Zhou, X.; Lin, B.; Chen, Y.; Sun, K.; Tian, X.; Town, J.; Cao, X.; Lin, F.; et al. A Short Nur77-Derived Peptide Converts Bcl-2 from a Protector to a Killer. *Cancer Cell* **2008**, *14*, 285–298. [CrossRef]
139. Nordström, R.; Malmsten, M. Delivery systems for antimicrobial peptides. *Adv. Colloid Interface Sci.* **2017**, *242*, 17–34. [CrossRef]
140. Braun, K.; Pochert, A.; Gerber, M.; Raber, H.F.; Lindén, M. Influence of mesopore size and peptide aggregation on the adsorption and release of a model antimicrobial peptide onto/from mesoporous silica nanoparticles in vitro. *Mol. Syst. Des. Eng.* **2017**, *2*, 393–400. [CrossRef]

141. Tenland, E.; Krishnan, N.; Rönnholm, A.; Kalsum, S.; Puthia, M.; Mörgelin, M.; Davoudi, M.; Otrocka, M.; Alaridah, N.; Glegola-Madejska, I.; et al. A novel derivative of the fungal antimicrobial peptide plectasin is active against Mycobacterium tuberculosis. *Tuberculosis* **2018**, *113*, 231–238. [CrossRef]
142. Heras, C.; Sanchez-Salcedo, S.; Lozano, D.; Peña, J.; Esbrit, P.; Vallet-Regi, M.; Salinas, A.J. Osteostatin potentiates the bioactivity of mesoporous glass scaffolds containing Zn 2+ ions in human mesenchymal stem cells. *Acta Biomater.* **2019**, *89*, 359–371. [CrossRef]
143. Pérez, R.; Sanchez-Salcedo, S.; Lozano, D.; Heras, C.; Esbrit, P.; Vallet-Regí, M.; Salinas, A.J. Osteogenic effect of ZnO-mesoporous glasses loaded with osteostatin. *Nanomaterials* **2018**, *8*, 592. [CrossRef] [PubMed]
144. Nayerossadat, N.; Ali, P.; Maedeh, T. Viral and nonviral delivery systems for gene delivery. *Adv. Biomed. Res.* **2012**, *1*, 27. [CrossRef] [PubMed]
145. Cha, W.; Fan, R.; Miao, Y.; Zhou, Y.; Qin, C.; Shan, X.; Wan, X.; Li, J. Mesoporous Silica Nanoparticles as Carriers for Intracellular Delivery of Nucleic Acids and Subsequent Therapeutic Applications. *Molecules* **2017**, *22*, 782. [CrossRef] [PubMed]
146. Zarei, H.; Kazemi Oskuee, R.; Hanafi-Bojd, M.Y.; Gholami, L.; Ansari, L.; Malaekeh-Nikouei, B. Enhanced gene delivery by polyethyleneimine coated mesoporous silica nanoparticles. *Pharm. Dev. Technol.* **2019**, *24*, 127–132. [CrossRef]
147. Xia, T.; Kovochich, M.; Liong, M.; Meng, H.; Kabehie, S.; George, S.; Zink, J.I.; Nel, A.E. Polyethyleneimine Coating Enhances the Cellular Uptake of Mesoporous Silica Nanoparticles and Allows Safe Delivery of siRNA and DNA Constructs. *ACS Nano* **2009**, *3*, 3273–3286. [CrossRef]
148. Wang, Y.; Shang, X.; Liu, J.; Guo, Y. ATP mediated rolling circle amplification and opening DNA-gate for drug delivery to cell. *Talanta* **2018**, *176*, 652–658. [CrossRef]
149. Wang, S.; Liu, F.; Li, X.-L. Monitoring of "on-demand" drug release using dual tumor marker mediated DNA-capped versatile mesoporous silica nanoparticles. *Chem. Commun.* **2017**, *53*, 8755–8758. [CrossRef]
150. Li, Z.; Zhang, L.; Tang, C.; Yin, C. Co-Delivery of Doxorubicin and Survivin shRNA-Expressing Plasmid Via Microenvironment-Responsive Dendritic Mesoporous Silica Nanoparticles for Synergistic Cancer Therapy. *Pharm. Res.* **2017**, *34*, 2829–2841. [CrossRef]
151. Sun, P.; Leidner, A.; Weigel, S.; Weidler, P.G.; Heissler, S.; Scharnweber, T.; Niemeyer, C.M. Biopebble Containers: DNA-Directed Surface Assembly of Mesoporous Silica Nanoparticles for Cell Studies. *Small* **2019**, *15*, 1900083. [CrossRef]
152. Li, Y.; Chen, Y.; Pan, W.; Yu, Z.; Yang, L.; Wang, H.; Li, N.; Tang, B. Nanocarriers with multi-locked DNA valves targeting intracellular tumor-related mRNAs for controlled drug release. *Nanoscale* **2017**, *9*, 17318–17324. [CrossRef]
153. Pascual, L.; Cerqueira-Coutinho, C.; García-Fernández, A.; de Luis, B.; Bernardes, E.S.; Albernaz, M.S.; Missailidis, S.; Martínez-Máñez, R.; Santos-Oliveira, R.; Orzaez, M.; et al. MUC1 aptamer-capped mesoporous silica nanoparticles for controlled drug delivery and radio-imaging applications. *Nanomed. Nanotechnol. Biol. Med.* **2017**, *13*, 2495–2505. [CrossRef]
154. Srivastava, P.; Hira, S.K.; Sharma, A.; Kashif, M.; Srivastava, P.; Srivastava, D.N.; Singh, R.A.; Manna, P.P. Telomerase Responsive Delivery of Doxorubicin from Mesoporous Silica Nanoparticles in Multiple Malignancies: Therapeutic Efficacies against Experimental Aggressive Murine Lymphoma. *Bioconjug. Chem.* **2018**, *29*, 2107–2119. [CrossRef] [PubMed]
155. Wang, J.; Zhu, R.; Gao, B.; Wu, B.; Li, K.; Sun, X.; Liu, H.; Wang, S. The enhanced immune response of hepatitis B virus DNA vaccine using SiO2@LDH nanoparticles as an adjuvant. *Biomaterials* **2014**, *35*, 466–478. [CrossRef] [PubMed]
156. Shen, J.; Kim, H.-C.; Su, H.; Wang, F.; Wolfram, J.; Kirui, D.; Mai, J.; Mu, C.; Ji, L.-N.; Mao, Z.-W.; et al. Cyclodextrin and Polyethylenimine Functionalized Mesoporous Silica Nanoparticles for Delivery of siRNA Cancer Therapeutics. *Theranostics* **2014**, *4*, 487–497. [CrossRef] [PubMed]
157. Prabhakar, N.; Zhang, J.; Desai, D.; Casals, E.; Gulin-Sarfraz, T.; Näreoja, T.; Westermarck, J.; Rosenholm, J. Stimuli-responsive hybrid nanocarriers developed by controllable integration of hyperbranched PEI with mesoporous silica nanoparticles for sustained intracellular siRNA delivery. *Int. J. Nanomed.* **2016**, *11*, 6591–6608. [CrossRef] [PubMed]
158. Ngamcherdtrakul, W.; Sangvanich, T.; Reda, M.; Gu, S.; Bejan, D.; Yantasee, W. Lyophilization and stability of antibody-conjugated mesoporous silica nanoparticle with cationic polymer and PEG for siRNA delivery. *Int. J. Nanomed.* **2018**, *13*, 4015–4027. [CrossRef]

159. Lio, D.C.S.; Liu, C.; Oo, M.M.S.; Wiraja, C.; Teo, M.H.Y.; Zheng, M.; Chew, S.W.T.; Wang, X.; Xu, C. Transdermal delivery of small interfering RNAs with topically applied mesoporous silica nanoparticles for facile skin cancer treatment. *Nanoscale* **2019**, *11*, 17041–17051. [CrossRef]
160. Wang, D.; Xu, X.; Zhang, K.; Sun, B.; Wang, L.; Meng, L.; Liu, Q.; Zheng, C.; Yang, B.; Sun, H. Codelivery of doxorubicin and MDR1-siRNA by mesoporous silica nanoparticles-polymerpolyethylenimine to improve oral squamous carcinoma treatment. *Int. J. Nanomed.* **2017**, *13*, 187–198. [CrossRef]
161. Shi, X.-L.; Li, Y.; Zhao, L.-M.; Su, L.-W.; Ding, G. Delivery of MTH1 inhibitor (TH287) and MDR1 siRNA via hyaluronic acid-based mesoporous silica nanoparticles for oral cancers treatment. *Colloids Surfaces B Biointerfaces* **2019**, *173*, 599–606. [CrossRef]
162. Pan, Q.-S.; Chen, T.-T.; Nie, C.-P.; Yi, J.-T.; Liu, C.; Hu, Y.-L.; Chu, X. In Situ Synthesis of Ultrathin ZIF-8 Film-Coated MSNs for Codelivering Bcl 2 siRNA and Doxorubicin to Enhance Chemotherapeutic Efficacy in Drug-Resistant Cancer Cells. *ACS Appl. Mater. Interfaces* **2018**, *10*, 33070–33077. [CrossRef]
163. Choi, E.; Lee, J.; Kwon, I.C.; Lim, D.-K.; Kim, S. Cumulative directional calcium gluing between phosphate and silicate: A facile, robust and biocompatible strategy for siRNA delivery by amine-free non-positive vector. *Biomaterials* **2019**, *209*, 126–137. [CrossRef] [PubMed]
164. Shahin, S.A.; Wang, R.; Simargi, S.I.; Contreras, A.; Parra Echavarria, L.; Qu, L.; Wen, W.; Dellinger, T.; Unternaehrer, J.; Tamanoi, F.; et al. Hyaluronic acid conjugated nanoparticle delivery of siRNA against TWIST reduces tumor burden and enhances sensitivity to cisplatin in ovarian cancer. *Nanomed. Nanotechnol. Biol. Med.* **2018**, *14*, 1381–1394. [CrossRef]
165. Zheng, G.; Shen, Y.; Zhao, R.; Chen, F.; Zhang, Y.; Xu, A.; Shao, J. Dual-Targeting Multifuntional Mesoporous Silica Nanocarrier for Codelivery of siRNA and Ursolic Acid to Folate Receptor Overexpressing Cancer Cells. *J. Agric. Food Chem.* **2017**, *65*, 6904–6911. [CrossRef] [PubMed]
166. Zheng, G.; Zhao, R.; Xu, A.; Shen, Z.; Chen, X.; Shao, J. Co-delivery of sorafenib and siVEGF based on mesoporous silica nanoparticles for ASGPR mediated targeted HCC therapy. *Eur. J. Pharm. Sci.* **2018**, *111*, 492–502. [CrossRef] [PubMed]
167. Morry, J.; Ngamcherdtrakul, W.; Gu, S.; Goodyear, S.M.; Castro, D.J.; Reda, M.M.; Sangvanich, T.; Yantasee, W. Dermal delivery of HSP47 siRNA with NOX4-modulating mesoporous silica-based nanoparticles for treating fibrosis. *Biomaterials* **2015**, *66*, 41–52. [CrossRef] [PubMed]
168. Vivero-Escoto, J.L.; Vadarevu, H.; Juneja, R.; Schrum, L.W.; Benbow, J.H. Nanoparticle mediated silencing of tenascin C in hepatic stellate cells: Effect on inflammatory gene expression and cell migration. *J. Mater. Chem. B* **2019**, *7*, 7396–7405. [CrossRef]
169. Pinese, C.; Lin, J.; Milbreta, U.; Li, M.; Wang, Y.; Leong, K.W.; Chew, S.Y. Sustained delivery of siRNA/mesoporous silica nanoparticle complexes from nanofiber scaffolds for long-term gene silencing. *Acta Biomater.* **2018**, *76*, 164–177. [CrossRef]
170. Mora-Raimundo, P.; Lozano, D.; Manzano, M.; Vallet-Regí, M. Nanoparticles to Knockdown Osteoporosis-Related Gene and Promote Osteogenic Marker Expression for Osteoporosis Treatment. *ACS Nano* **2019**, *13*, 5451–5464. [CrossRef]
171. Li, Y.; Duo, Y.; Bi, J.; Zeng, X.; Mei, L.; Bao, S.; He, L.; Shan, A.; Zhang, Y.; Yu, X. Targeted delivery of anti-miR-155 by functionalized mesoporous silica nanoparticles for colorectal cancer therapy. *Int. J. Nanomed.* **2018**, *13*, 1241–1256. [CrossRef]
172. Li, Y.; Duo, Y.; Zhai, P.; He, L.; Zhong, K.; Zhang, Y.; Huang, K.; Luo, J.; Zhang, H.; Yu, X. Dual targeting delivery of miR-328 by functionalized mesoporous silica nanoparticles for colorectal cancer therapy. *Nanomedicine* **2018**, *13*. [CrossRef]
173. Ahir, M.; Upadhyay, P.; Ghosh, A.; Sarker, S.; Bhattacharya, S.; Gupta, P.; Ghosh, S.; Chattopadhyay, S.; Adhikary, A. Delivery of dual miRNA through CD44-targeted mesoporous silica nanoparticles for enhanced and effective triple-negative breast cancer therapy. *Biomater. Sci.* **2020**. [CrossRef] [PubMed]
174. Yan, J.; Lu, X.; Zhu, X.; Hu, X.; Wang, L.; Qian, J.; Zhang, F.; Liu, M. Effects of miR-26a on Osteogenic Differentiation of Bone Marrow Mesenchymal Stem Cells by a Mesoporous Silica Nanoparticle-PEI-Peptide System. *Int. J. Nanomed.* **2020**, *15*, 497–511. [CrossRef] [PubMed]
175. Wang, Y.; Xie, Y.; Kilchrist, K.V.; Li, J.; Duvall, C.L.; Oupický, D. Endosomolytic and Tumor-Penetrating Mesoporous Silica Nanoparticles for siRNA/miRNA Combination Cancer Therapy. *ACS Appl. Mater. Interfaces* **2020**, *12*, 4308–4322. [CrossRef] [PubMed]

176. Maimaitiyiming, Y.; Hong, D.F.; Yang, C.; Naranmandura, H. Novel insights into the role of aptamers in the fight against cancer. *J. Cancer Res. Clin. Oncol.* **2019**, *145*, 797–810. [CrossRef] [PubMed]
177. Ingolotti, M.; Kawalekar, O.; Shedlock, D.J.; Muthumani, K.; Weiner, D.B. DNA vaccines for targeting bacterial infections. *Expert Rev. Vaccines* **2010**, *9*, 747–763. [CrossRef] [PubMed]
178. Darvishi, B.; Farahmand, L.; Majidzadeh-A, K. Stimuli-Responsive Mesoporous Silica NPs as Non-viral Dual siRNA/Chemotherapy Carriers for Triple Negative Breast Cancer. *Mol. Ther. Nucleic Acids* **2017**, *7*, 164–180. [CrossRef]
179. Lopes, C.F.B.; de Angelis, B.B.; Prudente, H.M.; de Souza, B.V.G.; Cardoso, S.V.; de Azambuja Ribeiro, R.I.M. Concomitant consumption of marijuana, alcohol and tobacco in oral squamous cell carcinoma development and progression: Recent advances and challenges. *Arch. Oral Biol.* **2012**, *57*, 1026–1033. [CrossRef]
180. Nishida, N.; Yano, H.; Nishida, T.; Kamura, T.; Kojiro, M. Angiogenesis in cancer. *Vasc. Health Risk Manag.* **2006**, *2*, 213–219. [CrossRef]
181. Richter, K.; Konzack, A.; Pihlajaniemi, T.; Heljasvaara, R.; Kietzmann, T. Redox-fibrosis: Impact of TGFβ1 on ROS generators, mediators and functional consequences. *Redox Biol.* **2015**, *6*, 344–352. [CrossRef]
182. Mora-Raimundo, P.; Manzano, M.; Vallet-Regí, M. Nanoparticles for the treatment of osteoporosis. *AIMS Bioeng.* **2017**, *4*, 259–274. [CrossRef]
183. Lozano, D.; Sánchez-Salcedo, S.; Portal-Núñez, S.; Vila, M.; López-Herradón, A.; Ardura, J.A.; Mulero, F.; Gómez-Barrena, E.; Vallet-Regí, M.; Esbrit, P. Parathyroid hormone-related protein (107–111) improves the bone regeneration potential of gelatin–glutaraldehyde biopolymer-coated hydroxyapatite. *Acta Biomater.* **2014**, *10*, 3307–3316. [CrossRef] [PubMed]
184. Ansari, A.S.; Santerre, P.J.; Uludağ, H. Biomaterials for polynucleotide delivery to anchorage-independent cells. *J. Mater. Chem. B* **2017**, *5*, 7238–7261. [CrossRef] [PubMed]
185. Gambari, R.; Brognara, E.; Spandidos, D.A.; Fabbri, E. Targeting oncomiRNAs and mimicking tumor suppressor miRNAs: New trends in the development of miRNA therapeutic strategies in oncology (Review). *Int. J. Oncol.* **2016**, *49*, 5–32. [CrossRef] [PubMed]
186. Bonneau, E.; Neveu, B.; Kostantin, E.; Tsongalis, G.J.; De Guire, V. How close are miRNAs from clinical practice? A perspective on the diagnostic and therapeutic market. *Electron. J. Int. Fed. Clin. Chem. Lab. Med.* **2019**, *30*, 114–127.
187. Song, G.; Wang, Q.; Wang, Y.; Lv, G.; Li, C.; Zou, R.; Chen, Z.; Qin, Z.; Huo, K.; Hu, R.; et al. A low-toxic multifunctional nanoplatform based on Cu9S5@mSiO2core-shell nanocomposites: Combining photothermal-and chemotherapies with infrared thermal imaging for cancer treatment. *Adv. Funct. Mater.* **2013**, *23*, 4281–4292. [CrossRef]
188. Salis, A.; Fanti, M.; Medda, L.; Nairi, V.; Cugia, F.; Piludu, M.; Sogos, V.; Monduzzi, M. Mesoporous Silica Nanoparticles Functionalized with Hyaluronic Acid and Chitosan Biopolymers. Effect of Functionalization on Cell Internalization. *ACS Biomater. Sci. Eng.* **2016**, *2*, 741–751. [CrossRef]
189. Popat, A.; Liu, J.; Lu, G.Q.; Qiao, S.Z. A pH-responsive drug delivery system based on chitosan coated mesoporous silica nanoparticles. *J. Mater. Chem.* **2012**, *22*, 11173–11178. [CrossRef]
190. Nairi, V.; Medda, S.; Piludu, M.; Casula, M.F.; Vallet-Regì, M.; Monduzzi, M.; Salis, A. Interactions between bovine serum albumin and mesoporous silica nanoparticles functionalized with biopolymers. *Chem. Eng. J.* **2018**, *340*, 42–50. [CrossRef]
191. Xi, J.; Qin, J.; Fan, L. Chondroitin sulfate functionalized mesostructured silica nanoparticles as biocompatible carriers for drug delivery. *Int. J. Nanomed.* **2012**, *7*, 5235–5247. [CrossRef]
192. Xu, X.; Lü, S.; Gao, C.; Bai, X.; Feng, C.; Gao, N.; Liu, M. Multifunctional drug carriers comprised of mesoporous silica nanoparticles and polyamidoamine dendrimers based on layer-by-layer assembly. *Mater. Des.* **2015**, *88*, 1127–1133. [CrossRef]
193. Radhakrishnan, K.; Tripathy, J.; Datey, A.; Chakravortty, D.; Raichur, A.M. Mesoporous silica—Chondroitin sulphate hybrid nanoparticles for targeted and bio-responsive drug delivery. *N. J. Chem.* **2015**, *39*, 1754–1760. [CrossRef]
194. Kavya, K.C.; Dixit, R.; Jayakumar, R.; Nair, S.V.; Chennazhi, K.P. Synthesis and characterization of chitosan/chondroitin sulfate/nano-SiO_2 composite scaffold for bone tissue engineering. *J. Biomed. Nanotechnol.* **2012**, *8*, 149–160. [CrossRef] [PubMed]

195. Porgham Daryasari, M.; Dusti Telgerd, M.; Hossein Karami, M.; Zandi-Karimi, A.; Akbarijavar, H.; Khoobi, M.; Seyedjafari, E.; Birhanu, G.; Khosravian, P.; SadatMahdavi, F. Poly-l-lactic acid scaffold incorporated chitosan-coated mesoporous silica nanoparticles as pH-sensitive composite for enhanced osteogenic differentiation of human adipose tissue stem cells by dexamethasone delivery. *Artif. Cells Nanomed. Biotechnol.* **2019**, *47*, 4020–4029. [CrossRef] [PubMed]
196. Cao, J.-F.; Xu, W.; Zhang, Y.-Y.; Shu, Y.; Wang, J.-H. Chondroitin sulfate-functionalized 3D hierarchical flower-type mesoporous silica with a superior capacity for selective isolation of low density lipoprotein. *Anal. Chim. Acta* **2020**, *1104*, 78–86. [CrossRef]
197. Argyo, C.; Cauda, V.; Engelke, H.; Rädler, J.; Bein, G.; Bein, T. Heparin-coated colloidal mesoporous silica nanoparticles efficiently bind to antithrombin as an anticoagulant drug-delivery system. *Chem. A Eur. J.* **2012**, *18*, 428–432. [CrossRef]
198. Dai, L.; Li, J.; Zhang, B.; Liu, J.; Luo, Z.; Cai, K. Redox-responsive nanocarrier based on heparin end-capped mesoporous silica nanoparticles for targeted tumor therapy in vitro and in vivo. *Langmuir* **2014**, *30*, 7867–7877. [CrossRef]
199. Wan, M.M.; Yang, J.Y.; Qiu, Y.; Zhou, Y.; Guan, C.X.; Hou, Q.; Lin, W.G.; Zhu, J.H. Sustained release of heparin on enlarged-pore and functionalized MCM-41. *ACS Appl. Mater. Interfaces* **2012**, *4*, 4113–4122. [CrossRef]
200. Qian, W.J.; Wan, M.M.; Lin, W.G.; Zhu, J.H. Fabricating a sustained releaser of heparin using SBA-15 mesoporous silica. *J. Mater. Chem. B* **2014**, *2*, 92–101. [CrossRef]
201. Wei, H.; Han, L.; Ren, J.; Jia, L. Anticoagulant surface coating using composite polysaccharides with embedded heparin-releasing mesoporous silica. *ACS Appl. Mater. Interfaces* **2013**, *5*, 12571–12578. [CrossRef]
202. Wu, F.; Xu, T.; Zhao, G.; Meng, S.; Wan, M.; Chi, B.; Mao, C.; Shen, J. Mesoporous Silica Nanoparticles-Encapsulated Agarose and Heparin as Anticoagulant and Resisting Bacterial Adhesion Coating for Biomedical Silicone. *Langmuir* **2017**, *33*, 5245–5252. [CrossRef]

7

Preparation and In Vitro Release of Total Alkaloids from *Alstonia Scholaris* Leaves Loaded mPEG-PLA Microspheres

Xiangyu Zheng [1], Hongli Li [1], Yi He [1], Mingwei Yuan [1], Meili Shen [2], Renyu Yang [1], Nianfeng Jiang [1], Minglong Yuan [1,*] and Cui Yang [1,*]

1 National and Local Joint Engineering Research Center for Green Preparation Technology of Biobased Materials, Yunnan Minzu University, Kunming 650500, China; zhengxiangyu1993@163.com (X.Z.); honglili@vip.163.com (H.L.); heyi_sichuan@163.com (Y.H.); yuanmingwei@163.com (M.Y.); yangrenyu1995@163.com (R.Y.); jnf1514@163.com (N.J.)

2 National and Local Joint Engineering Laboratory for Synthesis Technology of High Performance Polymer, Jilin University, Changchun 130012, China; sml199211@163.com

* Correspondence: yml@188.com (M.Y.); yangcui@ynni.edu.cn (C.Y.)

Abstract: Total alkaloids of *Alstonia scholaris* leaves (ASAs) are extracted from the lamp leaves, which have positive anti-inflammatory activity and remarkable effects in treating bronchitis. Due to its short half-life, we used a degradable mPEG-PLA to physically encapsulate the total alkali of the lamp stage, and prepared a sustained-release microsphere by double-emulsion method. The ASAs-loaded $mPEG_{10000}$-PLA microspheres were screened for better performance by testing the morphology, average particle size, embedding rate and drug loading of different molecular weight mPEG-PLA microspheres, which can stably and continuously release for 15 days at 37 °C. The results of cytotoxicity and blood compatibility indicated that the drug-loaded microspheres have beneficial biocompatibility. Animal experiments showed that the drug-loaded microspheres had a beneficial anti-inflammatory effect. These results all indicated that mPEG-PLA is a controlled release carrier material suitable for ASAs.

Keywords: total alkaloids from *Alstonia scholaris* leaves; mPEG-PLA; microspheres; drug release; biocompatibility

1. Introduction

Respiratory diseases are common and frequently occurring diseases whose incidence has increased in recent years. Inhalation of dust and irritating gases are the main causes of respiratory diseases, which cause tremendous harm to human health [1]. *Alstonia scholaris* leaves, a traditional Chinese medicine from the Dai nationality, are mainly used to treat chronic respiratory diseases [2]. *A. scholaris* leaves are also used as a traditional medicine to treat respiratory diseases in India, Malaysia, the Philippines, and Thailand [2]. *A. scholaris* leaf extracts, especially alkaloids, are widely used to treat bronchitis and have significant efficacy [3–7]. Luo et al. studied *A. scholaris* leaves and found an alkaloid component that beneficial effects respiratory diseases. This component has a positive effect on bronchitis and post-cold infections [8,9]; however, its half-life is short, which limits its clinical application.

Research and development of sustained-release formulations have always been a focus in drug research and have gradually begun to solve the problem of short half-lives. In recent years, polymer nanoparticles have shown to be efficient drug carriers for encapsulating drugs [10]. At present, designing and selecting drug nanocomposites has mainly focused on amphiphilic block copolymers. Polyethylene glycol (PEG) is often used in the hydrophilic segment of the copolymers, while many homopolymers, copolymers and derivatives of degradable polymers, such as polylactic acid (PLA), polyglycolic acid (PGA) and polycaprolactone (PCL), are used in the hydrophobic segment [11–14]. Methoxy poly(ethylene glycol)-poly(lactide) copolymer (mPEG-PLA) is an amphiphilic polymer formed by grafting mPEG onto PLA. mPEG-PLA has excellent biocompatibility, a low molecular weight, and many hydroxyl groups and is nontoxic and widely used as a coating material in drug-delivery systems [15,16]. PEG blocks can improve the polymer's hydrophilicity and flexibility, prevent protein adsorption and avoid recognition and phagocytosis by the reticuloendothelial system (RES). PEG encapsulates the drug to form the "core", while the "shell" is formed by the outside hydrophobic segment, which constitutes the typical "core-shell" structure, with great advantages for drug release [17–19]. Therefore, in this work, total alkaloids from *A. scholaris* leaves (ASAs) were studied, and mPEG-PLA with different molecular weights was used as the carrier material. A series of drug-loaded microspheres were prepared by the water-oil-water (W/O/W) double-emulsion technique. Based on the morphology, particle size, encapsulation efficiency (EE), drug-loading efficiency (LE), and in vitro drug release of the prepared microspheres, the best drug-loaded materials were screened out, and then the biological properties of its drug-loaded microspheres such as cytotoxicity, blood compatibility and anti-inflammatory activity were studied.

2. Materials and Methods

2.1. Materials

L-lactide was purchased from Purac Co., Ltd. (Shanghai, China). Dichloromethane (DCM), ethanol, tert-butyl methyl ether, and isopropanol were purchased from Tianjin Damao Chemical Reagent Co., Ltd. (Tianjin, China) and were all analytical grade. ASAs were purchased from Kunming Institute of Botany, Chinese Academy of Sciences, batch number 20180501 (Kunming, China). ASAs is a mixture of brown solid powder. Two of main active ingredients are Vallesamine and Picrinine, which were detected by HPLC with peak times of 43.133 min and 72.190 min. NaH_2PO_4, KH_2PO_4, and NaCl were purchased from Chengdu Chron Chemicals Co., Ltd. (Chengdu, China). Stannous octoate (95%, analytical grade) and polyvinyl alcohol (PVA; Mw = 75,000 Da and 88% alcoholysis degree) were purchased from Shanghai Jingchun Chemicals Co., Ltd. (Shanghai, China). mPEG (Mw 5000) was purchased from Shanghai Seebio Biotechnology Co., Ltd. (Shanghai, China). HL-7702 cells (normal human hepatocytes) were purchased from Procell Life Sciences and Technology Co., Ltd. (Wuhan, China). High glucose and 1640 medium were provided by HyClone Company. The 3-(4,5-dimethyl-2-thiazolyl)-2,5-diphenyl-2-H-tetrazolium bromide (MTT) was purchased from APExBIO (Houston, TX, USA). High-quality fetal bovine serum (FBS) was purchased from Shanghai ExCell Bio Co., Ltd. (Shanghai, China). Ethylenediaminetetraacetic acid (EDTA)-trypsin solution, cyan-streptomycin, and cisplatin were provided by Solarbio (Shanghai, China). Kunming mice, Sprague-Dawley (SD) rats, and rabbits were purchased from Kunming Medical University (Kunming, China). Dengtaiye Pian (DP) was purchased from Yunnan Datang Hanfang Pharmaceutical Co., Ltd. (Kunming, China). Aspirin was purchased from Bayer HealthCare Manufacturing Co., Ltd. (Beijing, China).

2.2. Preparation of mPEG-PLA

mPEG-PLA was prepared by ring-opening polymerization. L-LA (18 g) and mPEG (2 g) were putted in reaction flask as raw materials. Protected by nitrogen, catalyzed by stannous octoate (0.02 g), the mPEG-PLA was polymerized at 130–160 °C for 24 h. Using recrystallization, the product was precipitated by methylene chloride and ethanol. Product was filtered and washed with hot water to remove the mPEG bulk polymer. The obtained product was dried with P_2O_5 for 48 h to obtain a white copolymer. Figure 1 shows the synthesis process.

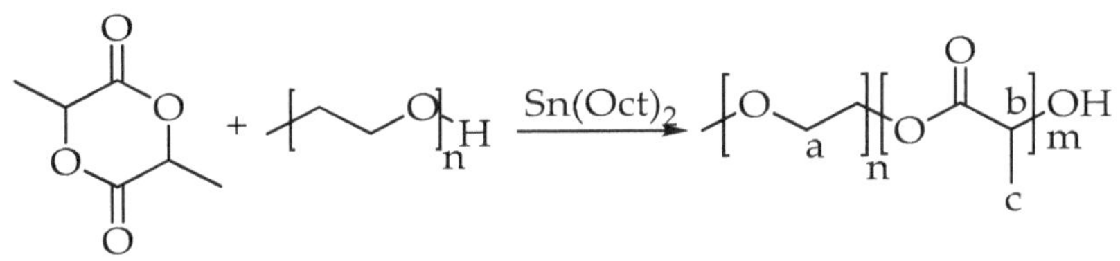

Figure 1. The synthesis process of mPEG-PLA.

2.3. Determination of Molecular Mass

3 mg copolymer were dissolved in 1 mL chromatography grade THF and was filtered by using a 0.45 μm nylon 66 filter membrane. Then using gel permeation chromatography (GPC) which was purchased from Waters Inc. (Milford, MA, USA) to define the molecular weight and distribution of the compounds, and THF was used as the eluent. The system is equipped with a column (7.8 × 300 mm, Waters Styragel, Waters Inc., Milford, MA, USA), a Waters 515 pump and a Waters 2414 refractive index detector. When the column temperature of GPC is 40 °C, the flow rate is 1 mL/min, and the baseline is smooth. The filtrate was pulled into an injection needle, and the sample was slowly and uniformly injected into the sampler when the air was removed. All data were obtained under the same standard curve.

2.4. Preparing the Blank and ASAs-Loaded mPEG-PLA Microspheres

The ASAs-loaded mPEG-PLA microspheres were prepared using the W/O/W double-emulsion technique. First, 100 mg of ASAs were dissolved in 1 mL methanol solution, which was the internal water phase (W_1). The 500-mg mPEG-PLA copolymer material was weighed and completely dissolved in 10 mL of methylene chloride as the oil phase (O). The external water phase (W_2) was a 2% PVA solution. Next, the ASAs solution was injected into the oil phase in an ice bath at a constant rate. The mixture was emulsified at high speed (21,000 rpm) for 2 min to form the first emulsion. Similarly, the first emulsion was continuously dropped into 20 mL of 2% PVA (W_2) in an ice bath and emulsified at high speed (21,000 rpm) for 2 min to form a double emulsion. The double emulsion was poured into 400 mL of 5% isopropanol solution and stirred at low speed at room temperature for 6 h. After the organic solvent had completely evaporated, the ASAs-loaded microsphere solution was obtained. Finally, the ASAs-loaded microsphere solution was centrifuged (6500 rpm, 10 min), and the supernatant was discarded. The microspheres were collected (white solid), washed with pure water 3 times, and lyophilized at −50 °C for 24 h. The obtained microspheres were dried at −20 °C. Blank microspheres were prepared by the same method.

2.5. Morphology, Particle size and Particle Size Distribution of the Microspheres

The morphological characteristics of the ASAs-loaded mPEG-PLA microspheres were observed using SEM (NOVA NANOSEM-450, FEI, Hillsboro, OR, USA). Conductive adhesive tape was applied to the surface of the loading platform. A few lyophilized microspheres (white powder) were evenly spread on a conductive adhesive, and the surface was sprayed with gold to observe. The particle size distribution of the microspheres was measured using a laser particle-size analyzer (Mastersizer 3500, Microtrac, Malvern, UK). A small portion of the microsphere suspension was diluted in a 15 mL centrifuge tube until the solution became nearly transparent. The particle size distribution of the microspheres was determined using a particle-size analyzer.

2.6. Measuring the EE of the Microspheres

Twenty milligrams of lyophilized microspheres were weighed, and 500 μL of methylene chloride was added to completely dissolve them. Next, 2 mL of methanol solution was added. After centrifugation, the supernatant was filtered through a 0.45-μm microfiltration membrane. Next,

20 μL of filtered solution was injected via HPLC, and the area normalization method was used to calculate the EE% and LE% using the following equations.

$$LE\% = \frac{\text{weight of ASAs in microspheres}}{\text{total weight of microspheres}} \times 100\%$$

$$EE\% = \frac{\text{weight of encapsulated drug}}{\text{weight of initial drug loading}} \times 100\%$$

2.7. In Vitro Microsphere Release

Fifty milligrams of lyophilized microspheres were weighed and placed in a 15 mL centrifuge tube, then 5 mL of phosphate buffer saline (PBS) was added and shaken in a thermostatic oscillator at 37 °C. The tube was removed at set time intervals and centrifuged at 5000 rpm for 6 min. Next, 1 mL of the release solution was removed from the supernatant, an equal amount of fresh PBS was added to the tube, and the tube was placed back in the thermostatic oscillator and shaken at 37 °C. The ASAs content in the release solution was determined by HPLC, and the cumulative drug release amount was calculated using the following formula [20]. The amount (%) of the released ASAs-loaded microspheres was plotted against the release time (t, in days) to obtain the in vitro release curve of the microspheres.

$$Q = C_n \times V_1 + V_2 \sum C_{n-1}$$

Q: cumulative drug release (μg);
C_n: concentration of the release solution (μg/mL) removed at time t;
V_1: volume of the released medium (mL);
V_2: volume of the medium to be withdrawn each time (mL).

2.8. In Vitro Microsphere Degradation

Fifty milligrams of lyophilized microspheres were weighed and placed in a 15 mL centrifuge tube, and then, 5 mL of PBS was added and shaken at 37 °C. The tube was removed at set time intervals and centrifuged at 5000 rpm. The supernatant was collected to determine the pH changes in the microspheres. Buffer salts on the microsphere surface were washed with pure water and frozen at −50 °C for 24 h. The microspheres were weighed using an analytical balance, and the dry weight loss of the degraded microspheres was calculated. The molecular weight of 3 mg of the lyophilized microspheres was measured via GPC. The pH value, the microsphere weight and the relative molecular weight (Mn) were separately plotted against degradation time to obtain the in vitro degradation curve of the microspheres.

2.9. Blood Compatibility Testing of The Microspheres

All the trials were approved by the laboratory animals Ethics Committee of Yunnan Minzu University and were registered on the Kunming Science and Technology Bureau (SYXK (Yunnan) K2017-0001, 16 January 2017).

2.9.1. Hemolysis Experiment

The samples were dissolved in deionized water (DI water), and the solutions were prepared at concentrations of 10.6 μg/mL, 1.06 mg/mL, and 0.106 mg/mL. Eight milliliters of fresh anticoagulated rabbit blood (blood mixed with sodium citrate at a volume ratio of 9:1) was diluted with 10 mL of 0.9% sodium chloride solution. Two hundred microliters of the sample was placed in a test tube, and 5 mL of 0.9% sodium chloride solution was added. The tube was then kept in a 37 °C water bath for 30 min. Next, 100 μL of diluted blood was added, and the mixture was gently mixed and incubated for 60 min. The positive control was treated with 5 mL DI water and 100 μL blood (D = 0.8 ± 0.3). The negative control was treated with 5 mL 0.9% NaCl solution and 100 μL blood. After centrifugation at 800 r/min for 5 min, the supernatant was transferred into a cuvette, and an ultraviolet (UV) spectrophotometer was used to measure the absorbance at 540 nm. Hemolysis of the sample was calculated per the formula below. The final sample concentrations were 40 μg/mL, 4 μg/mL, and 0.4 μg/mL. The material was considered hemolyzed when the hemolysis rate was above 5% [21–27].

$$\text{Hemolysis rate}(\%) = \frac{\text{Abs}_{\text{sample}} - \text{Abs}_{\text{negative control}}}{\text{Abs}_{\text{positive control}} - \text{Abs}_{\text{negative control}}} \times 100\%$$

2.9.2. Coagulation Experiment

The samples were dissolved in distilled water to prepare solutions with concentrations of 245.2 μg/mL, 24.52 μg/mL, and 2.452 mg/mL. The final concentrations were 40 μg/mL, 4 μg/mL, and 0.4 μg/mL. Next, 200 μL of the solution was placed in a 15-mL centrifuge tube and kept at 37 °C for 5 min. Fifty microliters of fresh anticoagulated rabbit blood was added to the samples, which were and kept at a constant temperature for 5 min. Ten microliters of aqueous calcium chloride solution (0.2 mL/L) was added to the blood sample, and the centrifuge tube was shaken to evenly mix the calcium chloride and blood and kept at a constant temperature for 5 min. The centrifuge tube was then removed, 12 mL of DI water was added to the solution, and the supernatant was collected. The blood was measured at 540 nm using a UV spectrophotometer. The optical absorbance (i.e., the optical density [OD] of the free hemoglobin remaining in the beaker containing 50 μL of whole blood treated with 12 mL of DI water) was used as a reference. The average of 5 measurements was taken. The sample's anticoagulant activity was expressed as the relative absorbance [28,29]:

$$\text{BCI} = \frac{I_o}{I_w} \times 100\%$$

I_o: relative absorbance of the mixture of blood and calcium chloride after contact with the sample for a set period of time;
I_w: relative absorbance of blood mixed with a certain amount of DI water.

2.10. Cytotoxicity of The Microspheres

2.10.1. Cell Culture

Normal human hepatocytes (HL-7702) were inoculated into culture flasks, and RPMI-1640 medium (containing 10% FBS, 100 U/mL penicillin, and 100 U/mL streptomycin) was added. Cells were cultured in a 5% CO_2 incubator at 37 °C. Cells grew as monolayers adherent to glass and were passaged once every 3–5 days using 0.25% trypsin.

2.10.2. MTT Assay of Sample Inhibition on Tumor Cell Proliferation

HL-7702 cells (180 μL; 5×10^4 cells/mL) in the logarithmic growth phase were inoculated in a 96-well plate, and 20 μL of the sample was added to each well after incubating overnight. Three concentration gradients were set with 3 wells per concentration. After a 48-h incubation, 20 μL of 5 mg/mL MTT was added to each well, and the cells were continuously cultured for 4 h. The culture medium was aspirated and discarded, and 150 μL dimethylsulfoxide (DMSO) was added to terminate the reaction. The plate was shaken for 15 min in a shaker. The OD value at 490 nm was measured in a microplate reader [30,31], and the inhibition rate was calculated [32]:

$$\text{Cell viability} = \frac{\text{ODsample}}{\text{ODnegative control}} \times 100\%$$

2.11. Anti-Inflammatory Activity Testing of The Microspheres

To determine the influence of xylene-induced auricle swelling on the mice [33], 35 Kunming mice (19–22 g) were randomly divided into 7 groups by body weight and sex, with 5 mice per group. Except for the aspirin group, only one intragastric administration on the day of the experiment, the other groups were pre-administered once daily for 3 consecutive days. The control group was administered the same volume of 1% CMC-Na (carboxymethyl cellulose-sodium). The gavage volume was 20 mL/kg per group. Thirty minutes after the last gastric gavage, 0.05 mL of xylene was evenly applied on both sides of each mouse's right ear, while the left ear was used as the control. The mice were sacrificed via cervical dislocation 1 h after inflammation. The same area of both ears was cut off using a 10-mm-diameter puncher, and the weight difference between the two ears was used as the swelling degree.

To determine the influence of the egg-white-induced pedal swelling in the rats, 35 male SD rats (170–220 g) were randomly divided into 7 groups by body weight, with 5 rats per group. All groups were intragastrically administered the microspheres once daily for 3 consecutive days, except the aspirin group, which received the microspheres via intragastric administration on the day of the experiment. The control group received the same volume of 1% CMC-Na (carboxymethyl cellulose-sodium). The gavage volume was 10 mL/kg per group. Thirty minutes after the last gastric gavage, 0.1 mL of fresh egg white was injected subcutaneously into the pedal of the right rear foot of each rat to induce inflammation. The foot areas before inflammation and at 0.5, 1, 2, 3, 4, and 5 h after inflammation were measured. The difference in the foot area before and after inflammation was determined as the degree of swelling, and the swelling rate was calculated.

$$\text{Swell rate} = \frac{A_{t1} - A_{t0}}{A_{t0}} \times 100\%$$

A_{t0}: foot area before administration
A_{t1}: foot area after administration

3. Results and Discussion

3.1. Characterization of Copolymer mPEG-PLA

Figure 2 shows the nuclear magnetic resonance (NMR) spectra of the mPEG-PLA copolymer. The ^{1}H NMR image shows the characteristic peaks of hydrogen in the mPEG-PLA. The peaks at 5.19 ppm and 1.5 ppm correspond to the PLA's methine and methyl peaks, respectively. The methylene peak at 3.6 ppm is the repeating unit in the PEG. The peak at 3.39 ppm corresponds to the hydrogen of the CH_3O- group of the mPEG at the end of the copolymer. NMR spectroscopy was performed at 25 °C (Bruker 400 MHz, Karlsruhe, Germany).

Figure 3 shows the mPEG-PLA gel permeation chromatography (GPC) curve with the different molecular weights of mPEG. Data were processed using different molecular weights of polystyrene as the reference material. Table 1 shows the weight-average molecular weight (Mw), number-average molecular weight (Mn) and polydispersity index of the molecular weight distribution (PDI) of the copolymer. The obtained copolymers have relatively small PDIs and relatively uniform molecular weights. Four copolymers with different molecular weights were prepared by copolymerization of four mPEG with the same amount of L-LA. The GPC curves show that the different molecular weights of the four mPEG-PLA, they all have a single peak, indicating that no other copolymers were formed. The copolymer synthesized from mPEG of different molecular weights, wherein the larger the molecular weight of mPEG, the higher the molecular weight of the obtained copolymer and the shorter the peak time of the copolymer, which is consistent with the results obtained by the GPC test.

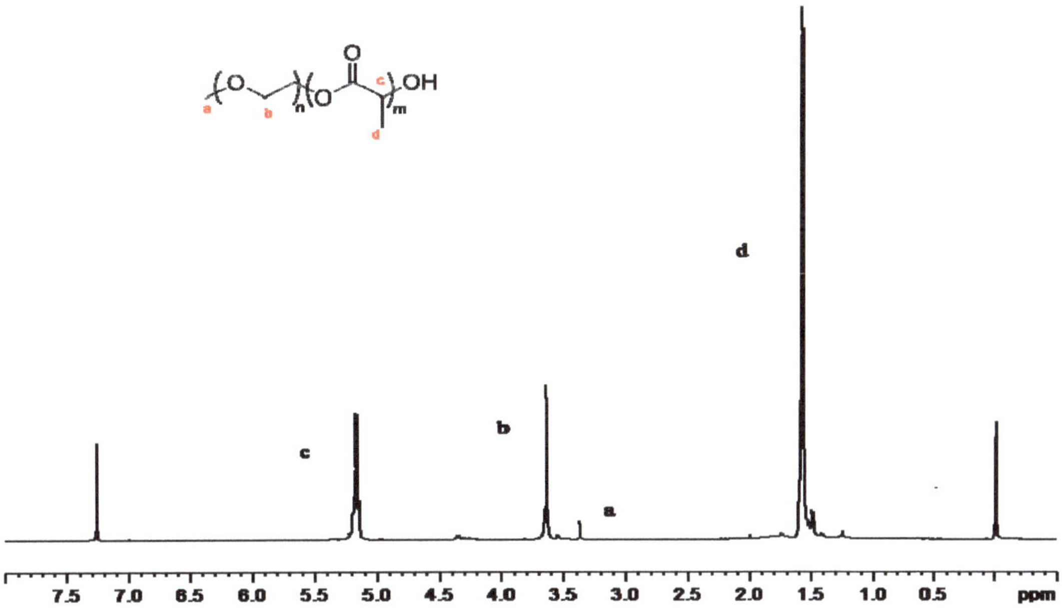

Figure 2. [1]H nuclear magnetic resonance (NMR) spectrum of mPEG-PLA.

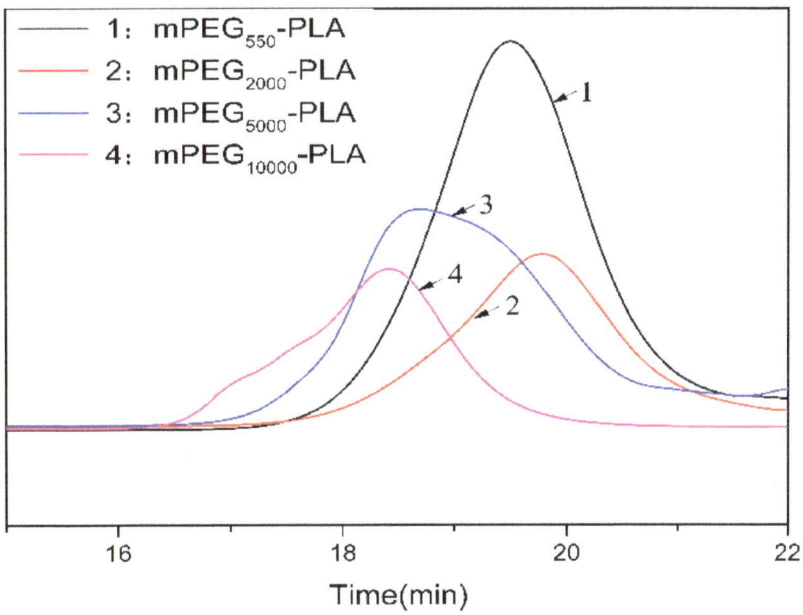

Figure 3. Gel permeation chromatography (GPC) of mPEG-PLA.

Table 1. The Mn, Mw and PDI of different molecular weight of mPEG-PLA.

Sample	Mn [1] ($g \cdot mol^{-1}$)	Mn [2] ($g \cdot mol^{-1}$)	Mw [1] ($g \cdot mol^{-1}$)	PDI [1]
$mPEG_{550}$-PLA	4013	4097	4540	1.13
$mPEG_{2000}$-PLA	5489	5504	6320	1.15
$mPEG_{5000}$-PLA	7378	7419	8637	1.17
$mPEG_{10000}$-PLA	11,307	11,416	12,889	1.14

[1] Determined by GPC via a universal calibration curve and appropriate Mark–Houwink parameters for THF.
[2] Calculated by ^{1}H NMR. Mn: The number-average molecular weight; Mw: The weight-average molecular weight; PDI: polydispersity index of the molecular weight distribution.

3.2. *Morphology and Size Distribution of the Microspheres*

Figure 4 shows the scanning electron microscopy (SEM) images of the mPEG-PLA microspheres loaded with ASAs. Figure 4A shows $mPEG_{550}$-PLA microspheres, which have a small particle diameter, a round smooth spherical shape, and no obvious adhesion. Figure 4B shows $mPEG_{2000}$-PLA microspheres with small pores on the surface and varied particle sizes. Figure 4C shows $mPEG_{5000}$-PLA microspheres with a few small pores on the surface and with different pore sizes and numbers. Figure 4D shows $mPEG_{10000}$-PLA microspheres. Compared with the $mPEG_{550}$-PLA, $mPEG_{2000}$-PLA, and $mPEG_{5000}$-PLA microspheres, the $mPEG_{10000}$-PLA's particle size is larger, its surface has few small pores and its shape is smooth. The adhesion is due to the relatively large molecular weight of the mPEG-PLA copolymer. The pores on the surface are caused by water molecule diffusion during lyophilization. Figure 5 shows the particle size distribution of the mPEG-PLA microspheres loaded with ASAs using a laser particle-size analyzer (Mastersizer 3500, Microtrac, Malvern, UK). The average diameter of the $mPEG_{550}$-PLA microspheres was 1.803 ± 0.21 μm, and the PDI was 0.15. The average diameter of the $mPEG_{2000}$-PLA microspheres was 2.083 ± 0.17 μm, and the PDI was 0.14. The average diameter of the $mPEG_{5000}$-PLA microspheres was 2.631 ± 0.2 μm, and the PDI was 0.20. The average diameter of the $mPEG_{10000}$-PLA microspheres was 3.84 ± 0.30 μm, and the PDI was 0.18(Table 2). These results are nearly the same as those shown in the SEM images. The experimental results showed that the diameters of the 4 microspheres were smaller than 5 μm, indicating that these microspheres are suitable for oral of drug delivery, which is consistent with the study by Wei et al. [34].

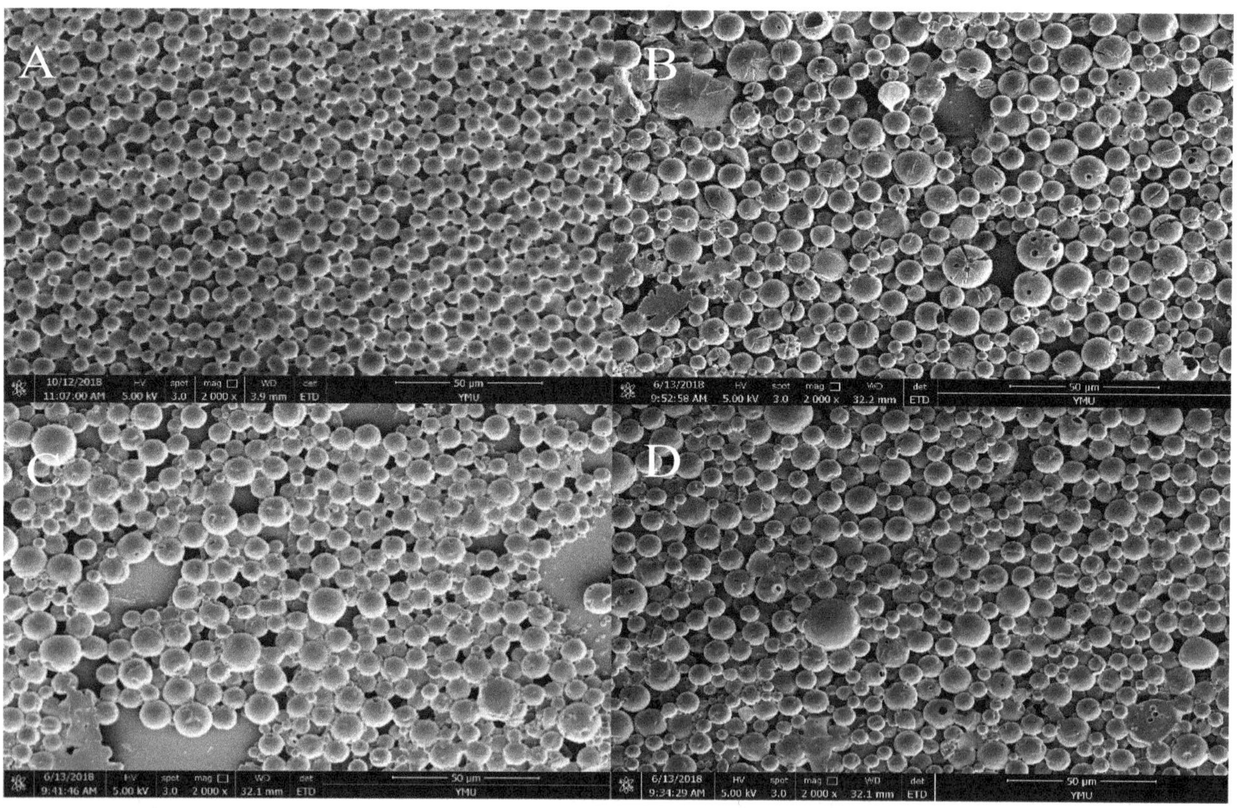

Figure 4. Scanning electron microscopy (SEM) images of mPEG-PLA microsphere. (**A**) mPEG 550-PLA, (**B**) mPEG 2000-PLA, (**C**) mPEG5000-PLA, (**D**) mPEG10000-PLA. The magnification of SEM image was 2000.

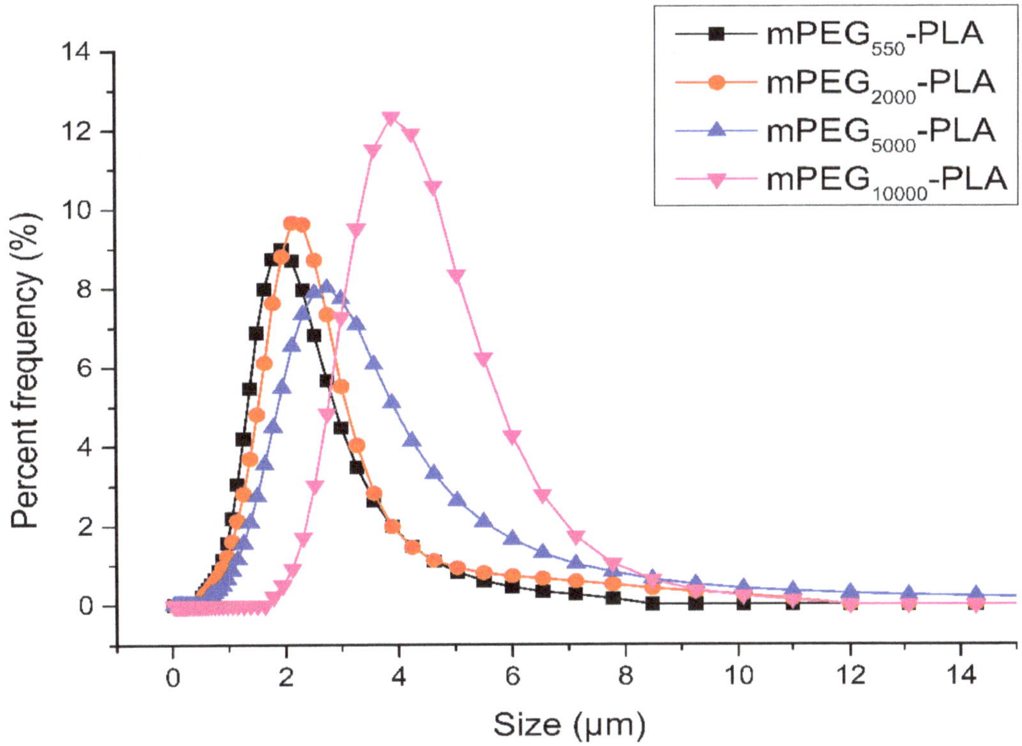

Figure 5. Size distribution of mPEG-PLA microsphere.

3.3. Drug Loads

mPEG-PLA microspheres loaded with ASAs were prepared using the W/O/W double-emulsion technique, and the EE and LE were measured by high-performance liquid chromatography (HPLC; Table 2). With the increased molecular weight, the microsphere's EE and LE increased, with trends similar to those of the mPEG-PLA microspheres loaded with recombinant human growth hormone (rhGH) prepared by Yi et al. [35]. While preparing the microspheres, a portion of the drug diffused into the external water phase due to solvent evaporation, resulting in drug loss. A copolymer with a high molecular weight has a large molecular gap, enabling the drug to diffuse outward, thus increasing drug loss.

Table 2. The average diameter, PDI, EE, LE of mPEG-PLA microspheres loaded ASAs.

Sample	Average Diameter (μm)	[1]PDI	[1]EE (%)	[1]LE (%)
$mPEG_{550}$-PLA	1.803 ± 0.21	0.15	53.97 ± 2.57	2.71 ± 0.21
$mPEG_{2000}$-PLA	2.083 ± 0.17	0.14	62.78 ± 3.44	3.05 ± 0.11
$mPEG_{5000}$-PLA	2.631 ± 0.20	0.20	70.28 ± 3.61	4.14 ± 0.12
$mPEG_{10000}$-PLA	3.840 ± 0.30	0.18	75.12 ± 4.25	5.17 ± 0.19

[1]PDI: polydispersity index of the particle size distribution. EE: encapsulation efficiency. LE: loading efficiency.

3.4. Analysis of In Vitro Microsphere Release

Figure 6 shows the release curve of mPEG-PLA microspheres loaded with ASAs in phosphate-buffered saline (PBS) (pH = 7.40). The cumulative amount of $mPEG_{550}$-PLA microspheres released on the first day was 24.32 ± 0.37%, and then, the release rate slowed, reaching 64.38 ± 1.21% after a two-week stable release. The cumulative amount of $mPEG_{2000}$-PLA microspheres released on the first day was 20.74 ± 0.29%, and then, the release rate slowed, reaching 57.09 ± 1.28% after a two-week stable release. The cumulative amount of $mPEG_{5000}$-PLA microspheres released on the first day was 19.54 ± 0.22%, and then, the release rate slowed, reaching 52.45 ± 1.28% after a two-week stable release. The cumulative amount of the $mPEG_{10000}$-PLA microspheres released on the first day was 15.03 ± 0.51%, and then, the release rate slowed, reaching 45.12 ± 1.04% after a two-week stable release. The relatively large amount of the drug released on the first day occurred because a small amount of the drug adhered to the microsphere surface when the microspheres encapsulated the drug. With the microsphere's increased molecular weight, in vitro release of the drug from the microspheres was relatively slow. The release time of the mPEG-PLA microspheres in this study was longer than that of the microspheres prepared by Zheng et al. [36] and Xiong et al. [37], indicating that the mPEG-PLA was well encapsulated on the ASAs.

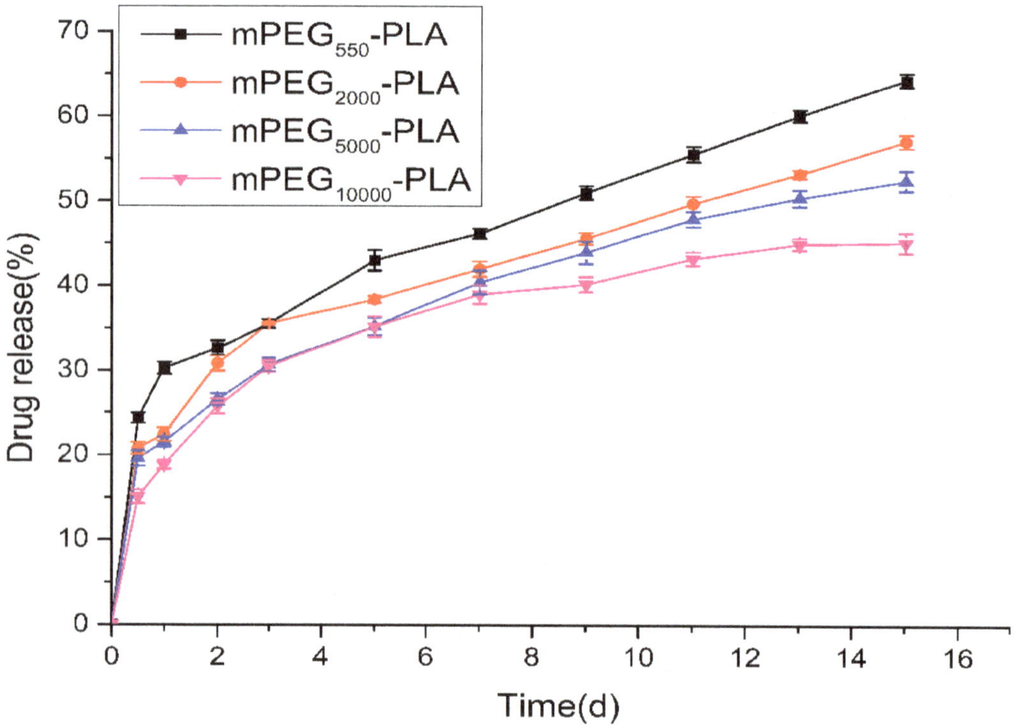

Figure 6. Release curve of mPEG-PLA microspheres loaded ASAs in PBS

3.5. Analysis of In Vitro Microsphere Degradation

Based on the morphology, particle size, EE, LE, and in vitro microsphere release, we selected $mPEG_{10000}$-PLA as the optimal microspheres for the study. Figure 7 shows the degradation process of the ASAs-loaded $mPEG_{10000}$-PLA microsphere. The figure shows the changes in the microsphere's dry weight, system pH and molecular weight over time. In PBS (pH = 7.40, 10 mM), the three curves all decreased with time. Within 60 days, the microspheric pH decreased from 7.40 to 5.89, the microspheres lost 47.16% of their dry weight, and their molecular weight dropped from 10307 Da to 8258 Da. As its degradation progressed, the mPEG-PLA was hydrolyzed to produce CO_2, which was dissolved in water to decrease the pH. mPEG-PLA is an amphiphilic material that absorbs water in PBS and breaks the hydrophilic segment, thus decreasing the molecular weight. As the hydrophilic segment breaks, the molecular weight of the copolymer decreases, resulting in a loss of copolymer quality. Li et al. [38] studied the degradation of mPEG-PLA nanoparticles and found that the mPEG-PLA degraded very slowly, and the Mn decreased by 27.6% within 30 days. Simone [39] et al. studied the polymer degradation conditions at pH and found that the pH decreased correspondingly over time, which is similar to the mPEG-PLA degradation trend in this study.

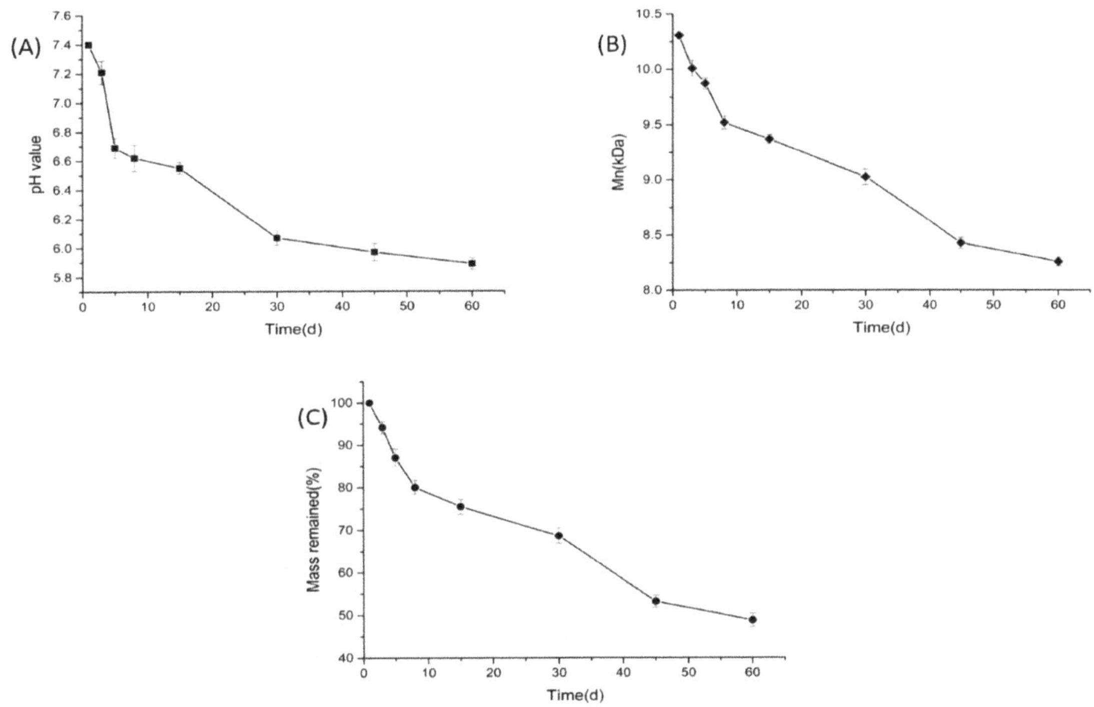

Figure 7. The degradation process of the ASAs-loaded $mPEG_{10000}$-PLA microspheres in the phosphate buffer saline (PBS) (pH = 7.40): the pH (**A**) Mn (**B**) and mass (**C**) changed with time.

3.6. Analysis of In Vitro Hemolytic Properties of Microspheres

Figure 8 shows the hemolysis and anticoagulation rates of the ASAs-loaded $mPEG_{10000}$-PLA microsphere, the $mPEG_{10000}$-PLA, and the ASAs. The hemolysis rates of the ASAs-loaded $mPEG_{10000}$-PLA microsphere, the $mPEG_{10000}$-PLA, and the ASAs increased as the concentration increased but did not exceed 5% at 40 μg/mL. Studies have shown that hemolysis rates below 5% indicate blood compatibility, which is consistent with the International Organization for Standardization (ISO) hemolysis standard, indicating applicability for intravenous injection. The anticoagulant chart shows that the blood clotting index (BCI) increases as the concentration increases, indicating that its anticoagulant activity increases as the sample concentration increases.

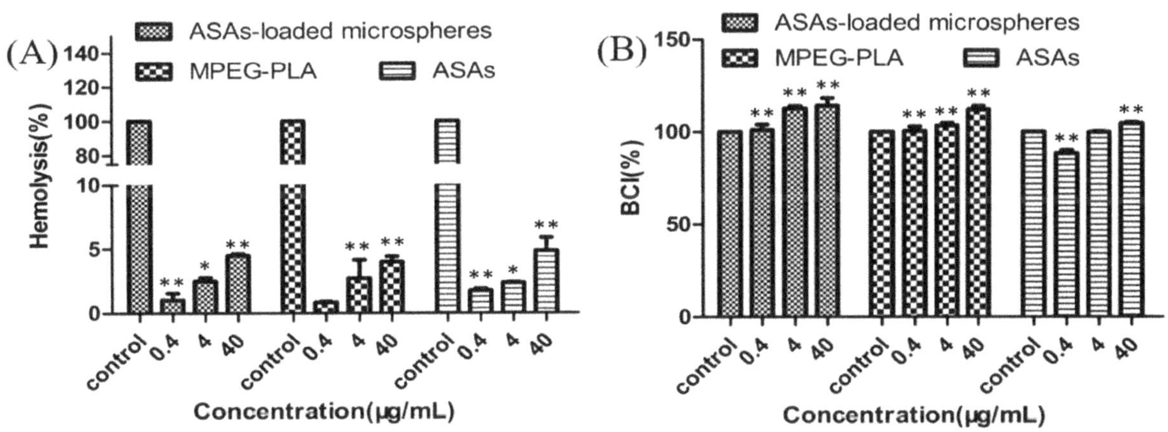

Figure 8. Hemolytic activity (**A**) and blood clotting index (**B**) of the ASAs-loaded $mPEG_{10000}$-PLA microsphere. * $P < 0.05$ and ** $P < 0.01$, compared with control, and the whole blood sample with the ASAs was used as a control.

3.7. *In Vitro Cytotoxicity Analysis of The Microspheres*

Figure 9 shows the cytotoxicity of the ASAs-loaded $mPEG_{10000}$-PLA microspheres, the $mPEG_{10000}$-PLA, and the ASAs to the HL-7702 (normal human hepatocyte) cell line. To study the cytotoxicity of the ASAs-loaded $mPEG_{10000}$-PLA microspheres, the 3-(4,5-dimethylthiazol-2-yl)-2,5-diphenyltetrazolium bromide (MTT) assay was used to detect HL-7702 cell viability under different concentrations of ASAs-loaded $mPEG_{10000}$-PLA microspheres, $mPEG_{10000}$-PLA, and ASAs. Figure 8 shows the toxicity at concentrations from 0.4 μg/mL to 40 μg/mL. The results showed that $mPEG_{10000}$-PLA microspheres could be used for drug loading. The microspheres prepared by Song et al. [40] showed that the HL-7702 cells were dose- and time-dependent, and as the concentration increased, the HL-7702 cell survival rate decreased, which is similar to the HL-7702 cell viability under the ASAs in this study.

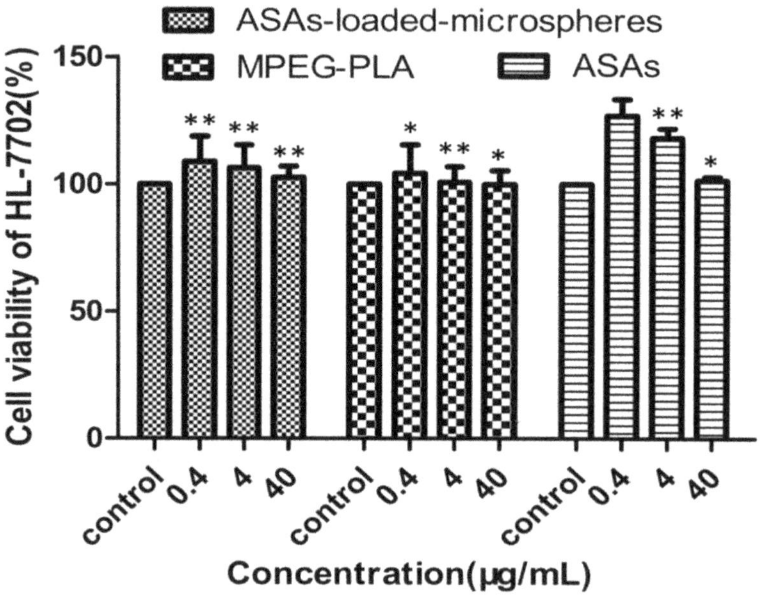

Figure 9. The cytotoxicity of the ASAs-loaded $mPEG_{10000}$-PLA microspheres, the $mPEG_{10000}$-PLA, and the ASAs to the HL-7702 cells. * $P < 0.05$ and ** $P < 0.01$, compared with control, and the whole blood sample with the ASAs was used as a control.

3.8. *Analysis of the Microspheric Anti-Inflammatory Activity*

Table 3 shows the effect of the ASAs on xylene-induced auricle swelling in mice. The ASAs-loaded microspheres significantly inhibited the xylene-induced auricle swelling in the mice. The effect of the ASAs-loaded microspheres at 10 mg/kg was comparable to that of the 0.3 g/kg DP, and the efficacies at 20 and 40 mg/kg were stronger than that of 10 mg/kg aspirin.

Table 3. Effect of the ASAs on xylene-induced auricle swelling in mice.

Group	Doses (/kg)	Auricular Swelling Degree ($\bar{x} \pm s$, mg)	Inhibition Rate (%)
Control	—	50.85 ± 3.61	—
Aspirin	10 mg	34.65 ± 2.90	31.86%
DP	0.3 g	37.65 ± 3.04	25.96%
ASAs	0.1 g	39.65 ± 0.78	22.03%
	10 mg	39.00 ± 2.69	23.30%
Loaded	20 mg	31.35 ± 6.86	38.35%
microspheres	40 mg	27.65 ± 7.57	45.62%

Table 4 shows the effect of the ASAs on egg-white-induced pedal swelling in rats. The ASAs-loaded microspheres significantly inhibited the egg-white-induced pedal swelling in the rats, and the action time of the ASAs-loaded microspheres at 20 mg/kg was longer than that of the DP, and the action time of ASAs-loaded microspheres at 80 mg/kg was similar to that of aspirin.

Table 4. Effect of the ASAs on egg-white-induced pedal swelling in rats.

Group	Doses (/kg)	Inhibitory Swelling Rate of Sole (%)				
		1h	2h	3h	4h	5h
Control	—	—	—	—	—	—
Aspirin	20 mg	66.77	62.07	57.02	52.17	49.55
DP	0.24 g	68.81	65.86	60.39	57.31	54.48
ASAs	0.16 g	78.97	69.99	68.29	60.14	57.87
Loaded microspheres	20 mg	51.73	47.12	43.72	38.97	35.14
	40 mg	59.62	55.47	46.64	44.61	41.78
	80 mg	75.37	73.22	65.14	58.07	55.27

4. Conclusions

ASAs-loaded mPEG-PLA microspheres were successfully prepared using the W/O/W double-emulsion technique. The comprehensive results for the microspheres, including particle size, EE, LE, in vitro release and other tests, showed that $mPEG_{10000}$-PLA microspheres performed excellently. The particle size of ASAs-loaded $mPEG_{10000}$-PLA microspheres was 3.84 ± 0.30 μm, the EE was 75.12 ± 4.25%, and the LE was 5.17 ± 0.19%. The microspheres sustained release for 15 days in a simulated human environment, with beneficial biocompatibility at 40 μg/mL, and showed no toxicity to HL-7702 cells. It significantly inhibited auricle swelling in mice and pedal swelling in rats. These results indicate that mPEG-PLA is a carrier material suitable for controlled ASAs release.

Author Contributions: M.Y. and C.Y. conceived and designed the experiments; X.Z., Y.H., R.Y. and N.J. performed the experiments; X.Z., M.S. and H.L. analyzed the data; M.Y., H.L. and M.Y. contributed reagents/materials/analysis tools; X.Z. wrote the paper. X.Z. and H.L. contributed equally to this work.

References

1. Mentese, S.; Mirici, N.A.; Otkun, M.T.; Bakar, C.; Palaz, E.; Tasdibi, D.; Cevizci, S.; Cotuker, O. Association between Respiratory Health and Indoor Air Pollution Exposure in Canakkale, Turkey. *Build. Environ.* **2015**, *93*, 72–83. [CrossRef]
2. Khyade, M.S.; Kasote, D.M.; Vaikos, N.P. *Alstonia scholaris* (L.) R. Br. and Alstonia macrophylla Wall. ex G. Don: A comparative review on traditional uses, phytochemistry and pharmacology. *J. Ethnopharmacol.* **2014**, *153*, 1–18. [CrossRef]
3. Atta-Ur-Rahman; Alvi, K.A. Indole alkaloids from *Alstonia scholaris*. *Phytochemistry* **1987**, *26*, 2139–2142. [CrossRef]
4. Atta-Ur-Rahman, A.; Asif, M.; Ghazala, M.; Fatima, J.; Alvi, K.A. Scholaricine, an alkaloid from *Alstonia scholaris*. *Phytochemistry* **1985**, *24*, 2771–2773. [CrossRef]
5. Xiang-Hai, C.; Zhi-Zhi, D.; Xiao-Dong, L. Unique monoterpenoid indole alkaloids from *Alstonia scholaris*. *Org. Lett.* **2007**, *9*, 1817–1820.
6. Cai, X.H.; Shang, J.H.; Tao, F.; Luo, X.D. Novel Alkaloids from *Alstonia scholaris*. *Zeitschrift Für Naturforschung B* **2010**, *65*, 1164–1168. [CrossRef]
7. Cai, X.H.; Tan, Q.G.; Liu, Y.P.; Feng, T.; Du, Z.Z.; Li, W.Q.; Luo, X.D. A cage-monoterpene indole alkaloid from *Alstonia scholaris*. *Org. Lett.* **2008**, *10*, 577–580. [CrossRef]
8. Zhao, Y.-L.; Shang, J.-H.; Pu, S.-B.; Wang, H.-S.; Wang, B.; Liu, L.; Liu, Y.-P.; Hong-Mei, S.; Luo, X.-D. Effect of total alkaloids from *Alstonia scholaris* on airway inflammation in rats. *J. Ethnopharmacol.* **2016**, *178*, 258–265. [CrossRef] [PubMed]
9. Shang, J.-H.; Cai, X.-H.; Zhao, Y.-L.; Feng, T.; Luo, X.-D. Pharmacological evaluation of *Alstonia scholaris*: Anti-tussive, anti-asthmatic and expectorant activities. *J. Ethnopharmacol.* **2010**, *129*, 293–298. [CrossRef] [PubMed]

10. Ho, D.; Leong, J.W.; Crew, R.C.; Norret, M.; House, M.J.; Mark, P.J.; Waddell, B.J.; Iyer, K.S.; Keelan, J.A. Maternal-placental-fetal biodistribution of multimodal polymeric nanoparticles in a pregnant rat model in mid and late gestation. *Sci. Rep.* **2017**, *7*, 2866. [CrossRef]
11. Anderson, J.M.; Shive, M.S. Biodegradation and biocompatibility of PLA and PLGA microspheres. *Adv. Drug Deliv. Rev.* **2012**, *64*, 72–82. [CrossRef]
12. Dong, C.M.; Guo, Y.Z.; Qiu, K.Y.; Gu, Z.W.; Feng, X.D. In vitro degradation and controlled release behavior of d, l-PLGA50 and PCL-b-d, l-PLGA50 copolymer microspheres. *J. Control. Release* **2005**, *107*, 53–64. [CrossRef]
13. Carreras, N.; Acuña, V.; Martí, M.; Lis, M.J. Drug release system of ibuprofen in PCL-microspheres. *Colloid Polym. Sci.* **2013**, *291*, 157–165. [CrossRef]
14. Yu, H.; Ping, L.; Chen, S.; Liu, Y.; Fu, D. The influence of hydrophilic mPEG segment on formation, morphology, and properties of PCL-mPEG microspheres. *Adv. Polym. Technol.* **2017**, *37*, 2281–2287.
15. Zheng, W.; Li, M.; Lin, Y.; Zhan, X. Encapsulation of verapamil and doxorubicin by MPEG-PLA to reverse drug resistance in ovarian cancer. *Biomed. Pharmacother.* **2018**, *108*, 565–573. [CrossRef]
16. Li, X.; Huang, Z. Advance of Preparation and Application of Polylactide and Its Copolymers. *Chin. Polym. Bull.* **1999**, *1*, 24–32.
17. Qing, X.; Yingying, Z.; Xu, C.; Haimei, L.; Evans, D.G.; Wensheng, Y. Nanosheet-based titania microspheres with hollow core-shell structure encapsulating horseradish peroxidase for a mediator-free biosensor. *Biomaterials* **2011**, *32*, 6588–6594.
18. Hou, X.; Hao, Y. *Fabrication of Polystyrene/Detonation Nanographite Composite Microspheres with the Core/Shell Structure via Pickering Emulsion Polymerization*; Hindawi Publishing Corp.: London, UK, 2013.
19. Hiraoka, S. Microspheres Having Core/Shell Structure. U.S. Patent 20100203151A1, 12 August 2010.
20. Keramati, M.; Ghasemi, I.; Karrabi, M.; Azizi, H.; Sabzi, M. Incorporation of surface modified graphene nanoplatelets for development of shape memory PLA nanocomposite. *Fibers Polym.* **2016**, *17*, 1062–1068. [CrossRef]
21. Qi, Y.; Geng, Y.; Ma, B.; Yun, H.; Cui, C. In vitro hemolytic properties' assessment of K2Ti6O13 nanowires. *Proc. Inst. Mech. Eng. Part N J. Nanoeng. Nanosyst.* **2014**, *229*, 201–205. [CrossRef]
22. Henkelman, S.; Rakhorst, G.; Blanton, J.; Oeveren, W.V. Standardization of incubation conditions for hemolysis testing of biomaterials. *Mater. Sci. Eng. C* **2009**, *29*, 1650–1654. [CrossRef]
23. Muthukumarasamyvel, T.; Rajendran, G.; Santhana, P.D.; Kasthuri, J.; Kathiravan, K.; Rajendiran, N. Role of Surface Hydrophobicity of Dicationic Amphiphile-Stabilized Gold Nanoparticles on A549 Lung Cancer Cells. *ACS Omega* **2017**, *2*, 3527–3538. [CrossRef]
24. Qiu, Y.Y.; Chen, Y.; Zhou, W.Y.; Xia, X.L.; Yang, X.J. Biocompatibility and security of calcium sulfate bone substitutes. *Chin. J. Tissue Eng. Res.* **2016**, *20*, 2317–2323.
25. Cao, Y.E.; Wang, H.; Yang, C.; Zhong, R.; Lei, Y.U.; Sun, K.; Liu, J. In vitro studies of PBT Nonwoven Fabrics adsorbent for the removal of low density lipoprotein from hyperlipemia plasma. *Appl. Surf. Sci.* **2011**, *257*, 7521–7528. [CrossRef]
26. Ciochină, A.D.; Bredeţean, O.; Dimitriu, D.C.; Iacob, G. Considerations on in vitro and in vivo magnetic nanoparticles hemocompatibility testing. *Revista Medico-Chirurgicala a Societatii de Medici si Naturalisti din Iasi* **2009**, *113*, 279–285.
27. Ren, B.R.; Liu, J.; Zhang, E.L.; Dong, H. Biocompatibility of a new titanium alloy containing copper. *Chin. J. Tissue Eng. Res.* **2015**, *1*, 5473–5479.
28. Archana, D.; Dutta, J.; Dutta, P.K. Evaluation of chitosan nano dressing for wound healing: Characterization, in vitro and in vivo studies. *Int. J. Biol. Macromol.* **2013**, *57*, 193–203. [CrossRef] [PubMed]
29. Lan, G.; Lu, B.; Wang, T.; Wang, L.; Chen, J.; Yu, K.; Liu, J.; Dai, F.; Wu, D. Chitosan/gelatin composite sponge is an absorbable surgical hemostatic agent. *Colloids Surf. B Biointerfaces* **2015**, *136*, 1026–1034. [CrossRef]
30. Chia-Jen, L.; Chia-Herng, Y.; Yu-Jie, L.; Yu-Yu, L.; Shao-Hsuan, K.; Jer-Yuh, L.; Yieng-How, C. Antitumor activity of acriflavine in lung adenocarcinoma cell line A549. *Anticancer Res.* **2014**, *34*, 6467–6472.
31. Kumar, S.P.; Birundha, K.; Kaveri, K.; Devi, K.T.R. Antioxidant studies of chitosan nanoparticles containing naringenin and their cytotoxicity effects in lung cancer cells. *Int. J. Biol. Macromol.* **2015**, *78*, 87–95. [CrossRef] [PubMed]
32. Ge, Y.; Cheng, R.; Zhou, Y.; Shen, J.; Peng, L.; Xu, X.; Dai, Q.; Liu, P.; Wang, H.; Ma, X. Cryptotanshinone induces cell cycle arrest and apoptosis of multidrug resistant human chronic myeloid leukemia cells by inhibiting the activity of eukaryotic initiation factor 4E. *Mol. Cell. Biochem.* **2012**, *368*, 17–25. [CrossRef] [PubMed]

33. Zhang, H.; Shi, X. Anti-inflammatory and analgesic effects of total flavonoids in flos sophorae immaturus. *Clin. Res. Pract.* **2018**, *11*, 4–6.
34. Wei, Y.; Wang, Y.; Kang, A.; Wang, W.; Ho, S.V.; Gao, J.; Ma, G.; Su, Z. A novel sustained-release formulation of recombinant human growth hormone and its pharmacokinetic, pharmacodynamic and safety profiles. *Mol. Pharm.* **2012**, *9*, 2039. [CrossRef] [PubMed]
35. Yi, W.; Xia, W.Y.; Wei, W.; Ho, S.V.; Feng, Q.; Guang Hui, M.; Guo, S.Z. Microcosmic mechanisms for protein incomplete release and stability of various amphiphilic mPEG-PLA microspheres. *Langmuir* **2012**, *28*, 13984–13992.
36. Zheng, X.L.; Kan, B.; Gou, M.L.; Fu, S.Z.; Zhang, J.; Men, K.; Chen, L.J.; Luo, F.; Zhao, Y.L.; Zhao, X. Preparation of MPEG–PLA nanoparticle for honokiol delivery in vitro. *Int. J. Pharm.* **2010**, *386*, 262–267. [CrossRef] [PubMed]
37. LizhiXiong; ZeqiangHe, Preparation and In-Vitro Properties of mPEG/PLA Microspheres Loaded 5-Fluorouracil for Controlled Release. *J. Macromol. Sci. Part D Rev. Polym. Process.* **2013**, *52*, 268–272.
38. Yuan, L.; Rong, Q.X.; Yoshie, M.; Tsuneji, N. PEG-PLA diblock copolymer micelle-like nanoparticles as all-trans-retinoic acid carrier: In vitro and in vivo characterizations. *Nanotechnology* **2009**, *20*, 055106.
39. Simone, E.A.; Dziubla, T.D.; Francheska, C.G.; Discher, D.E.; Muzykantov, V.R. Effect of polymer amphiphilicity on loading of a therapeutic enzyme into protective filamentous and spherical polymer nanocarriers. *Biomacromolecules* **2007**, *8*, 3914–3921. [CrossRef]
40. Song, X.L.; Bo, L.; Xu, K.; Liu, J.; Wen, J.; Wang, J.; Liu, X.D.; Li, J.; Qi, Y.F. Cytotoxicity of water-soluble mPEG-SH-coated silver nanoparticles in HL-7702 cells. *Cell Biol. Toxicol.* **2012**, *28*, 225–237. [CrossRef] [PubMed]

8

Particle-Size-Dependent Delivery of Antitumoral miRNA Using Targeted Mesoporous Silica Nanoparticles

Lisa Haddick [1], Wei Zhang [2], Sören Reinhard [2], Karin Möller [1], Hanna Engelke [1], Ernst Wagner [2] and Thomas Bein [1,*]

1 Department of Chemistry and Center for NanoScience, University of Munich (LMU), Butenandtstrasse 5-13, 81377 Munich, Germany; lisa.haddick@cup.lmu.de (L.H.); K.Moeller@lmu.de (K.M.); hanna.engelke@cup.lmu.de (H.E.)

2 Pharmaceutical Biotechnology and Center for NanoScience, University of Munich (LMU), Butenandtstrasse 5-13, 81377 Munich, Germany; wei.zhang@cup.uni-muenchen.de (W.Z.); reinhard.soeren@cup.uni-muenchen.de (S.R.); Ernst.Wagner@cup.uni-muenchen.de (E.W.)

* Correspondence: bein@lmu.de

Abstract: Multifunctional core-shell mesoporous silica nanoparticles (MSN) were tailored in size ranging from 60 to 160 nm as delivery agents for antitumoral microRNA (miRNA). The positively charged particle core with a pore diameter of about 5 nm and a stellate pore morphology allowed for an internal, protective adsorption of the fragile miRNA cargo. A negatively charged particle surface enabled the association of a deliberately designed block copolymer with the MSN shell by charge-matching, simultaneously acting as a capping as well as endosomal release agent. Furthermore, the copolymer was functionalized with the peptide ligand GE11 targeting the epidermal growth factor receptor, EGFR. These multifunctional nanoparticles showed an enhanced uptake into EGFR-overexpressing T24 bladder cancer cells through receptor-mediated cellular internalization. A luciferase gene knock-down of up to 65% and additional antitumoral effects such as a decreased cell migration as well as changes in cell cycle were observed. We demonstrate that nanoparticles with a diameter of 160 nm show the fastest cellular internalization after a very short incubation time of 45 min and produce the highest level of gene knock-down.

Keywords: mesoporous silica nanoparticles; core-shell; surface functionalization; cell targeting; size-dependent delivery; antitumoral microRNA (miRNA); confocal microscopy

1. Introduction

A novel modality in cancer therapy emerged over the past two decades in the form of gene therapy and in this context, small interfering RNA (siRNA) and micro RNA (miRNA) are promising alternatives to common anti-cancer medications [1,2]. Both nucleotide oligomers mediate the process of RNA interference (RNAi) in which cells use these short RNA strands of 19-24 nucleotides to recognize messenger RNA (mRNA) with a complementary sequence, induce their destruction and thus inhibit the translation into proteins. To provide cancer therapy, synthetically produced siRNA and miRNA mimics can be used that target and silence specific oncogenes. Recent studies have identified a number of cancer-related genes as potential targets for RNAi-based therapy [3–5]. One of these tumor suppressor miRNA is miR200c, which targets the proto-oncogene KRAS. It regulates cell differentiation, proliferation and survival [6], the epithelial to mesenchymal transition [7] and suppresses chemoresistance [8].

However, a major challenge for a widespread therapeutic application of RNAi is creating appropriate delivery vehicles to safely and effectively deliver and release siRNA and miRNA into the cytosol of disease-causing cells. Several excellent reviews summarize the requirements for siRNA delivery and comprehensively report on the efficiencies of gene silencing achieved with various delivery materials [9–11].

Some promising results were recently obtained from ongoing clinical trials concerning RNA delivery vehicles and in 2018 Alnylam's Onpattro (Patisiran) has been FDA-approved as the first ever RNAi drug against nerve damage caused by the rare hereditary disease, transthyretin amyloidosis [12]. However, Patisiran is a lipid-based nanocarrier system that does not actively target the cancer tissue, and most of the administered drug accumulates passively in the liver instead. Therefore, robust and specifically targeted carrier systems are needed for an efficient delivery of siRNA and miRNA to prevent a premature degradation of the unstable RNA. For this purpose, nanoparticles have attracted much attention because they provide a stable, nontoxic, and highly flexible platform.

Mesoporous silica nanoparticles (MSN) are emerging as potential nanocarriers for a variety of anti-cancer cargos including nucleic acids [13,14]. The properties that have rendered them specifically suitable for siRNA and miRNA delivery include a high surface area and pore volume, a controllable biodegradability [15,16], the tunability of particle size and pore size, their variable morphology and importantly, the possibility to create core-shell particles constructed of spatially separated regions with different surface functionalization [17,18].

This tunability of MSNs opens the possibility to systematically study the influence of the carrier properties on the gene silencing efficacy. Multiple parameters can affect successful gene silencing using carrier agents, e.g., the adsorption and release kinetics of the nucleic acid in the drug carrier, the dependence of cellular uptake or endosomal escape on nanoparticle size, surface characteristics such as charge and/or the attachments of functional residues, to name a few, but systematic studies addressing these issues are rare [19].

For the adsorption and release kinetics of nucleic acids using MSNs, the pore size, pore morphology and surface charge are important parameters. High loadings of nucleic acid were achieved by using large pore MSNs with a pore diameter of around 10–20 nm [20] and when pores were modified with cationic functional groups—aminopropyltriethoxysilane (APTES) or polylysine—to create a cationic layer for nucleic acid adsorption [14,21]. However, some of these systems suffer from poor release kinetics associated with low knockdown efficacies because of either the high affinity of polycations towards nucleic acid or because of a bottleneck-type pore morphology that features smaller pore openings than pore diameters, which both might decrease an efficient release of the highly charged nucleic acid molecules. Based on these findings, our group introduced novel medium-pore MSNs (pore diameter of around 5 nm) with stellate pore morphology, which were able to adsorb an exceptionally high amount of siRNA of 380 $\mu g\ mg^{-1}$ and which enabled a mainly electrostatically driven fast and efficient RNA desorption, resulting in a high silencing efficacy [21].

Cellular internalization of the nanocarrier is another factor that influences gene silencing efficacy. The relationship between shape and size of MSNs [22–25] or other nanocarriers [26,27] and cellular internalization is important as nanoparticle size may affect the uptake efficiency and kinetics and the internalization mechanism [28]. One of the great advantages of MSNs is that they can be designed to feature different sizes and shapes. For MSNs [22,29] as well as for Au [30], polystyrene [31] and iron oxide nanoparticles [32], a size-dependent uptake in cells was observed with a maximum uptake at a particle diameter of 30–50 nm. However, as size is only one among several parameters controlling cellular uptake of nanoparticles, optimal sizes may vary for different surfaces and different surface functionalizations. Additionally, targeting ligands were shown to improve selective cellular uptake and a better accumulation in tumor tissue [33,34]. The effect of particle size on gene transfection efficiency using silica-based nanoparticles with diameters from 125 to 570 nm as nanocarriers for plasmid DNA was studied by Yu et al. Here, the transfection efficiency was found to be a compromise between binding capacity of the nanocarriers and cellular uptake. Smaller particles showed higher cellular uptake but less binding capacity for plasmid DNA. Particles with a diameter of 330 nm showed the best gene transfection efficacy [35].

Gene silencing mediated by delivery of siRNA and miRNA with MSN nanocarriers is strongly dependent on the escape of siRNA or miRNA from the endosomes into the cytosol. To trigger this reaction, the surface of particles is often decorated with cationic polymers, which are known to support an endosomal escape. Polyethylenimine (PEI) is one well-studied polymer exhibiting good endosomal escape capability when used at high dosage, attributed to a 'proton sponge' effect, however, it has a poor toxicity profile [36]. For instance, the group of Gu showed very good knockdown efficacies when PEI was attached to the outside of their particles [37,38].

A systematic study of the correlation between gene knockdown efficacy and endosomal escape kinetics was performed by Wang et al. [39]. They used magnetic MSNs capped with PEI at low concentrations to avoid toxic effects, resulting in poor endosomal escape ability. When endosomal escape was induced by a chloroquine treatment at early transfection times they could still see a high gene silencing efficacy. In contrast, when applied at later stages, a low gene-silencing efficacy was found, presumably because the released RNA was already degraded within the endosome.

Although MSNs have shown great potential as an efficient carrier system for siRNA and miRNA delivery, systematic studies about particle properties and corresponding gene-silencing efficacy remain rare. Herein, we present a systematic investigation of the particle size-dependent delivery of miRNA using core-shell MSNs for gene silencing in T24 cells. A series of MSNs with uniform sizes ranging from 60 to 160 nm with an average pore diameter of around 5–6 nm was used to encapsulate an antitumoral microRNA mimic (miR200c) or a control RNA with a scrambled sequence (Ctrl). The core of these particles was functionalized with APTES to yield a positively charged inner surface to accommodate the negatively charged miRNA, while a thinner surface layer was enriched with mercaptosilane, forming a negatively charged shell to enable binding of the capping agent. This consisted of an amino-acid block-copolymer 454 (see Figure 1) to aid endosomal escape and which was further linked via polyethylene glycol (PEG) to the peptide GE11, targeting the epidermal growth factor receptor [40]. This vector is abbreviated as MSN-454-GE11. An alternative construct for the delivery of this miRNA was studied before by Müller et al. using RNA-encapsulating polyplexes consisting of the same copolymer 454 functionalized with GE11 [41]. Their particles, featuring a size of 120–150 nm, successfully showed antitumoral effects with two different therapeutic RNAs.

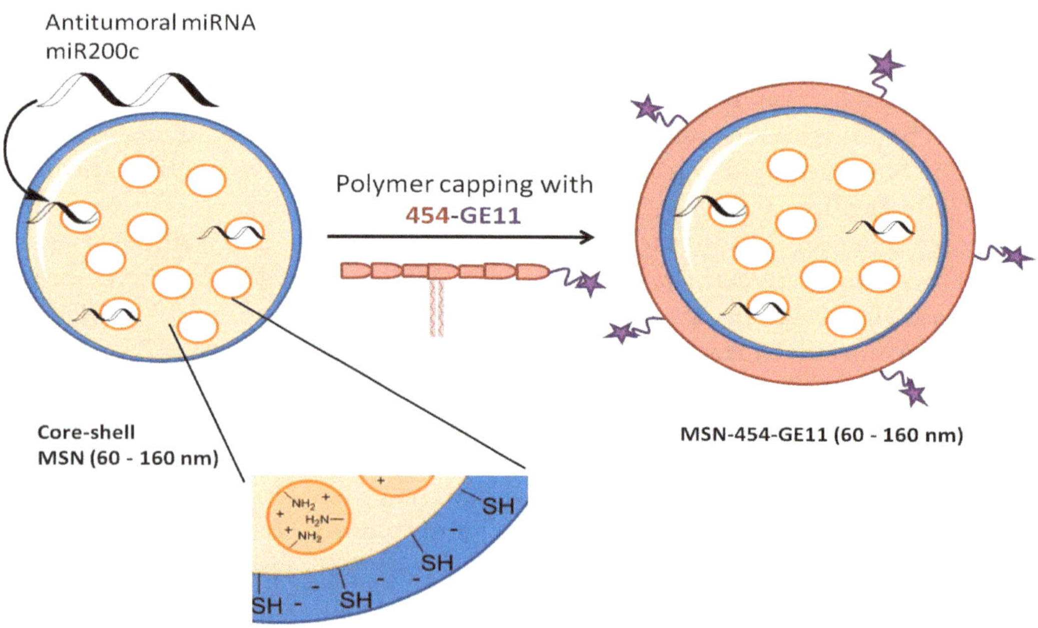

Figure 1. Schematic overview of the structure of core-shell mesoporous silica nanoparticles (MSN), the loading of miR200c and the polymer capping resulting in the MSN-454-GE11 vector. The positively

charged core in core-shell MSN enables a high loading capacity for miRNA. The mercapto-lined MSN shell associates with a positively charged block copolymer carrying the targeting ligand GE11, thus acting simultaneously as capping, endosomal release and targeting agent.

Our series of MSN-454-GE11 particles covers a broad size range but still provides comparable properties for each sample, including surface chemistry, surface charge, pore size and miRNA concentration to enable a conclusive study of the particle-size effect on miRNA delivery. Here, we show that good gene-silencing and antitumoral effects are obtained when miR200c is delivered by the largest MSN-454-GE11 particles in this sequence.

2. Materials and Methods

2.1. *Reagents and Materials*

2-(*N*-morpholino)ethanesulfonic acid (MES, Sigma-Adrich, Darmstadt, Germany), 3-aminopropyltriethoxysilane (APTES, Sigma-Adrich), 3-mercaptopropyl triethoxysilane (MPTES, >95%, Sigma-Adrich), ammonium fluoride (NH_4F, >98% Fluka, Darmstadt, Germany), Atto 633-carboxy dye (Atto-Tec, Siegen, Germany), 4′,6-diamidino-2-phenylindole (DAPI, Thermo Fisher, Schwerte, Germany), block copolymer surfactant (Pluronic F127 ($EO_{106}PO_{70}EO_{106}$), Sigma-Aldrich), cetyltrimethyl-ammonium chloride (CTAC, 25% in H_2O, Sigma-Adrich), *N*-(3-dimethylaminopropyl)-*N*′-ethylcarbodiimide hydrochloride (EDC, >97%, Sigma-Adrich), *N*-hydroxysulfosuccinimide (sulfo-NHS, 98%, Sigma-Adrich), octadecyltrimethylammonium bromide ($C_{18}Br$, Sigma-Adrich), propidium iodide, tetraethylorthosilicate (TEOS, >98%, Sigma-Aldrich), triethanolamine (TEA, 98%, Fluka), triisopropylbenzene (TiPB, 96%, Sigma-Adrich). Oligomer 454 [42] and Mal-PEG-GE11 [41] were synthesized as described before. siRNA and miRNA duplexes were purchased from Axolabs GmbH (Kulmbach, Germany): control RNA (sense: 5-AuGuAuuGG ccuGuAuuAGdTsdT-3′, antisense: 5′-CuAAuAcAGGcAAuAcAUdTsdT-3), miR200c (sense: 5′-UCCAUCAUUACCCGGCAGUAUUA-3, antisense: 5′-UAAUACUGCCGGGUAAUGAUGGA-3).

2.2. *Synthesis of MSN-NH2in-Shout*

Two slightly different synthesis methods were used to prepare core-shell functionalized MSN containing 4.5% amino groups in the core and 2% thiol groups on the shell (MSN-NH_{2in}-SH_{out}).

Procedure A: Core-shell MSN particles were prepared by a co-condensation reaction according to our previous reports [17,43]. Early reports from our group showed that a consistent decrease in particle size can be obtained by decreasing the amount of TEA serving as organic base. This concept was applied for the synthesis of samples MSN160 nm, MSN130 nm and MSN100 nm [44]. A mixture of TEA (14 g, 93.8 mmol/10 g, 67 mmol/4 g, 26.8 mmol, respectively), tetraethylorthosilicate (TEOS, 1.74 mL, 7.84 mmol) and 3-aminopropyltriethoxysilane (APTES, 89 μL, 0.38 mmol) in a polypropylene reactor was heated in an oil bath at 90 °C for 20 min without stirring. A second solution was prepared consisting of water (2.41 mL, 1.21 mol), CTAC (2.71 mL, 1.83 mmol), TiPB (2.97 mL, 12 mmol) and ammonium fluoride (NH_4F, 100 mg, 2.7 mmol) and was heated to 60 °C under stirring. The second solution was subsequently added to the first solution under strong stirring. The whole mixture was further stirred at room temperature for 20 min. After this time, four portions of TEOS (4 × 51 μL, 0.92 mmol) were added in three minute intervals and the solution was stirred for another 30 min. To prepare the shell layer, a premixed solution of TEOS (42 μL, 0.190 mmol) and mercaptopropyl triethoxysilane (MPTES) (42 μL, 0.22 mmol) was added to the whole mixture. The condensation reaction was allowed to continue over night at room temperature.

Procedure B: MSN80 nm and MSN60 nm were prepared using the tri-block copolymer F127 as a particle growth inhibitor/dispersant. The procedure is based on an adapted recipe reported in the literature [45]. First, a mixture of TEA (7 g, 46.8 mmol/4 g, 26.7 mmol, respectively), TiPB (1.5 mL, 6.2 mmol), F127 (100 mg, 8 μmol) TEOS (2 mL, 9 mmol), and APTES (89 μL, 0.38 mmol) was prepared in a polypropylene reactor and heated at 90 °C for 20 min. Separately, NH_4F (100 mg, 2.7 mmol) and $C_{18}Br$

(0.35 g, 0.9 mmol) were dissolved in H_2O. This solution was heated to 90 °C under static conditions for 30 min and was then added under strong stirring to the first solution at once. The combined solutions were further heated at 60 °C for 30 min. The ingredients for the shell layer, TEOS (42 μL, 0.190 mmol) and MPTES (42 μL, 0.22 mmol), were mixed, preheated to 60 °C and added to the reaction mixture. Heating at 60 °C was continued for 30 min, and then the reaction mixture was allowed to cool down to room temperature under stirring and was continuously stirred overnight.

2.3. Template Extraction

Agglomerates were removed from the as- synthesized samples by centrifugation for a short time at low speed (7197 rcf, 5 min). The pellet was discarded and the remaining particles in the supernatant were collected via centrifugation (7197 rcf, 20 min) for template extraction. After centrifugation, the particles were resuspended in a solution containing 2 g ammonium nitrate in 100 mL ethanol and heated for 45 min under reflux (90 °C), cooled and collected by centrifugation (7197 rcf, 20 min). The first reflux treatment was followed by a second extraction step for 45 min under reflux (90 °C) using a solution of 10 mL concentrated hydrochloric acid in 90 mL ethanol. The MSNs were collected by centrifugation for 20 min (7197 rcf) and washed with ethanol (3 × 70 mL). Finally, MSNs were dispersed in 15 mL ethanol and used for further characterization.

2.4. Characterization

For transmission electron microscopy (TEM), samples were prepared by drying a diluted ethanolic suspension of MSN on a carbon-coated copper grid at room temperature for several hours. The measurements were performed on a Tecnai G2 20 S-Twin instrument operated at 200 kV with a TVIPS TemCam-F216 camera.

Dynamic light scattering (DLS) and zeta potential measurements were performed with a Malvern Zetasizer Nano instrument equipped with a 4 mW He-Ne-Laser (633 nm). For DLS data, a diluted colloidal suspension of the particles was measured in PMMA cuvettes at 25 °C. For zeta potential measurements, the additional Zetasizer titration system (MPT-2) was used based on diluted NaOH and HCl as titrants. For this purpose, a colloidal suspension of MSNs in water at a concentration of 0.1 mg mL^{-1} was prepared.

Raman spectroscopy was performed on a Bruker Equinox 55 with FRA-106 Raman attachment with a ND:YAG laser (1064 nm) and a laser power of 100 mW. Infrared spectra of dried sample powder were recorded on a ThermoScientific Nicolet iN10 IRmicroscope in reflection–absorption mode with a liquid-N_2 cooled MCT-A detector.

A Quantachrome Instrument NOVA 4000e was used for nitrogen sorption analysis at −196 °C. Sample outgassing was performed for 12 h at 120 °C and at a vacuum of 13.3×10^{-3} mbar. A quenched solid density functional theory (QSDFT) equilibrium model of N_2 on silica at a relative pressure $p/p_0 = 0.8$ was used to calculate the pore size and pore volume, based on the adsorption and desorption branch of the isotherm. A BET model in the range $p/p_0 = 0.05$–0.2 was used to determine the specific surface area.

Thermogravimetric analysis (TGA) of the powder samples (10 mg) was performed on a Netzsch STA 440 C TG/DSC using a heating rate of 10 °C/min up to 900 °C with a stream of synthetic air of about 25 mL·min^{-1}. siRNA concentrations were determined by UV measurements performed with the Nanodrop 2000c spectrometer (Thermo Scientific).

2.5. Loading of Ctrl and miR200c for Gene Silencing

In all experiments, 100 μL Ctrl or miR200c solution (c = 50 ng μL^{-1}) in MES buffer (pH = 5) was added to 100 μg MSN-NH_{2in}-SH_{out} samples, resulting in a final RNA concentration of 50 μg mg^{-1} of MSN carrier. Samples were vortexed and shaken at 37 °C for 30 min to complete adsorption. Particles were washed via centrifugation and were resuspended in 100 μL HEPES buffer. The supernatant was collected to verify complete adsorption of RNA.

2.6. Loading of Fluorescent Dye for Cellular Internalization Studies

A total of 1 mL MSN-NH_{2in}-SH_{out} samples (pH = 5; 1 mg mL^{-1} MES buffer) was mixed with 2 μL Atto-633 carboxy (2 mg mL^{-1} in anhydrous DMSO), 10 μL EDC and a catalytic amount of sulfo-NHS. The samples were vortexed and shaken for 4 h, were washed multiple times afterwards with MES and HEPES buffer (1 mL, respectively) (centrifugation steps: 10 min, 16,900 rcf) and were redispersed in 1 mL MES buffer.

2.7. Capping with 454-GE11

For capping of MSN-NH_{2in}-SH_{out} samples, 10 μL Mal-PEG-GE11 reagent (5 mg mL^{-1} in H_2O) was added to 100 μL 454 solution (5 mg mL^{-1} in H_2O) and shaken for 2 h at 37 °C. Then, 454-GE11 was mixed with 1 mL MSN suspension (1 mg mL^{-1} in HEPES buffer) and again shaken for 2 h at 37 °C. Resulting MSN-454-GE11 samples were centrifuged (16,900 rcf, 10 min) and washed with water and HEPES buffer. The samples were redispersed in 2 mL HEPES buffer.

2.8. miRNA Binding Assay

For the miRNA binding assay, a 2.5% agarose gel was prepared by dissolving agarose in TBE buffer (Trizma base 10.8 g, boric acid 5.5 g, disodium EDTA 0.75 g, and 1 L of water) and by heating to 100 °C. GelRed® (1:10,000) was added and the agarose gel was cast in the electrophoresis unit. MSN-454-GE11 samples loaded with Ctrl RNA were mixed with 4 μL loading buffer (6 mL glycerol, 1.2 mL of 0.5 M EDTA, 2.8 mL H_2O, 0.02 g bromophenol blue) and placed into the gel sample pockets. Electrophoresis was run at 120 V for 90 min.

2.9. Cell Culture

HeLa, T24 or T24/eGFPLuc-200cT (authenticated by DSMZ, Braunschweig, Germany) cells, stably expressing an eGFP-luciferase fusion gene under the control of the CMV promoter and with a target site for miR200c, were cultivated in Dulbecco's modified Eagle's medium (DMEM) supplemented with 10% fetal bovine serum (FBS), 100 U mL^{-1} penicillin and 100 U mL^{-1} streptomycin.

2.10. Cell Viability Determined by MTT Assay

MTT assay was performed in triplicate in 96-well plates. One day prior to transfection, T24 cells were seeded at 3500 cells/well. Before transfection, medium was replaced by 80 μL fresh medium. MSN samples (20 μL) loaded with or without RNA were added at different concentrations in HEPES buffer and incubated for 45 min at 37 °C followed by a medium exchange. Subsequently, cells were returned to the incubator and 48 h after transfection a viability assay was performed. For this, an MTT solution (100 μL/well; 0.5 mg mL^{-1} in DMEM) was added for 2 h. Then, the supernatant was removed and cells were lysed by freezing at −80 °C. DMSO (100 μL) was added and plates were incubated at 37 °C under shaking. Absorption at 590 nm against a reference wavelength of 630 nm was measured using a SpectraFluorTM Plus microplate reader S4 (Tecan, Groeding, Austria). Cell viability was calculated as percentage of absorption compared to wells treated with HEPES buffer.

2.11. Cellular Adhesion Determined by Flow Cytometry

T24/eGFPLuc-200cT cells were seeded 24 h before transfection on 24-well plates with a density of 5×10^5 cells per well in 1000 μL growth medium. After 24 h, the medium was replaced by 400 μL fresh medium. A total of 100 μL MSN, MSN-454-PEG and MSN-454-GE11 samples loaded with fluorescent dye (500 μg mL^{-1} MSN in HEPES buffer) were added and incubated for 45 min at 37 °C. After incubation time, the cells were washed three times with PBS, 500 I.U. heparin to remove particles non-specifically associated to the cell surface and were detached with trypsin/EDTA, taken up in growth medium, centrifuged and resuspended in PBS containing 10% FBS. Cellular internalization of the MSN samples was assayed by flow cytometry at an Atto-633 carboxy fluorescent dye excitation wavelength of 635 nm and detection of emission at 665 nm. Cells were gated by forward/sideward scatter and pulse width for exclusion of doublets. DAPI (4′,6-diamidino-2-phenylindole) was used to discriminate between viable and dead cells. Data were recorded by BD LSRFortessa™ (BD Biosciences, USA) and analyzed by FlowJo® 7.6.5 flow cytometric analysis software. All experiments were performed in triplicate.

2.12. Confocal Fluorescence Microscopy

Fluorescence microscopy was performed with a Zeiss Observer SD spinning disk confocal microscope using a Yokogawa CSU-X1 spinning disc unit and an oil objective (63× magnification) and BP 525/50 (WGA488) and LP 690/50 (Atto633) emission filters. A 488 nm and a 639 nm laser were used for excitation. At 24 h prior to transfection, 3500 T24 cells per well were seeded in 8-well plates in 280 μL growth medium. A total of 20 μL MSN-454-GE11 covalently labeled with Atto-633 carboxy (200 μg mL^{-1} MSN in HEPES buffer) were added to each well and incubated for 45 min or 6 h, respectively, at 37 °C followed by addition of WGA-488 to the medium for cell membrane staining. Cells were washed with PBS and after addition of 300 μL fresh medium, cells were directly imaged.

The cellular uptake of nanoparticles was quantified using the ImageJ macro "Particle_in_Cell-3D" developed by Adriano A. Torrano and Julia Blechinger, Department of Chemistry and Center for NanoScience (CeNS, University of Munich (LMU), Munich, Germany. http://imagejdocu.tudor.lu/doku.php?id=macro:particle_in_cell-3d)

2.13. Luciferase Gene Silencing

In all experiments, siRNA and miRNA delivery was performed in 96-well plates in triplicate. 3500 T24/eGFPLuc-200cT cells per well were seeded 24 h prior to transfection in 100 μL growth medium. Before transfection, medium was replaced with 80 μL fresh growth medium. 20 μL MSN, MSN-454-PEG and MSN-454-GE11 for RNA delivery (500 μg mL^{-1} MSN in HEPES buffer) were added to each well and incubated for 45 min at 37 °C followed by a medium exchange. Cells were then incubated with 100 μL fresh medium for an additional 48 h following transfection. After this time, cells were treated with 100 μL cell lysis buffer (Promega (Mannheim, Germany)). Luciferase activity in cell lysate (35 μL) was measured using a luciferin-LAR (1 M glycylglycine, 100 mM $MgCl_2$, 500 mM EDTA, DTT, ATP, coenzyme A) buffer solution on a luminometer for 10 s (Centro LB 960 plate reader luminometer, Berthold Technologies, Bad Wildbad, Germany).

2.14. Cell Cycle Analysis

At 24 h prior to transfection, 3.5×10^4 T24 cells per well were seeded in a 12-well plate in 1000 μL growth medium and then medium was replaced by 400 μL fresh medium. A total of 100 μL MSN-160 nm-454-GE11 (500 μg mL^{-1} in HEPES buffer) loaded with Ctrl RNA or miR200c was added and incubated at 37 °C for 4 h. After a selected incubation time, the medium was replaced with fresh medium and cells were incubated for an additional 72 h. Afterwards, cells were washed with PBS and detached with trypsin/EDTA. Cells were washed with PBS twice and suspended in 100 μL PBS. The cell suspension was added dropwise to 0.9 mL cold 70% ethanol and incubated at 4 °C for 2 h. Then, cell pellets were suspended in 1 mL PBS after centrifugation and incubated for 15 min at room temperature for counting. A total of 1×10^5 cells of each sample was incubated in 300 μL propidium iodide/TritonX-100 containing RNase solution for 15 min at 37 °C. For cell cycle analysis, the cells were analyzed by flow cytometry at an excitation wavelength of 488 nm and detection of emission with a 613/20 bandpass filter. Data were recorded by BD LSRFortessa™ (BD Biosciences, USA) and analyzed by FlowJo® 7.6.5 flow cytometric analysis software. All experiments were performed in triplicate.

2.15. Scratch Assay

At 24 h prior to transfection, 1×10^5 T24 and MDA-MB 231 cells per well were seeded in a 6-well plate in 2000 μL of growth medium. The medium was replaced by 800 μL fresh medium and 200 μL

MSN160 nm-454-GE11 (500 μg mL^{-1} in HEPES buffer) loaded with Ctrl RNA or miR200c was added. Cells were incubated with MSN160 nm-454-GE11 for 4 h, then the medium was changed. After 24 h additional incubation time, the cell layer was broken by a scratch using a 200 μL Eppendorf tip. Cells were washed with PBS and microscope (Axiovert 200, Zeiss, Oberkochen, Germany) pictures were taken after 24 h.

3. Results

3.1. Particle Synthesis

We synthesized a series of core-shell MSNs with uniform size, ranging from 60 to 160 nm via a delayed co-condensation method [17]. The core of all MSNs was functionalized with 4.5 mol% APTES (with respect to total silica) carrying amino groups in order to create a positively charged inner void volume capable of encapsulating the negatively charged RNA by electrostatic interaction. The outer surface was functionalized with 2 mol% mercaptopropyl triethoxysilane (MPTES) carrying a thiol functionalization to act as regiospecific linker for external binding of polymer and targeting ligand.

Two slightly different approaches were used to modulate the particle size of MSNs and to prepare a series of MSNs with uniform sizes over a range from 60 to 160 nm. Larger particles with average particle sizes of 160, 130 and 100 nm (MSN160 nm, MSN130 nm and MSN100 nm) were synthesized based on our previous reports using a decreasing amount of the base triethanolamine (TEA) in order to reduce the particle size (experimental details are described in the Materials and Methods section) [43,44,46]. Briefly, to prepare the core of our core-shell particles, a preheated solution containing cetyltrimethylammonium chloride (CTAC) as template and triisopropylbenzene (TiPB) as pore-expanding agent was mixed with a preheated solution containing TEA, tetraethoxysilane (TEOS) and APTES at an elevated temperature for 20 min. This was then followed by addition of the ingredients for the surface layer containing TEOS and MPTES. To prepare smaller particles with average particle sizes of 80 and 60 nm (MSN80 nm and MSN60 nm), we applied a slightly different procedure, additionally using F127 as growth inhibitor/pore expanding agent according to published reports [45]. The particle size and core-shell structure were then established as above, again by changing the molar ratio of TEOS:TEA. Hereby, a preheated solution of octadecyltrimethylammonium bromide ($C_{18}Br$) as template was mixed with a second preheated solution of TiPB, F127, TEA, TEOS and APTES, and stirred at 60 °C for 30 min. Afterwards, premixed TEOS and MPTES were added to form the negatively charged shell layer.

3.2. Characterization

The particles were characterized using a number of techniques including transmission electron microscopy (TEM), dynamic light scattering (DLS), thermogravimetric analysis (TGA), zeta potential measurements, Raman and IR spectroscopy. The particle size and the morphology were analyzed with TEM and DLS. All MSN samples show a spherical particle morphology with a disordered, wormlike pore structure, independent of size (Figure 2). Figure 2a,b shows a size distribution around 160 nm (sample MSN160 nm) for particles obtained with the CTAC synthesis using a molar ratio of TEOS:TEA = 1:10. As the molar ratio of TEOS:TEA was decreased to TEOS:TEA = 1:5 and 1:3, the average particle size decreased to 128 nm (sample MSN130 nm, Figure 2c,d) and 100 nm (sample MSN100 nm, Figure 2e,f), respectively. Particles obtained by the F127 synthesis show a mean particle size of 80 nm (sample MSN80 nm, TEOS:TEA = 1:5, Figure 2g,h). The smallest particles with a mean particle size of 60 nm (sample MSN60 nm, Figure 2i,j) were obtained with F127 and a TEOS:TEA ratio of 1:3. DLS measurements of suspended particles show slightly larger hydrodynamic diameters ranging from 90 to 250 nm (Figure S1) but clearly illustrate the same trend of a decreasing particle size with decreasing TEA concentration.

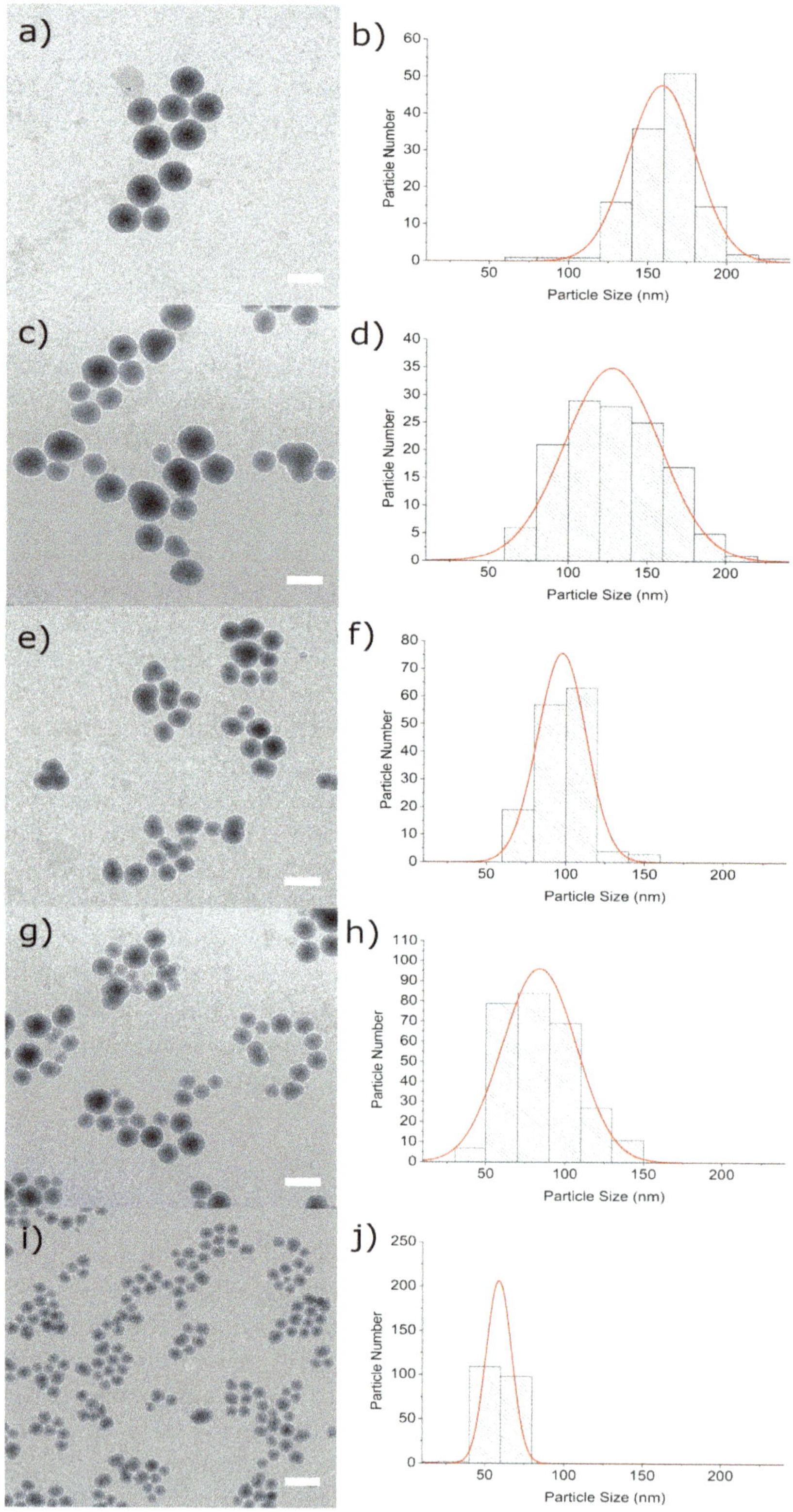

Figure 2. TEM micrographs of (**a**) MSN160 nm, (**c**) MSN130 nm, (**e**) MSN100 nm, (**g**) MSN80 nm, (**i**) MSN60 nm and corresponding particle size distribution histograms obtained from TEM images (**b**,**d**,**f**,**h**,**j**). Scale bar represents 150 nm.

Nitrogen sorption measurements resulted in typical type IV isotherms for all samples, as expected for MSNs (Figure 3a). Surface analysis indicates higher surface areas for particles prepared by the CTAC synthesis (samples MSN160 nm, MSN130 nm and MSN100 nm) ranging between 742–960 m^2/g, and shows a similar pore size of about 4.8 nm. Slightly smaller surface areas but larger pore sizes were obtained for particles prepared by the F127 synthesis (MSN80 nm, MSN60 nm; 660–685 m^2/g; pore size 6.0 nm, Figure 3b). Table 1 summarizes the properties of the particles obtained by the different synthesis methods.

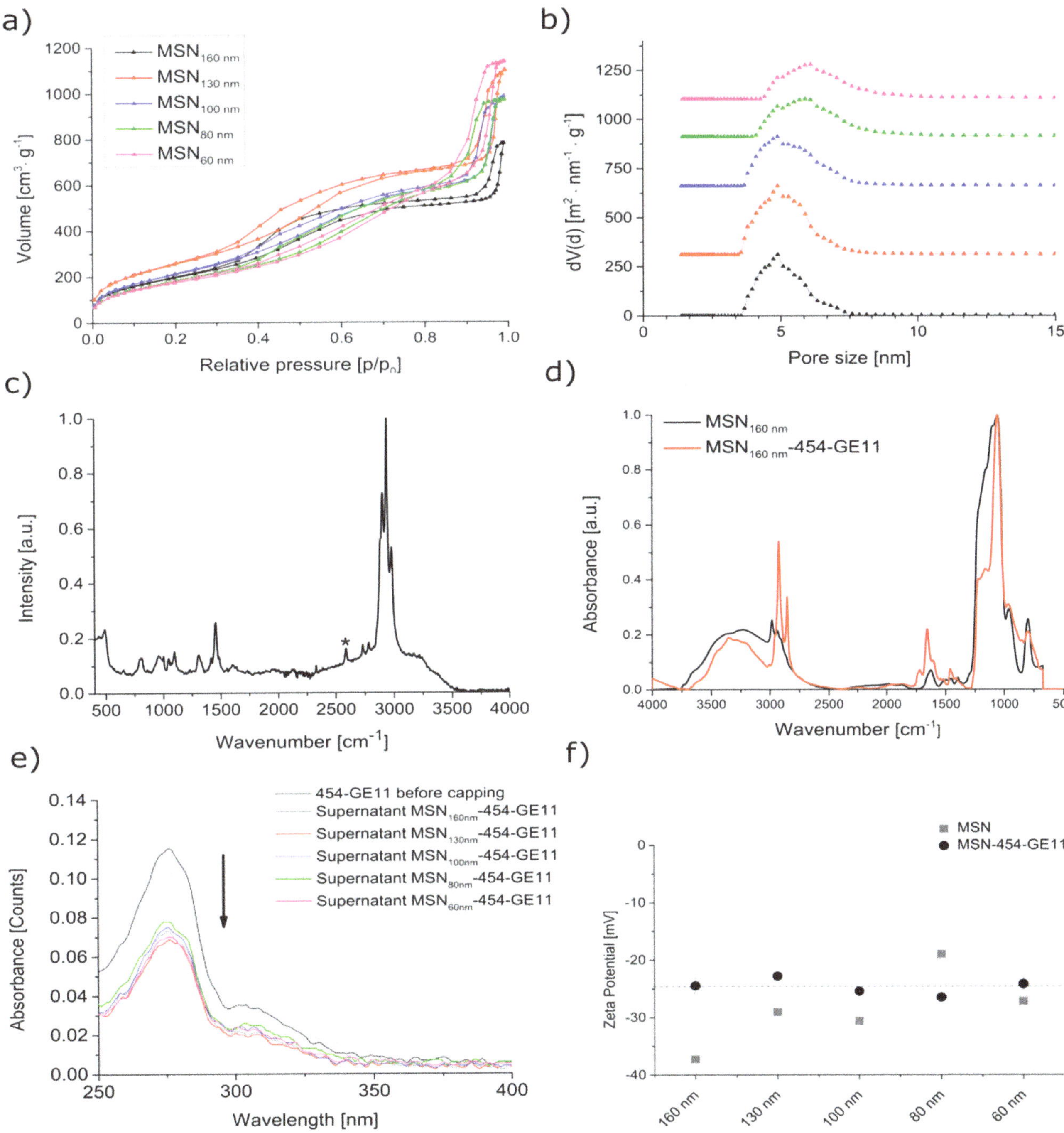

Figure 3. Characterization of MSN and MSN-454-GE11. (**a**) Nitrogen sorption isotherms and (**b**) corresponding pore size distributions. For clarity, the pore size distribution curves in panel b are shifted along the *y*-axis. (**c**) Raman spectrum of MSN160 nm. The signal at 2580 cm^{-1} (indicated by *) indicates the presence of thiol groups. (**d**) IR spectra, (**e**) UV VIS spectra of the capping solution before capping (black line) and the supernatants after capping, and (**f**) zeta potential measurements of MSN and MSN-454-GE11 at pH = 7.3.

Table 1. Synthesis and properties of MSN samples.

Name	Synthesis Method	Diameter TEM [a] [nm]	A_{BET} [m^2/g]	Pore Volume [b] [cc/g]	Pore Size [c] [nm]
MSN160 nm	CTAC Synthesis; TEOS:TEA = 1:10	159 ± 21	742	0.80	4.8
MSN130 nm	CTAC Synthesis; TEOS:TEA = 1:5	128 ± 30	961	1.06	4.8
MSN100 nm	CTAC Synthesis; TEOS:TEA = 1:3	100 ± 37	811	0.95	4.8
MSN80 nm	F127 Synthesis; TEOS:TEA = 1:5	84 ± 23	685	0.95	6.0
MSN60 nm	F127 Synthesis; TEOS:TEA = 1:3	59 ± 8	660	1.00	6.0

[a] The average particle size was obtained from TEM micrographs by measuring the diameter of around 200 particles of respective samples. [b] The total pore volume was determined at $p/p_0 = 0.9$ to exclude contributions of textural porosity. [c] Data were acquired from the adsorption branch of the nitrogen isotherm.

The presence of the amino and thiol groups originating from functionalization was verified with Raman and IR spectroscopy as well as with TGA. Representative results for sample MSN160 nm are shown in Figure 3c,d, respectively. Raman spectroscopy shows the S–H stretching mode of the thiol groups in the particle shell at 2580 cm^{-1} (Figure 3c), while the primary amines from core functionalization are seen at 1630 cm^{-1} with IR spectroscopy (MSN160 nm, black line, Figure 3d). TGA confirms the inclusion of organic functional groups by a weight loss of 20% (Figure S2). The decomposition of aminopropyl and successively, the mercaptopropyl groups starts at 290 °C.

3.3. *Polymer Capping with 454-PEG and 454-GE11 and Targeting*

The surface of the MSNs was capped with a modularly designed block copolymer 454 to prevent a premature release of the cargo and to enhance endosomal escape for intracellular delivery of miRNA. The structure of the copolymer 454 is shown in Figure S3. This T-shaped polymer 454 consists of a hydrophobic domain in the center made of two oleic acids attached to lysine units. Branched off at each side from the center are two succinyl-tetraethyl-pentamine (Stp) units [47], providing the polymer with a cationic charge. Each end contains a tyrosine trimer coupled to a terminal cysteine unit, potentially allowing additional functionalization. The combination of the central Stp and oleic acid units in 454 is assumed to facilitate interactions with the endosomal membrane, resulting in endosomal destabilization and thus enabling the nucleic acid cytosolic delivery. This block copolymer was successfully used for the formulation of INF-7-polyplex/siRNA vehicles [48] and was further essential for the highly efficient delivery of siRNA using MSNs, reported previously [21].

An anticancer therapy can potentially be improved by implementing cancer-cell-specific targeting molecules to the external surface of a carrier system. It is well known that EGF receptors (EGFR) are concentrated on many cancer cells. The small peptide GE11 has been used successfully before to specifically address EGFR-expressing cells [41,49,50]. Here, we exploit the mercapto residues of the cysteine groups in the capping polymer 454 for binding GE11 via a PEG linker to study the targeted, particle-size-dependent delivery of the miR200c.

For anchoring GE11 to the cysteine units in the block copolymer, we used a mercapto-reactive maleimide-PEG moiety consisting of 28 ethylene glycol monomer units that was previously linked to the GE11 ligand (Mal-PEG-GE11 reagent). The Mal-PEG-GE11 reagent was then mixed with the 454 block-copolymer (454-GE11). Only 0.1 equivalents (eq.; relative to 454-polymer) of the targeting ligand were used for 454-functionalization to maintain free thiol groups at the end of 454. The latter can potentially undergo a disulfide bridging with the terminal mercapto-groups on the outer surface of the MSNs, thus creating a stable copolymer capping. The attachment of the cationic polymer 454 to the surface is additionally electrostatically favored since zeta potential measurements of our pure MSNs reveal a negative surface charge for all samples at a pH higher than 5.5 (Figure S4). To perform the attachment of the premixed 454-GE11 to the surface of MSN, a suspension of MSN at pH 7.3 was mixed with 454-GE11 and the successful capping was confirmed using UV–VIS, IR, and zeta potential measurements. IR spectroscopy shows a significant increase of the CH stretching vibrations between 2850 and 2930 cm^{-1} and of the C-H bending vibrations of 1460 cm^{-1} as compared to the bare MSN particles (red graph in Figure 3d). Furthermore, the MSN-454-GE11 spectrum shows an increase of the N–H bending vibrations at 1650 cm^{-1} and a new signal at 1720 cm^{-1} related to a C=O stretching mode, indicating the multiple amide bonds of the copolymer. UV–VIS measurements were further used to quantify the amount of the 454-GE11 capping agent, which was similar in all samples and ranged from 17 to 20 wt% (Figure 3e, calibration curve Figure S5 and capping amount of different samples, Table S1).

Figure 3f shows the zeta potential measurements of all MSN samples before and after attachment of the 454-GE11 linker (MSN-454-GE11) at pH = 7.3. Besides the size of the nanoparticles, their surface charge is an important parameter for cellular internalization. Our pure MSN samples display a negative surface charge between −37 and −20 mV, as expected for mercapto-covered MSNs. The zeta potential of all capped MSN-454-GE11 samples is very comparable and has increased to about −24 mV when measured at pH 7.3. The observed difference before and after capping can be seen as an additional indication for a successful attachment of the targeted copolymer. The polymer capping did not affect the particle size distribution in water for most of the MSN-454-GE11 samples when measured by DLS. Only the sample with a mean particle size of 60 nm showed some moderate agglomeration (Figure S6).

3.4. Cell Internalization

As documented above, we have now established that our MSN carrier system shows physical properties such as surface area, pore size, zeta potential and capping concentration that are all very comparable, thus, leaving solely the particle size as a distinct variable. First, flow cytometry and confocal fluorescence microscopy data were used to investigate how the targeting ligand concentration as well as particle size might influence the cell internalization of the fully assembled MSN-454-GE11 samples.

Figure 4 shows the cellular internalization of the MSNs by T24 cells as examined via flow cytometry after a 45 min incubation time. MSN-454-GE11 samples were labeled with the Atto-633-carboxy fluorescent dye, which was covalently bound to the amino groups in the core of the particles. In order to investigate the best targeting concentration, we mixed different weight equivalents of targeting ligand GE11 with the 454 polymer in the range from 0.1 to 1 eq. before attaching the polymer to the MSN samples. Maleimide-PEG without ligand was used as negative control for polymer capping without targeting ligand (sample MSN-454-PEG). A significant targeting effect can be seen in Figure 4a when 0.1 eq. of the targeting ligand was used, while only a minor improvement is observed at higher concentrations.

Figure 4b documents the particle-size-dependent association of MSN-454-GE11 to cells as investigated via flow cytometry. Flow cytometry showed a similar degree of cell association for all samples, while a slight trend towards stronger association can be seen for smaller particles (quantification and statistical analysis can be found in SI, Figure S7). Since flow cytometry is not able to differentiate internalization from externally adhering particles, we followed this process also with confocal fluorescence microscopy as shown in Figure 5 (for enlarged images with additional orthogonal views of each image showing the particle internalization, see Figure S8, Supplementary Materials). Images were subsequently analyzed via the digital method 'Particle_in_Cell-3D' to quantify the cellular uptake of the differently sized MSN vectors. After imaging cells directly after an incubation time of 45 min, we found that only MSN160 nm-454-GE11 particles had penetrated through the cell membrane and were truly internalized. Other smaller MSN-454-GE11 particles were only attached to the outer cell membrane at this time. In contrast, all particle sizes were internalized after a 6 h incubation time. However, also after this time, MSN160 nm-454-GE11 particles showed the highest number of internalized particles of all samples (Figure S9).

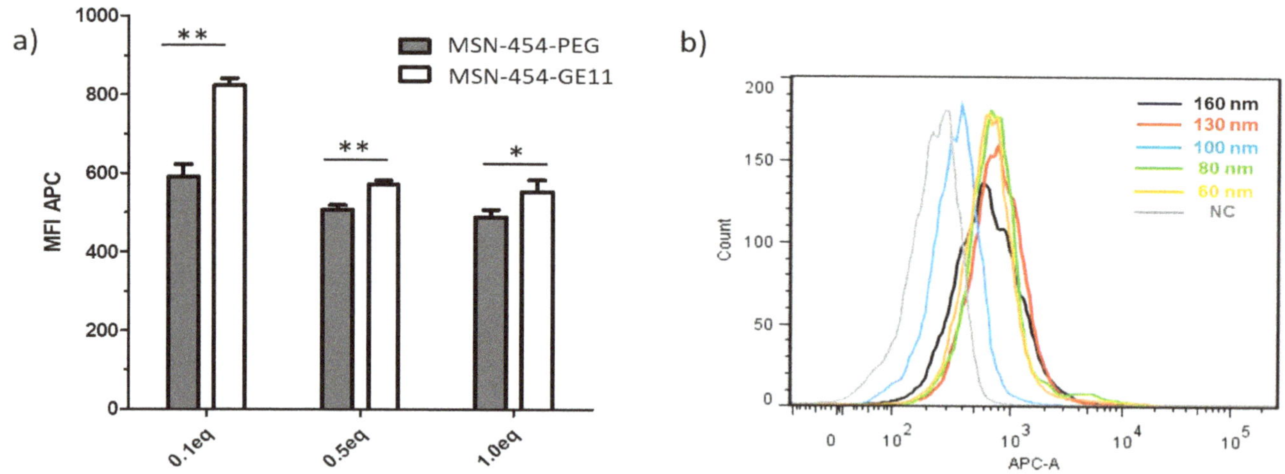

Figure 4. Cellular internalization determined by flow cytometry. Cells were incubated for 45 min, washed and analyzed. (**a**) MSN160 nm-454-PEG was used for passive and MSN160 nm-454-GE11 for receptor-mediated uptake. 454 was functionalized with different equivalents of Mal-PEG (454-PEG) and Mal-PEG-GE11 reagent (454-GE11), respectively, in the range from 0.1 to 1 eq. The mean fluorescence intensity of the Atto-633 signal (MFI APC) represents the amount of internalized nanoparticles. A high MFI corresponds to a large cell uptake of MSN. For statistical analysis, a two-tailed t-test was performed (n = 3, mean ± SD, * $p < 0.05$, ** $p < 0.01$) (**b**) Histograms of cellular internalization of Atto-633 labeled MSN-454-GE11 after 45 min incubation with particle sizes in the range of 160 nm to 60 nm and negative control (NC). The Atto-633 intensity (APC-A channel) is plotted against the number of events detected ('count'). 'Count' represents cumulative counts of cells with indicated Atto-633 fluorescence after appropriate gating by forward/sideward scatter and pulse width. For statistical analysis, see Figure S7.

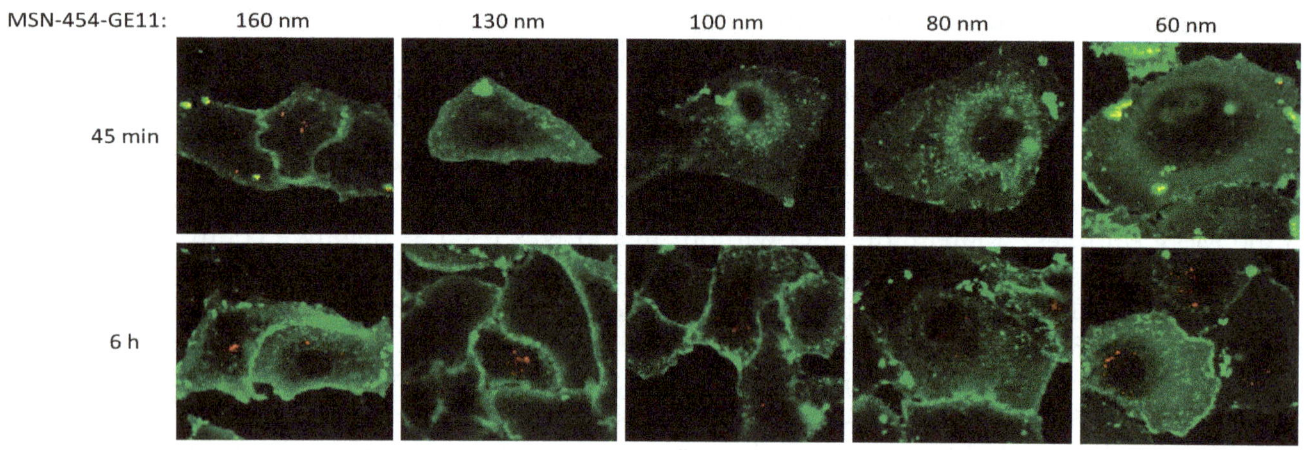

Figure 5. Representative confocal fluorescence microscopy images of Atto-633 labeled MSN-454-GE11 (red) with particle sizes in the range of 160 nm to 60 nm after 45 min (upper panel) and 6 h (lower panel) incubation on WGA488-stained T24 cells (green). For a statistical evaluation of particle-size-dependent uptake, see Figure S9, SI.

3.5. Loading of RNA

Loading of the genetic material into our MSN samples was performed with all samples prior to the attachment of the block copolymer. The adsorption of the miRNA is mainly driven by electrostatic interactions with the cationic, amino-functionalized core of the MSNs. The negatively charged thiol groups at the particle periphery are expected to minimize any external adsorption. For the best results, we performed the RNA adsorption in MES buffer at pH = 5. The MSN particles show a positive zeta potential at this pH due to protonation of the amino groups (zeta potential titration, see Figure S4).

Here, aliquots of 50 μg mg^{-1} RNA/MSN were used for loading and the actual uptake was calculated by difference measurements by determining the remaining RNA concentration in the supernatant. All samples were able to adsorb the amount offered, as no residual RNA could be detected in the supernatant after loading times as short as 30 min. The samples were subsequently capped with 454-GE11 to obtain the final MSN-454-GE11 samples used for subsequent experiments. The stable binding of RNA in these samples is reflected in gel shift results, as shown in Figure 6a). Only little RNA elution is visible upon applying a voltage of 100 V for 1 h to the gel.

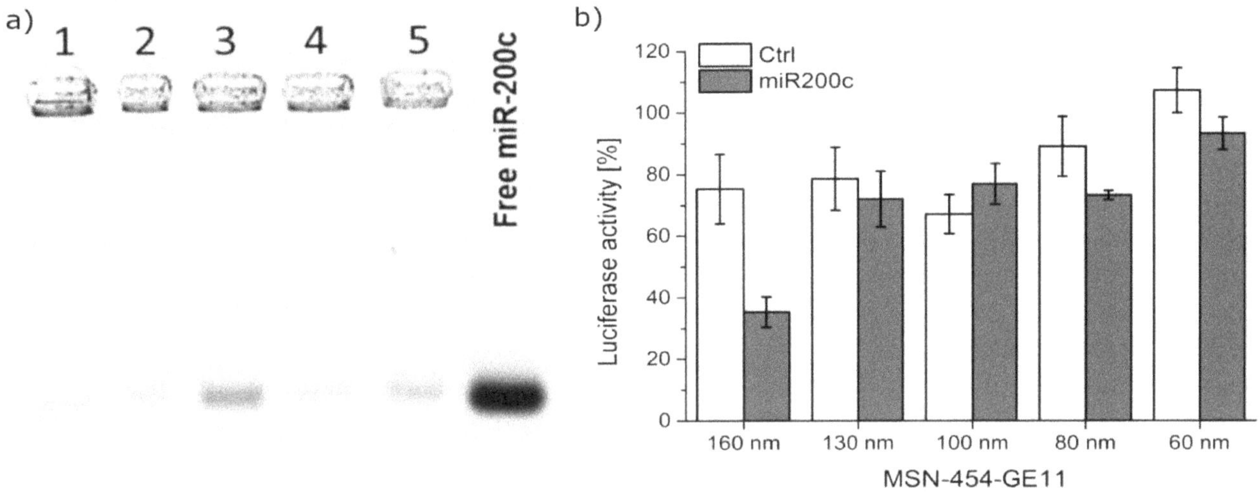

Figure 6. (**a**) Gel electrophoresis of samples MSN160 nm-454-GE11 (1), MSN130 nm-454-GE11 (2), MSN100 nm-454-GE11 (3), MSN80 nm-454-GE11 (4), and MSN60 nm-454-GE11 (5). (**b**) Gene silencing of T24/eGFPLuc-200cT cells transfected with MSN-454-GE11 containing either Ctrl (white) or miR200c (grey). After an incubation time of 45 min, cells were washed. At 48 h after transfection, gene-silencing effects were analyzed.

3.6. Gene Silencing

As a proof of concept, the gene silencing of the eGFP-luciferase reporter gene was performed using T24/eGFPLuc-200cT cells. This cell line stably expresses the eGFP-luciferase fusion protein, while simultaneously featuring a miR200c target site on the expressed mRNA. Therefore, the gene expression of eGFP-luciferase fusion protein can be blocked by the delivery of miR200c. The luciferase signal was thus used to evaluate the gene-silencing efficacy of miR200c. In order to simulate the dynamic conditions of drug delivery and to avoid a prolonged overexposure of the cells with particles suspended in the medium, we have used extremely short incubation times of 45 min. Cells were subsequently washed by exchanging the medium and the effect of this short exposure was then analyzed after time spans referred to as transfection time in the following. Cells were transfected with MSN and MSN-454-GE11 of different sizes loaded with either a synthetic miR200c mimic or a control siRNA without any target gene (Ctrl, Figure 6b). Gene silencing was never observed with the pure MSN samples (missing the 454 polymer construct) loaded with miR200c for silencing (Figure S10a). This might be caused by a premature release of the RNA or by endosomal trapping of the MSN samples missing the 454 polymer.

Similarly, none of the smaller sized MSN-454-GE11 samples showed any significant silencing efficacy. In contrast, with the larger 160 nm targeted polymer-capped MSN160 nm-454-GE11 sample, a luciferase gene knockdown of up to 65% was observed. These findings are in good agreement with the confocal fluorescence microscopy images, which showed the fastest internalization for particles with a size of 160 nm.

Flow cytometry data showed an improved cellular internalization of the targeted MSN160 nm-454-GE11 vector in comparison with the non-targeted control MSN-454-PEG when 0.1 eq. of the targeting ligand was used. This targeted vector showed a higher silencing efficacy compared to the non-targeted control, which is in good agreement with the increased uptake observed via flow cytometry.

As expected, the same sample loaded with just scrambled RNA (Ctrl) did not show a significant unspecific knockdown, thus excluding major toxic effects induced by the carrier system itself. Systematic cell viability studies using an MTT assay also show a good tolerance of the cells towards these samples (Figure S11).

These results show that a particle size of about 160 nm in combination with the copolymer 454 enables the fastest cell internalization and also the best transfection efficacy when short incubation times of only 45 min are used. Inhibition experiments addressing specific endocytic pathways were inconclusive with respect to a preferred mechanism for a certain particle size. However, endocytosis was substantially more blocked for the larger particles as compared to the 60 nm particles (see Figure S12, Supplementary Materials). Our data also confirm the endosomolytic activity of the 454 polymer since cell adherence/uptake was observed for all pure MSN samples (flow cytometry of pure MSN samples in Figure S13), but no transfection occurred without the 454 polymer (see Figure S10a). As described above, we further found that only MSN160 nm-454-GE11 showed gene-silencing activity, while all smaller MSN-454-GE11 samples were not active after the short incubation period applied here. Confocal fluorescence microscopy showed that MSN160 nm-454-GE11 particles were already internalized after 45 min, while all other MSN-454-GE11 samples needed much longer incubation times to achieve internalization. Thus, particle internalization of the smaller particles is likely too slow and prevents a larger efficacy.

Recently, miR200c was delivered by some of us using GE11 modified 454 polyplexes with a similar size of 120–150 nm [41]. The gene silencing efficiency achieved in the same T24/eGFPLuc-200cT cells with these polyplexes was around 60%, which is in the same range as the knockdown efficiency of the MSN-454-GE11 constructs presented here. This comparison suggests that the size of the targeted constructs is a determining feature controlling the knockdown efficiency. As MSN160 nm-454-GE11 constructs were shown to offer the best cellular-uptake behavior and gene-silencing efficiency, they were used for the following cell migration and cell cycle experiments.

3.7. *Antitumoral Effects*

The tumor suppressor miR200c inhibits the epithelial–mesenchymal transition, a process involved in metastasis by enhancing the motility and migration of tumor cells, by targeting ZEB1 and ZEB2. ZEB1 and ZEB2 are transcriptional repressors, which downregulate the marker E-cadherin [7,51]. Furthermore, Kopp et al. reported that one of the most prominent oncogenes KRAS is targeted by miR200c, which results in an altered cell cycle of the cancer cells [6]. Notably, they could show that miR200c inhibits cell cycle progression by decreasing the G1-population. We have performed direct investigations of these antitumoral effects through tumor cell migration and cell cycle analysis on two different EGFR overexpressing cell lines, T24 bladder cancer and HeLa cervical cancer cells using miR200c loaded MSN-454-GE11 samples.

Cell migration was studied using a scratch assay, as shown in Figure 7. T24 cells and HeLa cells were incubated with MSN-454-GE11 for 4 h (5 μg miR200c/well), then the medium was changed. After additional 24 h, the cell layer was broken by a scratch using a 200 μL Eppendorf pipette tip. The closure of the scratch, which is an indicator for cell migration, was measured at indicated time points. In both cell lines, the scratch was almost completely closed after 48 h when MSN-454-GE11 was loaded with Ctrl-RNA (88% scratch closure for T24 and 82% closure for HeLa cells). In contrast, with MSN-454-GE11 particles loaded with miR200c, a scratch closure of only 48% (for T24) and 53% (for HeLa cells) was observed after this time. Hence, miR200c delivered by MSN-454-GE11 significantly hinders cell migration.

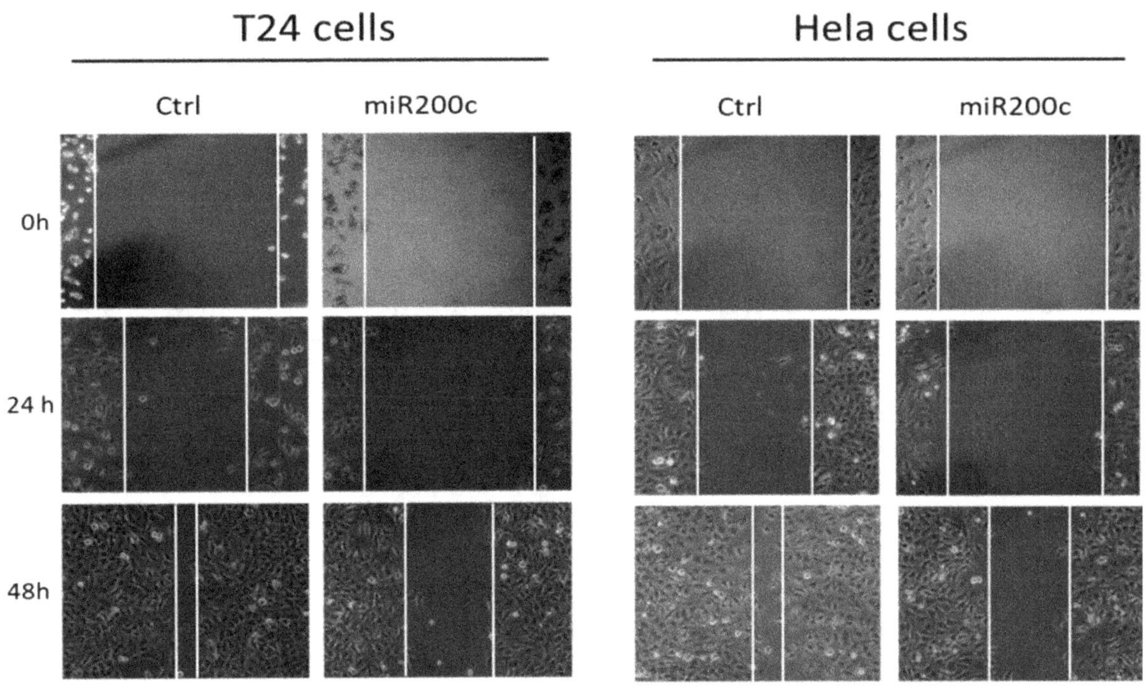

Figure 7. Inhibition of tumor cell migration. Images of a scratch assay of T24 and HeLa cells. Cells were treated with MSN160 nm-454-GE11 loaded with miR200c. The cell layer was broken after 24 h through a scratch and the closure was monitored for 48 h.

In addition, the effect of miR200c on the cell cycle was studied. Cells were transfected with MSN-454-GE11 loaded with miR200c or with the control RNA Ctrl and incubated for 4 h (Figure 8). A significant decrease in the number of cells in the G1 phase is observed when exposed to miR200C delivered by MSN, in combination with an increase in the number of cells in the S-phase. Thus, tumor cells transfected with MSN-454-GE11 loaded with miR200c showed the expected decreased migration and changes in the cell cycle.

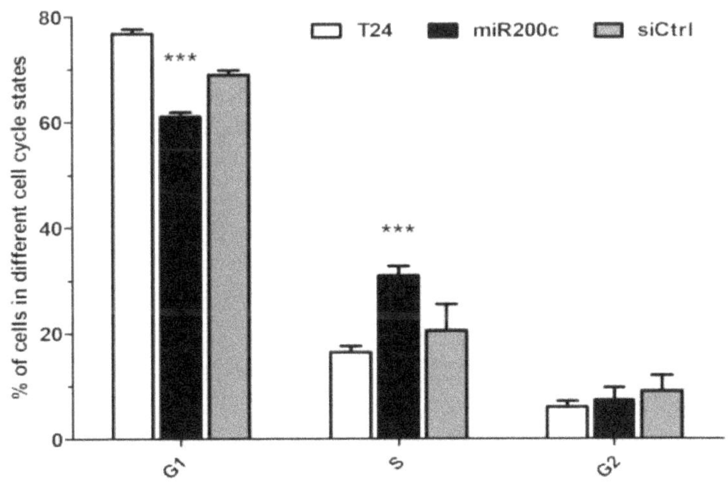

Figure 8. Cell cycle analysis via flow cytometry of cell stages G1, S and G2 of T24 cells at 72 h after treatment. For statistical analysis, a two-tailed t-test was performed ($n = 3$, mean ± SD, *** $p < 0.01$)

4. Conclusions

In this study, we exploited the tunability of MSNs to synthesize a series of core-shell MSNs with different particle sizes between 60 to 160 nm for studying the size effect of these carriers on antitumoral miRNA delivery. All other properties of the delivery vehicles, including surface area, pore size and zeta potential were kept comparable. The nanoparticles were capped with a positively charged block copolymer 454 equipped with the targeting agent Mal-PEG-GE11. Since gene silencing was only observed after capping the nanocarriers with this 454 polymer, we conclude that it is essential for the endosomal escape by destabilizing the endosomal membrane. It was shown that the targeting ligand GE11 enhances a receptor-mediated uptake. After capping, the MSN-454-GE11 vehicles were used for a systematic investigation of size-dependent gene silencing. While smaller particles did not lead to significant effects, MSN-454-GE11 with a size of 160 nm showed a remarkable gene knockdown efficacy and antitumoral effects such as a decreased migration and changes in cell cycle. Overall, we observed the fastest cellular internalization as well as the best knock-down efficacies with MSN-454-GE11 sized 160 nm. In contrast to FACS results that indicated a particle association with the cells independent of MSN particle size, we found with statistically evaluated image analysis that only the largest particles are truly internalized in the cells after short incubation times. Thus, cell studies as performed here, aiming to simulate dynamic conditions of in vivo drug delivery by washing the incubated cells after a short incubation time, might discriminate against all particles that are not well attached to the cell surface. Fast internalized particles are thus the winner. We hypothesize that due to their size, they expose a larger contact area to the cell membrane and simultaneously a larger number of targeting ligands, which, when spaced just right, allow for a maximum degree of endocytosis. Our study shows that fast cellular internalization is essential for a successful downregulation. In summary, the nanoscale MSN160 nm-454-GE11 vehicles show the most promising potential for future in vivo biomedical applications.

Supplementary Materials:
Figure S1: DLS measurements of MSN samples, Figure S2: TGA, Figure S3: Structure of copolymer 454, Figure S4: Zeta potential titration curves of pure MSN samples, Figure S5: 454-GE11 calibration curve, Figure S6: DLS measurements of MSN-454-GE11 samples, Figure S7: Quantification of FACS data shown in Figure 4b, Figure S8: Confocal fluorescence microscopy images, Figure S9: Quantification of the cellular uptake of MSN-454-GE11, Figure S10: Gene-silencing assay, Figure S11: MTT cell viability study, Figure S12: Inhibition results, Figure S13: FACS of internalization of untargeted nanoparticles, Table S1: Estimated capping amount of 454-GE11 for different MSN samples.

Author Contributions: Conceptualization, T.B., E.W., K.M.; Measurements and Data Analysis, L.H., W.Z., S.R., H.E.; Writing—Original Draft Preparation, L.H.; Writing—Review & Editing, K.M., T.B. All authors have read and agreed to the published version of the manuscript.

References

1. Elbashir, S.M.; Harborth, J.; Lendeckel, W.; Yalcin, A.; Weber, K.; Tuschl, T. Duplexes of 21-Nucleotide Rnas Mediate RNA Interference in Cultured Mammalian Cells. *Nature* **2001**, *411*, 494. [CrossRef] [PubMed]
2. McCaffrey, A.P.; Meuse, L.; Pham, T.-T.T.; Conklin, D.S.; Hannon, G.J.; Kay, M.A. RNA Interference in Adult Mice. *Nature* **2002**, *418*, 38. [CrossRef] [PubMed]
3. Xin, Y.; Huang, M.; Guo, W.W.; Huang, Q.; Zhang, L.Z.; Jiang, G. Nano-Based Delivery of RNAi in Cancer Therapy. *Mol. Cancer* **2017**, *16*, 134. [CrossRef] [PubMed]
4. Friedman, R.C.; Farh, K.K.-H.; Burge, C.B.; Bartel, D.P. Most Mammalian mRNAs Are Conserved Targets of Micrornas. *Genome Res.* **2009**, *19*, 92–105. [CrossRef]
5. Lee, S.J.; Kim, M.J.; Kwon, I.C.; Roberts, T.M. Delivery Strategies and Potential Targets for siRNA in Major Cancer Types. *Adv. Drug Deliv. Rev.* **2016**, *104*, 2–15. [CrossRef]
6. Kopp, F.; Wagner, E.; Roidl, A. The Proto-Oncogene KRAS Is Targeted by Mir-200c. *Oncotarget* **2013**, *5*, 185–195. [CrossRef]
7. Hurteau, G.J.; Carlson, J.A.; Spivack, S.D.; Brock, G.J. Overexpression of the MicroRNA hsa-miR-200c Leads to Reduced Expression of Transcription Factor 8 and Increased Expression of E-Cadherin. *Cancer Res.* **2007**, *67*, 7972–7976. [CrossRef]
8. Kopp, F.; Oak, P.S.; Wagner, E.; Roidl, A. Mir-200c Sensitizes Breast Cancer Cells to Doxorubicin Treatment by Decreasing Trkb and Bmi1 Expression. *PLoS ONE* **2012**, *7*, e50469. [CrossRef]
9. Kim, H.J.; Kim, A.; Miyata, K.; Kataoka, K. Recent Progress in Development of siRNA Delivery Vehicles for Cancer Therapy. *Adv. Drug Deliv. Rev.* **2016**, *104*, 61–77. [CrossRef]

10. Kim, B.; Park, J.-H.; Sailor, M.J. Rekindling RNAi Therapy: Materials Design Requirements for in Vivo siRNA Delivery. *Adv. Mater.* **2019**, *31*, 1903637. [CrossRef]
11. Revia, R.A.; Stephen, Z.R.; Zhang, M. Theranostic Nanoparticles for Rna-Based Cancer Treatment. *Acc. Chem. Res.* **2019**, *52*, 1496–1506. [CrossRef] [PubMed]
12. Adams, D.; Gonzalez-Duarte, A.; O'Riordan, W.D.; Yang, C.C.; Ueda, M.; Kristen, A.V.; Tournev, I.; Schmidt, H.H.; Coelho, T.; Berk, J.L.; et al. Patisiran, an RNAi Therapeutic, for Hereditary Transthyretin Amyloidosis. *New Engl. J. Med.* **2018**, *379*, 11–21. [CrossRef] [PubMed]
13. Chen, Y.; Gu, H.; Zhang, D.S.-Z.; Li, F.; Liu, T.; Xia, W. Highly Effective Inhibition of Lung Cancer Growth and Metastasis by Systemic Delivery of siRNA Via Multimodal Mesoporous Silica-Based Nanocarrier. *Biomaterials* **2014**, *35*, 10058–10069. [CrossRef] [PubMed]
14. Hartono, S.B.; Gu, W.; Kleitz, F.; Liu, J.; He, L.; Middelberg, A.P.J.; Yu, C.; Lu, G.Q.; Qiao, S.Z. Poly-L-Lysine Functionalized Large Pore Cubic Mesostructured Silica Nanoparticles as Biocompatible Carriers for Gene Delivery. *ACS Nano* **2012**, *6*, 2104–2117. [CrossRef] [PubMed]
15. Möller, K.; Bein, T. Degradable Drug Carriers: Vanishing Mesoporous Silica Nanoparticles. *Chem. Mater.* **2019**, *31*, 4364–4378. [CrossRef]
16. Braun, K.; Pochert, A.; Beck, M.; Fiedler, R.; Gruber, J.; Linden, M. Dissolution Kinetics of Mesoporous Silica Nanoparticles in Different Simulated Body Fluids. *J. Sol.-Gel. Sci. Technol.* **2016**, *79*, 319–327. [CrossRef]
17. Kecht, J.; Schlossbauer, A.; Bein, T. Selective Functionalization of the Outer and Inner Surfaces in Mesoporous Silica Nanoparticles. *Chem. Mater.* **2008**, *20*, 7207–7214. [CrossRef]
18. Möller, K.; Bein, T. Talented Mesoporous Silica Nanoparticles. *Chem. Mater.* **2017**, *29*, 371–388.
19. Wang, J.; Lu, Z.; Wientjes, M.G.; Au, J.L.S. Delivery of siRNA Therapeutics: Barriers and Carriers. *AAPS J.* **2010**, *12*, 492–503. [CrossRef]
20. Gao, F.; Botella, P.; Corma, A.; Blesa, J.; Dong, L. Monodispersed Mesoporous Silica Nanoparticles with Very Large Pores for Enhanced Adsorption and Release of DNA. *J. Phys. Chem. B* **2009**, *113*, 1796–1804. [CrossRef]
21. Möller, K.; Müller, K.; Engelke, H.; Bräuchle, C.; Wagner, E.; Bein, T. Highly Efficient siRNA Delivery from Core–Shell Mesoporous Silica Nanoparticles with Multifunctional Polymer Caps. *Nanoscale* **2016**, *8*, 4007–4019.
22. Jin, Y.; Lohstreter, S.; Pierce, D.T.; Parisien, J.; Wu, M.; Hall, C.; Zhao, J.X. Silica Nanoparticles with Continuously Tunable Sizes: Synthesis and Size Effects on Cellular Contrast Imaging. *Chem. Mater.* **2008**, *20*, 4411–4419. [CrossRef]
23. Gan, Q.; Dai, D.; Yuan, Y.; Qian, J.; Sha, S.; Shi, J.; Liu, C. Effect of Size on the Cellular Endocytosis and Controlled Release of Mesoporous Silica Nanoparticles for Intracellular Delivery. *Biomed. Microdevices* **2012**, *14*, 259–270. [CrossRef] [PubMed]
24. Huang, X.; Teng, X.; Chen, D.; Tang, F.; He, J. The Effect of the Shape of Mesoporous Silica Nanoparticles on Cellular Uptake and Cell Function. *Biomaterials* **2010**, *31*, 438–448. [CrossRef] [PubMed]
25. Zhu, J.; Tang, J.; Zhao, L.; Zhou, X.; Wang, Y.; Yu, C. Ultrasmall, Well-Dispersed, Hollow Siliceous Spheres with Enhanced Endocytosis Properties. *Small* **2010**, *6*, 276–282. [CrossRef]
26. Chono, S.; Tanino, T.; Seki, T.; Morimoto, K. Uptake Characteristics of Liposomes by Rat Alveolar Macrophages: Influence of Particle Size and Surface Mannose Modification. *J. Pharm. Pharmacol.* **2007**, *59*, 75–80. [CrossRef]
27. Osaki, F.; Kanamori, T.; Sando, S.; Sera, T.; Aoyama, Y. A Quantum Dot Conjugated Sugar Ball and Its Cellular Uptake. On the Size Effects of Endocytosis in the Subviral Region. *J. Am. Chem. Soc.* **2004**, *126*, 6520–6521. [CrossRef]
28. Shang, L.; Nienhaus, K.; Nienhaus, G.U. Engineered Nanoparticles Interacting with Cells: Size Matters. *J. Nanobiotechnology* **2014**, *12*, 5. [CrossRef]
29. Lu, F.; Wu, S.-H.; Hung, Y.; Mou, C.-Y. Size Effect on Cell Uptake in Well-Suspended, Uniform Mesoporous Silica Nanoparticles. *Small* **2009**, *5*, 1408–1413. [CrossRef]
30. Chithrani, B.D.; Ghazani, A.A.; Chan, W.C.W. Determining the Size and Shape Dependence of Gold Nanoparticle Uptake into Mammalian Cells. *Nano Lett.* **2006**, *6*, 662–668. [CrossRef]
31. Varela, J.A.; Bexiga, M.G.; Åberg, C.; Simpson, J.C.; Dawson, K.A. Quantifying Size-Dependent Interactions between Fluorescently Labeled Polystyrene Nanoparticles and Mammalian Cells. *J. Nanobiotechnology* **2012**, *10*, 39. [CrossRef] [PubMed]
32. Huang, J.; Bu, L.; Xie, J.; Chen, K.; Cheng, Z.; Li, X.; Chen, X. Effects of Nanoparticle Size on Cellular Uptake and Liver MRI with Polyvinylpyrrolidone-Coated Iron Oxide Nanoparticles. *ACS Nano* **2010**, *4*, 7151–7160. [CrossRef] [PubMed]

33. Goel, S.; Chen, F.; Hong, H.; Valdovinos, H.; Hernandez, R.; Shi, S.; Barnhart, T.; Cai, W. Vegf121-Conjugated Mesoporous Silica Nanoparticle: A Tumor Targeted Drug Delivery System. *ACS Appl. Mater. Interfaces* **2014**, *6*, 21677–21685.
34. Chen, F.; Nayak, T.R.; Goel, S.; Valdovinos, H.F.; Hong, H.; Theuer, C.P.; Barnhart, T.E.; Cai, W. In Vivo Tumor Vasculature Targeted Pet/Nirf Imaging with Trc105(Fab)-Conjugated, Dual-Labeled Mesoporous Silica Nanoparticles. *Mol. Pharm.* **2014**, *11*, 4007–4014. [CrossRef]
35. Yu, M.; Niu, Y.; Zhang, J.; Zhang, H.; Yang, Y.; Taran, E.; Jambhrunkar, S.; Gu, W.; Thorn, P.; Yu, C. Size-Dependent Gene Delivery of Amine-Modified Silica Nanoparticles. *Nano Res.* **2016**, *9*, 291–305. [CrossRef]
36. Nayak, T.R.; Krasteva, L.K.; Cai, W. Multimodality Imaging of RNA Interference. *Curr. Med. chem.* **2013**, *20*, 3664–3675. [CrossRef]
37. Li, X.; Chen, Y.; Wang, M.; Ma, Y.; Xia, W.; Gu, H. A Mesoporous Silica Nanoparticle – Pei – Fusogenic Peptide System for siRNA Delivery in Cancer Therapy. *Biomaterials* **2013**, *34*, 1391–1401. [CrossRef]
38. Chen, Y.; Wang, X.; Liu, T.; Zhang, D.S.-Z.; Wang, Y.; Gu, H.; Di, W. Highly Effective Antiangiogenesis Via Magnetic Mesoporous Silica-Based siRNA Vehicle Targeting the Vegf Gene for Orthotopic Ovarian Cancer Therapy. *Int. J. Nanomed.* **2015**, *10*, 2579–2594.
39. Wang, M.; Li, X.; Ma, Y.; Gu, H. Endosomal Escape Kinetics of Mesoporous Silica-Based System for Efficient siRNA Delivery. *Int. J. Pharm.* **2013**, *448*, 51–57. [CrossRef]
40. Li, Z.; Zhao, R.; Wu, X.; Sun, Y.; Yao, M.; Li, J.; Xu, Y.; Gu, J. Identification and Characterization of a Novel Peptide Ligand of Epidermal Growth Factor Receptor for Targeted Delivery of Therapeutics. *Faseb. J.* **2005**, *19*, 1978–1985. [CrossRef]
41. Müller, K.; Klein, P.M.; Heissig, P.; Roidl, A.; Wagner, E. EGF Receptor Targeted Lipo-Oligocation Polyplexes for Antitumoral siRNA and Mirna Delivery. *Nanotechnology* **2016**, *27*, 464001. [CrossRef] [PubMed]
42. Troiber, C.; Edinger, D.; Kos, P.; Schreiner, L.; Kläger, R.; Herrmann, A.; Wagner, E. Stabilizing Effect of Tyrosine Trimers on PDNA and siRNA Polyplexes. *Biomaterials* **2013**, *34*, 1624–1633. [CrossRef]
43. Cauda, V.; Schlossbauer, A.; Kecht, J.; Zürner, A.; Bein, T. Multiple Core–Shell Functionalized Colloidal Mesoporous Silica Nanoparticles. *J. Am. Chem. Soc.* **2009**, *131*, 11361–11370. [CrossRef] [PubMed]
44. Möller, K.; Kobler, J.; Bein, T. Colloidal Suspensions of Nanometer-Sized Mesoporous Silica. *Adv. Funct. Mater.* **2007**, *17*, 605–612. [CrossRef]
45. Gu, J.; Huang, K.; Zhu, X.; Li, Y.; Wei, J.; Zhao, W.; Liu, C.; Shi, J. Sub-150nm Mesoporous Silica Nanoparticles with Tunable Pore Sizes and Well-Ordered Mesostructure for Protein Encapsulation. *J. Colloid Interface Sci.* **2013**, *407*, 236–242. [CrossRef] [PubMed]
46. Kobler, J.; Möller, K.; Bein, T. Colloidal Suspensions of Functionalized Mesoporous Silica Nanoparticles. *ACS Nano* **2008**, *2*, 791–799. [CrossRef]
47. Schaffert, D.; Badgujar, N.; Wagner, E. Novel Fmoc-Polyamino Acids for Solid-Phase Synthesis of Defined Polyamidoamines. *Org. Lett.* **2011**, *13*, 1586–1589. [CrossRef]
48. Zhang, W.; Muller, K.; Kessel, E.; Reinhard, S.; He, D.; Klein, P.M.; Hohn, M.; Rodl, W.; Kempter, S.; Wagner, E. Targeted siRNA Delivery Using a Lipo-Oligoaminoamide Nanocore with an Influenza Peptide and Transferrin Shell. *Adv. Healthc. Mater.* **2016**, *5*, 1493–1504. [CrossRef]
49. Genta, I.; Chiesa, E.; Colzani, B.; Modena, T.; Conti, B.; Dorati, R. Ge11 Peptide as an Active Targeting Agent in Antitumor Therapy: A Minireview. *Pharmaceutics* **2017**, *10*, 2. [CrossRef]
50. Biscaglia, F.; Rajendran, S.; Conflitti, P.; Benna, C.; Sommaggio, R.; Litti, L.; Mocellin, S.; Bocchinfuso, G.; Rosato, A.; Palleschi, A.; et al. Enhanced EGFR Targeting Activity of Plasmonic Nanostructures with Engineered Ge11 Peptide. *Adv. Healthc. Mater.* **2017**, *6*, 1700596. [CrossRef]
51. Korpal, M.; Lee, E.S.; Hu, G.; Kang, Y. The miR-200 Family Inhibits Epithelial-Mesenchymal Transition and Cancer Cell Migration by Direct Targeting of E-Cadherin Transcriptional Repressors Zeb1 and Zeb2. *J. Biol. Chem.* **2008**, *283*, 14910–14914. [CrossRef] [PubMed]

9

Hydrogels as Potential Nano-, Micro- and Macro-Scale Systems for Controlled Drug Delivery

Adam Chyzy †, Monika Tomczykowa † and Marta E. Plonska-Brzezinska *

Department of Organic Chemistry, Faculty of Pharmacy with the Division of Laboratory Medicine, Medical University of Bialystok, Mickiewicza 2A, 15-222 Bialystok, Poland; adam.chyzy24@gmail.com (A.C.); monika.tomczyk@umb.edu.pl (M.T.)

* Correspondence: marta.plonska-brzezinska@umb.edu.pl

† These authors contributed equally to this work.

Abstract: This review is an extensive evaluation and essential analysis of the design and formation of hydrogels (HGs) for drug delivery. We review the fundamental principles of HGs (their chemical structures, physicochemical properties, synthesis routes, different types, etc.) that influence their biological properties and medical and pharmaceutical applications. Strategies for fabricating HGs with different diameters (macro, micro, and nano) are also presented. The size of biocompatible HG materials determines their potential uses in medicine as drug carriers. Additionally, novel drug delivery methods for enhancing treatment are discussed. A critical review is performed based on the latest literature reports.

Keywords: hydrogel; drug delivery; polymer; biocompatibility; immobilization of drug

1. Introduction

Drug delivery systems grounded on hydrogels (HGs) are interesting because of their high biocompatibility and biodegradability. These properties are especially relevant for materials used for biomedical engineering applications, an example of which may be drug delivery or tissue engineering [1–3]. HGs are water-swollen polymeric networks containing chemical or physical cross-links able to absorb large quantities of water or biological fluids [4]. HGs have a variety of structures, architectures, sizes (from centimetres to sub-nanometres), and functions, and together with other properties, these variables determine HG use for drug delivery [1–3,5].

HGs can be prepared from one polymer (homo-polymeric HG), two or more polymers (multi-polymeric HG); they may also contain other nanostructures/nanoparticles in a polymeric network [6–9]. These polymeric networks can be chemically and physically modified imparting new and unusual properties [9–11]. Chemical structures, compositions, biodegradability, biological functions and different physicochemical properties (e.g., mechanical, rheological, spectral, thermosensitive, pH stability) can be modified [2,6,9,12]. These variations influence the performances of HGs and affect loading and releasing properties for drugs [7,9,11–15].

HGs can be used to form microparticles, nanoparticles, micelles and films [15,16]. For HG particles, the particle size (macro, micro and nano) determines the route by which HGs can be delivered into the human body [17–21]. For micro- or nano-sized HGs, the effects of various physical and chemical factors on drug release should be considered [15,21]. Therefore, drug immobilization in a polymer matrix should be considered in the context of controlled release at target sites. Various in vivo and in vitro drug application techniques have been developed with various therapeutic properties [12,22–24], including antifungal [25–27], antibacterial [28–32], antitumor [33–36], anti-inflammatory [37,38], immunomodulatory [39–41], anti-glycemic [42], antioxidant [32,37,43], tissue repair and regeneration [14,16,44].

The objective of this review is to explore the potential use of HG particles in drug delivery systems with respect to their size (macro, micro and nano). This review also attempts to identify the effects of HG particle size and physicochemical properties on biological performance and medical applications. Finally, novel drug delivery methods for enhancing treatments are discussed.

2. Types of Hydrogels

A gel is a liquid treated with gelling substances, including natural polymers (e.g., agar, alginates, and dextran), semi-synthetic polymers (cellulose derivatives) or synthetic polymers (acrylic and methacrylic acid derivatives) [45]. Lipophilic gels (oleogels) are obtained using oil as the dispersing phase. Hydrophilic gels (hydrogels) are obtained using water as the dispersing phase [46–48]. Due to their similarity to living human tissues, HGs with controlled drug release are widely used in pharmaceuticals. By modifying their compositions and physicochemical properties (e.g., to impart hydrophilic or hydrophobic character), HGs can be used as drug carriers for external or internal use [49].

HGs are classified using different criteria [50]. The simplest criterion is origin, i.e., natural or synthetic [50,51]. Natural HGs are biocompatible, biodegradable [1] and support cell activity. However, natural HGs have low mechanical strength and large inter-batch variety. Proteins such as collagen or polysaccharides (e.g., chitosan, dextran, and alginate) are examples of natural HGs [52–55]. Synthetic HG polymers are prepared from polymerizable monomers, including vinyl acetate, acrylamide, ethylene glycol and lactic acid (made from plants, mostly from corn and sugarcane) [56–59]. Synthetic HGs can be precisely controlled and tailored to achieve desired properties. However, synthetic HGs typically lack bioactivity and have low biodegradability. Hybrid HGs consist of chemically, functionally and morphologically different units [60–65]. Biologically active proteins, peptides, nano/microstructures are constituent parts of hybrid HGs and are connected with each other by physical or chemical forces [60–66]. Because of their construction, hybrid HGs derive their bioactivity from natural materials; furthermore, the easy control over physical and chemical properties of hybrid HGs are due to synthetic material properties [66].

2.1. *Physical and Chemical Hydrogels*

HGs can be classified into two groups based on the type of interactions involved in the creation of the network structure. The first group includes chemical solids [47,51,67,68], wherein HGs form three-dimensional (3D) networks with polymer chains are connected by permanent covalent bonds via cross-linking reactions [69]. Characteristic features of chemical HGs include their ability to swell resulting from interactions among the polymer network, water and the density of connections between polymer chains. Chemical HGs are not homogeneous due to the hydrophobic aggregation of cross-linking agents and high cross-link-density clusters [60].

The second group includes physical (reversible) HGs [51,67,68]. These HGs have chains connected by weak hydrogen bonds, ionic bonds and dipolar or hydrophobic interactions excluding those that dissolve before use [68]. These forces result in non-homogeneous HGs [60]. Examples of physical HG are solutions of agar, gelatine, and polyvinyl alcohol [70,71].

These two types of HGs encompass a wide variety of macromolecular structures formed from cross-linked and entangled linear homopolymers and linear, block or graft copolymers [72–74]. The HG networks can be stabilized by reactions of monovalent and polyvalent ions, multiple monovalent ions or complexes containing hydrogen bonds. The properties and applications of these HGs are closely related to cross-linking density, which determines swelling behaviour and the combined properties of solid and liquid phases [51,68,75].

2.2. *Conventional and Stimuli-Responsive Hydrogels*

HGs are also classified as conventional and stimuli-responsive. Conventional HGs comprise loosely connected hydrophilic, mostly non-ionic polymers with significant degrees of swelling in water without dissolution [76]. Stimuli-responsive HGs respond to various factors, such as small changes in temperature, ionic strength, pH, electric field, mechanical stress, light and selected substances (Figure 1a) [49,51,77–80]. Stimuli-responsive HGs can be tailored to react to various types of stimuli in the body, including ionic strength, pH and temperature, to act as potential drug carriers [49,51,77].

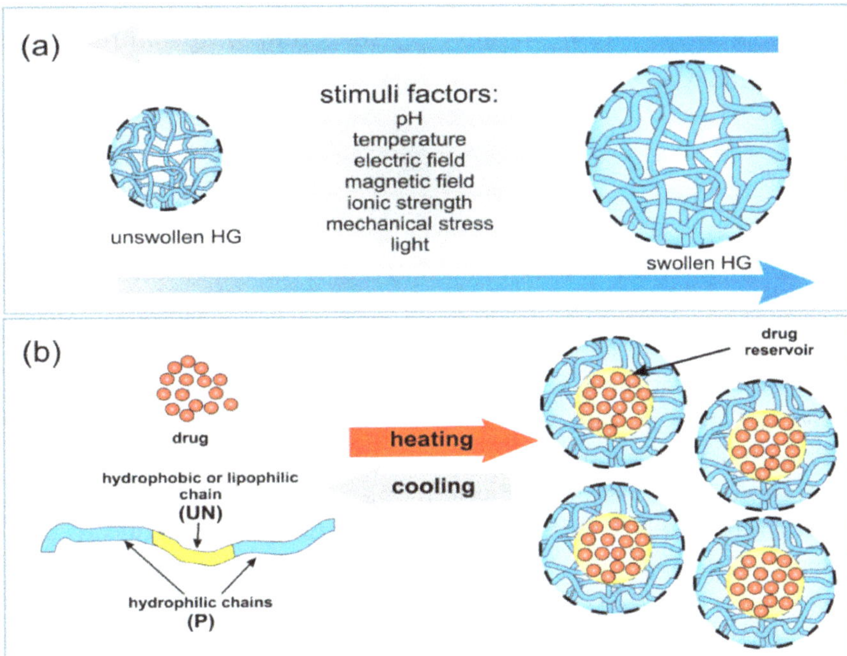

Figure 1. (**a**) Types of stimuli causing HG swelling. (**b**) Schematic illustration of a thermo-reactive HG formation loaded with a drug that uses temperature as a stimulus.

2.2.1. Thermosensitive Hydrogels

Thermosensitive HGs have a specific balance between a hydrophilic polymer gel and water molecules. In these systems, even small changes in temperature can disturb this balance and cause a phase change from sol to gel [50]. Such phase transitions often occur when the temperature changes from room temperature to physiological temperature of the human body [46]. This is because temperature influences interactions among water molecules and the hydrophilic and hydrophobic segments of the HG polymer [81].

HGs comprise hydrophilic (P) and hydrophobic (UN) segments arranged in the sequence: P-UN-P or UN-P-UN (Figure 1b). The hydrophilic segments used in HG formulations are characterized by high swelling properties, water solubility and biocompatibility [46]. The hydrophobic segments increase the loading capacity of other hydrophobic molecules, such as drugs, due to the micellization of nanoparticles (Figure 1b) [6,82].

For the proper design of thermosensitive HGs, the phase transition temperature should be identified [83]. The temperature at which the polymer solution separates into two phases is called the critical solution temperature (CST) [46] and is used to classify thermosensitive HGs as positive or negative temperature responsive systems [84,85]. The CST is typically lower for HG polymers with higher molecular weight or hydrogen-bonding interactions. Thermo-responsive HG polymers with lower CST (LCST) remain liquid at low temperature and are called negative temperature HGs. At temperatures lower than the LCST, these HGs swell [86]. When the temperature increases these HGs undergo a sol-gel transition and become insoluble upon heating. The opposite phenomenon is observed for HG polymers with upper CST (UCST, positive temperature HGs), which become soluble upon heating [46]. At temperatures lower than the UCST, positive temperature HGs dehydrate [87]. LCST HGs are used in the medical field because they form gels in situ at physiological temperatures, i.e., 30–37 °C (Table 1) [88]. Examples of synthetic polymers used to develop LCST HGs include copolymer blocks of poly(ethylene oxide) and poly(pentapeptide), poly(*N*-isopropylacrylamide) (PNIPAM), and poly(*N*,*N*-diethyl acrylamide) (PDEAM) [88]. Natural LCST polymers include cellulose derivatives, chitosan and gellan gum (Table 1) [88–90].

Table 1. Phase transition temperatures for selected polymers with LCST and UCST.

Polymer Name	Abbreviation	Transition Temperature (in Water)	Refs.
Poly(*N*-isopropylacrylamide)	PNIPAM	30–34 °C	[88]
Poly(*N*,*N*-diethylacrylamide)	PDEAM	32–34 °C	[88]
Poly(methyl vinyl ether)	PMVE	37 °C	[91]
Polyvinyl chloride	PVC	30–50 °C	[92,93]
Gellan gum	-	50–60 °C	[88]
Methylcellulose	-	40 °C	[94,95]
Acrylamide and acrylic acid	AAm and AAc	15–25 °C	[96]

2.2.2. Photo-Responsive Hydrogels

Light-responsive HGs are subjected to sol-gel changes under the influence of light at different wavelengths: infrared (IR), ultraviolet (UV), or visible (VIS) [50]. The initiation of sol-gel phase transitions in photo-responsive HGs using light is straightforward and non-invasive making these HGs a potential source of functional material in biomedicine, e.g., for drug delivery [50,97,98]. To prepare a photo-responsive HG, a light-responsive chromophore group is attached to HG polymers [99,100]. Incident light initiates swelling/deswelling processes or sol-gel phase transition to release drugs at desired locations. UV-light-responsive HGs undergo photopolymerization or photocleavage depending on the exposure length [101,102]. Light wavelength is also extremely important because it affects the drug release control process [103].

2.2.3. pH-, Electric- and Magnetic-Responsive Hydrogels

pH-responsive HGs have specific pH-dependent physicochemical properties [104]. These HGs have acidic and alkaline groups associated with HG polymer chains [50,105]. The human body is a dynamic environment with different tissues having different pH ranges, which provides delivery means for in vivo pH-responsive HGs in pharmaceutical and biomedical applications [106–108].

Ionizable groups embedded in the polymer network of pH-responsive HGs accept or donate protons in response to pH change, resulting in changes to the structure and solubility of the HGs and consequently, swelling or deswelling (Figure 1a). The most frequently used synthetic monomer with acidic characteristics are acrylic acid, methacrylic acid, maleic anhydride, *N*,*N*-dimethylaminoethyl methacrylate and sulphonamide-containing polymers [2,18,20,91,109]. Weak synthetic polybases, such as aromatics 4-vinylpyridine, 2-vinylpyridine, poly(vinyl imidazole), poly(*N*,*N*-dimethyl aminoethyl methacrylate), and poly(*N*,*N*-diethyl aminoethyl methacrylate), accept protons at low pH [50,110,111]. There is also a large group of natural polymers used in pH-responsive HGs that has advantages over synthetic polymers due to their degradability within the human body, making them excellent biocompatible components in drug delivery [9,33,88,112].

There are also HGs that respond to external physical stimuli, like electric and magnetic fields [52,105]. Magnetic or electrically responsive HG networks have been developed for drug-delivery applications. The influence of an electric field causes electro-responsive HGs to swell or de-swell, which can be adapted for drug delivery systems [113]. Similar applications have been determined for magnetic field-based stimuli, especially high frequency fields, which are much safer for humans than electric fields or UV light [114]. Magnetic and electrical stimuli-responsive HGs allow for the study of cell behaviour by altering hydrogel properties in situ. These stimuli-responsive HGs can serve in potential drug delivery systems for targeting and localizing to delivery sites for controlled drug release upon application of electric or magnetic fields [115–117].

2.3. Other Classifications for Hydrogels

HGs could also be classified by the substrates used for their production. Polymer networks may be synthesized from linking monomers to form high-molecular weight polymers. Hydrophilic monomers, such as polyphenylene oxide (PPO) or polyethylene glycol (PEG), are copolymerised with crosslinkers to form networks for drug delivery [118,119]. When prepolymers (oligomers) are used as synthetic substrates, different types of HGs are obtained. A series of model networks consisting of PEG, tetra-PEG gels, have been prepared by Sakai et al. [119,120]. Small-angle neutron scattering measurements confirmed, that network structure is extremely uniform, even in the presence of different functional groups at the ends, i.e., amine group and succinimidyl ester group [121,122]. Additionally, the modified with ionic liquid form of tetra-PEG gels possesses high ion conductivity and high mechanical properties [123,124]. For example, polyurethane-based HGs are used in the fabrication of flexible medical devices, prosthetics for example [125]. Other substrate-specific HGs are those with network structures made by crosslinking hydrophilic polymer chains, e.g., chitosan crosslinked with glutaraldehyde [75].

Due to large differences in their chemical compositions, HGs are sometimes broadly classified [51,126]. For example, in terms of the types of monomers used to prepare HGs (polymeric composition), three groups of HGs are recognized: (i) homopolymeric HGs (consisting of one type of hydrophilic monomer); (ii) copolymeric HGs (two or more monomer types of which at least one is hydrophilic), and (iii) multipolymer HGs (obtained from more than one type of polymer).

Multipolymer interpenetrating polymeric (IPN) HGs represent a class of HGs made of two independent cross-linked synthetic and/or natural polymers [51,75,127–129]. HGs there are two polymer networks, one of which is polymerized around and within the on the second polymer network, and what is very important, there are no covalent linkages between those two polymeric networks.

HGs may take significantly different morphological forms, which can be a criterion for their division depending on the state of aggregation (physical form) [17,105,129]: (i) solid (amorphous, semicrystalline or crystalline); (ii) semisolid (for example shear-thinning HGs), and (iii) liquid [17,51,75,130]. Solid HGs can be useful in formation of functional tissues [75,131]. At room temperature they are solid in nature with strong cross-linked network structure [17]. Solid HGs swell in the presence of water or other hydrophilic solutions like buffers or biological fluids. Semisolid HG consists of two types components where at least one possess biological nature, e.g., plant resins or gums [17]. The shear-thinning HGs also belong to this group [17,132,133]. These HGs can be pre-gelled outside of the body and injected by applying shear stress and flow like low-viscosity fluids. The shear-thinning behaviour is a result of reversible physical cross-links. That group of HGs is often called bio- or muco-adhesive HGs according to their specific adhesive properties [16,75,134]. Liquid HGs are injected in liquid form and a sol-gel transition is performed inside the human body [19,109,135–137]. The resulting HGs takes the shape of space available at the injection site which allows to achieve the sol–gel transition with variety of strategies. Slow-gelling systems based on gelation mechanisms (charge interaction, stereocomplexation, click chemistry, etc.), termo- or pH-responsive systems are good representatives of this group.

It is also possible to classify HG based on ionic charges into the following four groups: (i) neutral (no charge, e.g., dextran); (ii) anionic (negative charge) like carrageenan; (iii) cationic (with positive charge) such as chitosan, and (iv) amphiphilic (having the ability to strongly interact with both polar and nonpolar solvent molecules—such as collagen) [17,138–143].

3. Types of Physical Appearance of Hydrogels

HGs have a number of properties, such as oxygen and nutrient permeability and the ability to bind, transport and control drug delivery and release, attractive for use in biological applications. Different tissues have different requirements and would be better served using different types of HGs [144]. HGs can be formed in almost any shape and size [145], e.g., as a matrix, a film, microparticles, nanoparticles, macro-beads, membranes, or coatings, depending on the polymerization technique [46,51,82,146]. HGs are altered to improve their compatibility with hydrophobic or hydrophilic compounds or drugs with different properties [147,148].

Polymeric HGs are classified as macro-, micro- and nanogels with respect to particle size [17,149]. Microgels, cross-linked structure is large, usually from millimetres to centimetres [150]. A group of gels called microgels, whose particles are smaller, separate and cross-linked, having a size between 1 μm and 100 nm [151]. Nanogels are those gels whose particles have a size smaller than 100 nm [49,106,152]. It should be noted that gels with particle sizes only slightly larger than 100 nm were called quasi-nanogels [153].

Microgel is a submicron- or micron-sized network polymer which is highly swellable but insoluble in water [154]. Cross-linked microgel particles possess special kind of control over particle shape and size, which is probably due to specific extensive swelling pattern [155]. Microgels are obtained in two ways. One of them is molecular assembly of existing polymer molecules in aqueous solutions. The other one, particle-forming polymerization, includes two types of polymerization: precipitation and inverse emulsion polymerization [154,156].

Nanogels are prepared in water by self-aggregation of polymers, mostly of natural origin; natural polysaccharides (dextran, pullulan) or cholesterol-containing polysaccharide [14,157]. The dimensions of these HGs are usually of 20–30 nm. Such a small size causes the use of nanogels for cell targeting, because swelling caused by pH changes in the surrounding environment is the reason to release the entrapped drug [158]. Nanogels react to the external stimuli changes much quicker than macrogels. The reason for this is probably their small size and short relaxation time [159,160]. Swelling and deswelling properties and small size of biocompatible and biodegradable nanogel particles are the cause of easy crossing the blood brain barrier [21,149,153].

Obtaining a specific shape of HG at a nanoscale is difficult. HG nanofibers, for example, can be obtained by the by electrostatic spinning method [161]. HGs are also given the form of microcapsules and microspheres, whose size is 1–1000 μm. This allows more protection of substances enclosed in the interior of microcapsules and microspheres. HGs can form micelles in an aqueous environment, as a result of aggregation of amphiphilically connected blocks or end-modified polymers. It is often difficult to differentiate micelles from reversible HGs, because HGs can form micelles above a appropriate concentration called the micelle gel concentration [162]. Similarly, biodegradable nanoparticles of HGs are classified as nanocapsules or nanospheres having drug molecules adsorbed on the surface or closed inside [163,164].

There also exist the group of in situ-gelling HGs, which undergo a sol-gel transition inside the human body [165]. That group of HG always adapts to the free space with its shape. An example of such HGs are shear-thinning HGs. Because of reversible physical cross-links shear-thinning hydrogels pre-gelled outside of the human body, after shear stress injection can regain its initial stiffness.

Despite of many nano- and microgels advantages, it should remember about the possibility of using macroporous HGs and the benefits resulting from it. Macroporous HGs can mechanically collapse at up to 90% and recover reversibly almost immediately after injection in the human body. Such macroporous HGs allow for the preparation of highly defined shapes for drug delivery [151].

4. Immobilization of Drugs in Hydrogel

4.1. HG Structure and Physical Properties

A physical and chemical properties, including structural parameters, swelling behaviour, diffusive characteristics, and surface properties, determine the biomedical and pharmaceutical applications of HGs [5]. After the creation of porous HG structures, different drug molecules may be incorporated into the scaffolding (post-loading) or in the network during formation (in situ loading); these drugs are subsequently released from the hydrophilic matrix to biological media. Thus, network mesh size (or pore size) is a major parameter which determines the sizes of the drug system that can be immobilized in the porous matrix of the HG. The network mesh size (ξ) indicates the distance between adjacent junctions, cross-links and tie points. Cross-links may be chemical (mainly covalent bonds) or physical (e.g., electrostatic, hydrophobic and dipole-dipole) [5].

The cross-linking density (ρ_x) of HGs, which refers to the number of cross-links in a given volume, is a parameter that defines the structural properties of HGs [5,166,167]. Relationships between cross-linking density and HG properties (e.g., shear modulus, equilibrium swelling ratio, drug diffusivity) are presented in Figure 2 [5]. These parameters allow for the prediction of HG release behaviour.

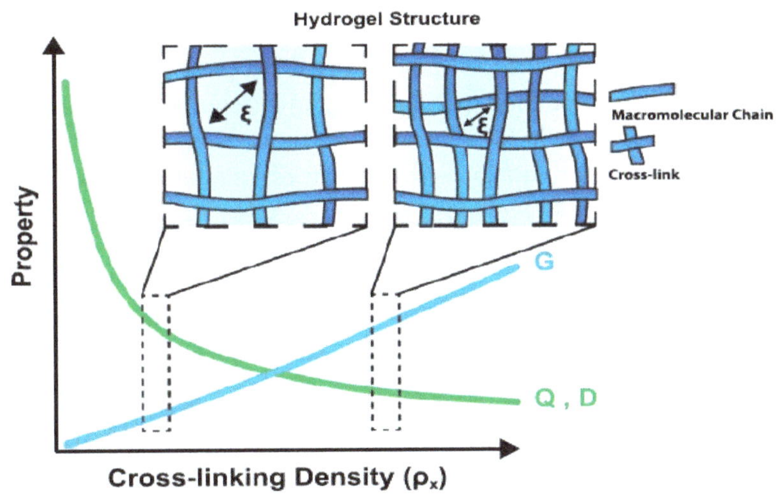

Figure 2. Relationship between the cross-linking density and HG properties. Two network structures representative of low and high cross-linking densities are depicted to demonstrate the relationship between the cross-linking density and basic HG properties of highly swollen, non-ionic gels, including shear modulus (G), equilibrium volumetric swelling ratio (Q) and diffusivity (D). As the cross-linking density increases, the mesh size (ξ) decreases, which is a measure of the space available between macromolecular chains for the diffusion. Reprinted with permission from Ref. [5].

From experimentally measured volumetric swelling ratios of HGs (Q), the average molecular weight can be calculated between cross-links ($\overline{M}_c$) and the equilibrium polymer volume fraction (v_2) of a given network [167]. There are many equations describing the relationship between the network structure and its physical properties, which allow the calculation and prediction of transport properties of homogenous porous materials:

$$\xi = v_2^{-\frac{1}{3}} \left(\overline{r_0^2}\right)^{\frac{1}{2}} \tag{1}$$

$$\frac{D_g}{D_0} = \left(1 - \frac{r_s}{\xi}\right) \exp\left(-Y\left(\frac{v_2}{1 - v_2}\right)\right) \tag{2}$$

$$Q \sim \left(\overline{M_c}\right)^{3/5} \tag{3}$$

where ξ is the mesh size; $\left(\overline{r_0^2}\right)^{\frac{1}{2}}$ describes the root-mean-squared end-to-end distance of the polymer chains in the unperturbated state; D_g means the solute diffusivity in e swollen gel; D_0 means the diffusivity of the solute in the swelling solvent; r_s is a sign of the radius of the solute; Y is the proportion of the critical volume needed for a successful translational motion of the solute molecule to a medium free volume attributable per molecule of the liquid [167–169]. After some simplification, these equations can be used to find the correlation between all mentioned parameters (Equation (4)) for highly swollen, non-ionic HGs, and scale with $\overline{M}_c$:

$$1 - \frac{D_g}{D_0} = \frac{r_s}{\xi} \sim \left(\overline{M_c}\right)^{-\frac{7}{10}} \tag{4}$$

The HG network structure is also important in determining the mechanical properties of porous material. The network structure controls swelling behaviour and drug release in biological environment. Swelling behaviour is defined as the ratio of the volume of the water-swollen gel to the volume of dry polymer and is indicative of the water content of the swollen HG. However, higher water content resulting from high network porosity is more beneficial for immobilizing active substances and can simultaneously lead to polymer degradation and prevent the controlled delivery of drugs. In this context, the cross-linking density must be high enough to allow for the immobilization of the active substance in the polymer matrix. Beyond the structural properties, the chemical composition of HGs regulates the final biochemical properties, e.g., charge, hydrophilicity and bioactivity.

In this brief discussion, we highlighted the structural properties of macroscale HGs. These HGs have consistent physicochemical properties throughout, and drugs can be distributed homogeneously in "bulk HGs" (Figure 3a). Macroscopic HGs have dimensions of millimetres to centimetres and are typically surgically implanted or arranged in contact with the patient's body to achieve transepithelial drug delivery [17,137].

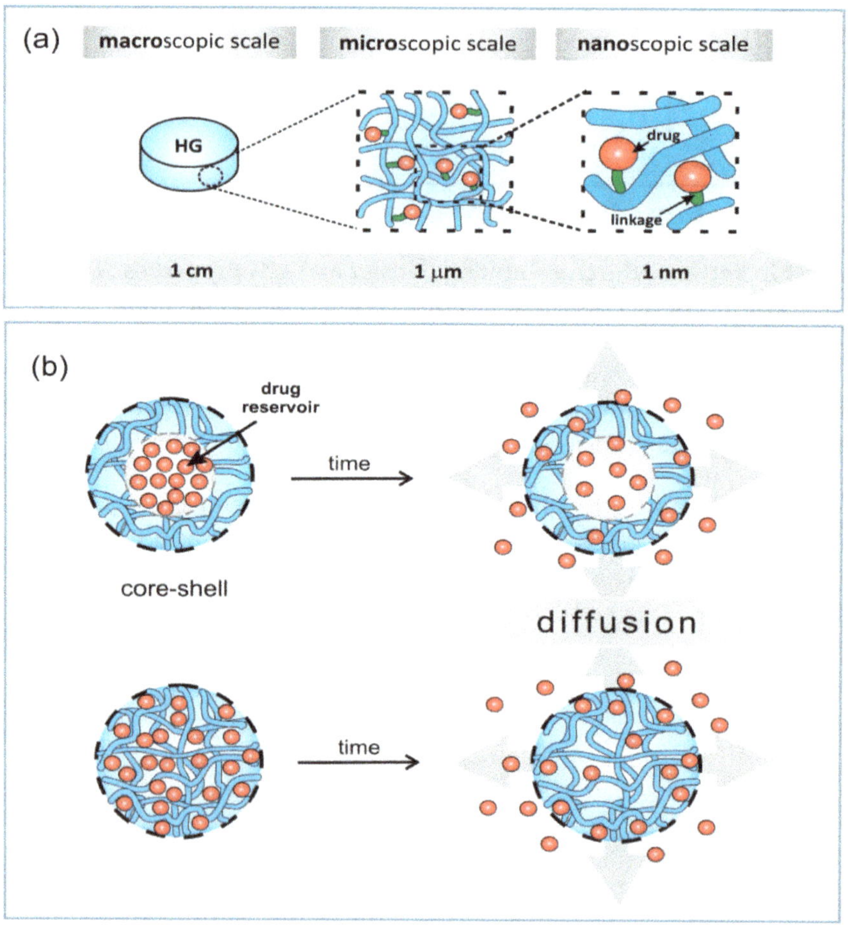

Figure 3. (**a**) Macroscopic design of HGs including the size and porous structure. (**b**) Schematic structures of micro- and nanogels showing the release of drugs.

Other structures, e.g., micro- and nanogels, draw attention to their use as injection materials (Figures 3 and 4). Their relative scale (1 μm to 100 nm microgels and 10–100 nm nanogels) determines the course by which HGs can be delivered to the human body [17–20]. Small HG particles are needle-injectable, provide large surfaces for bioconjugation and enhance penetration through tissue barriers [135,136,170,171].

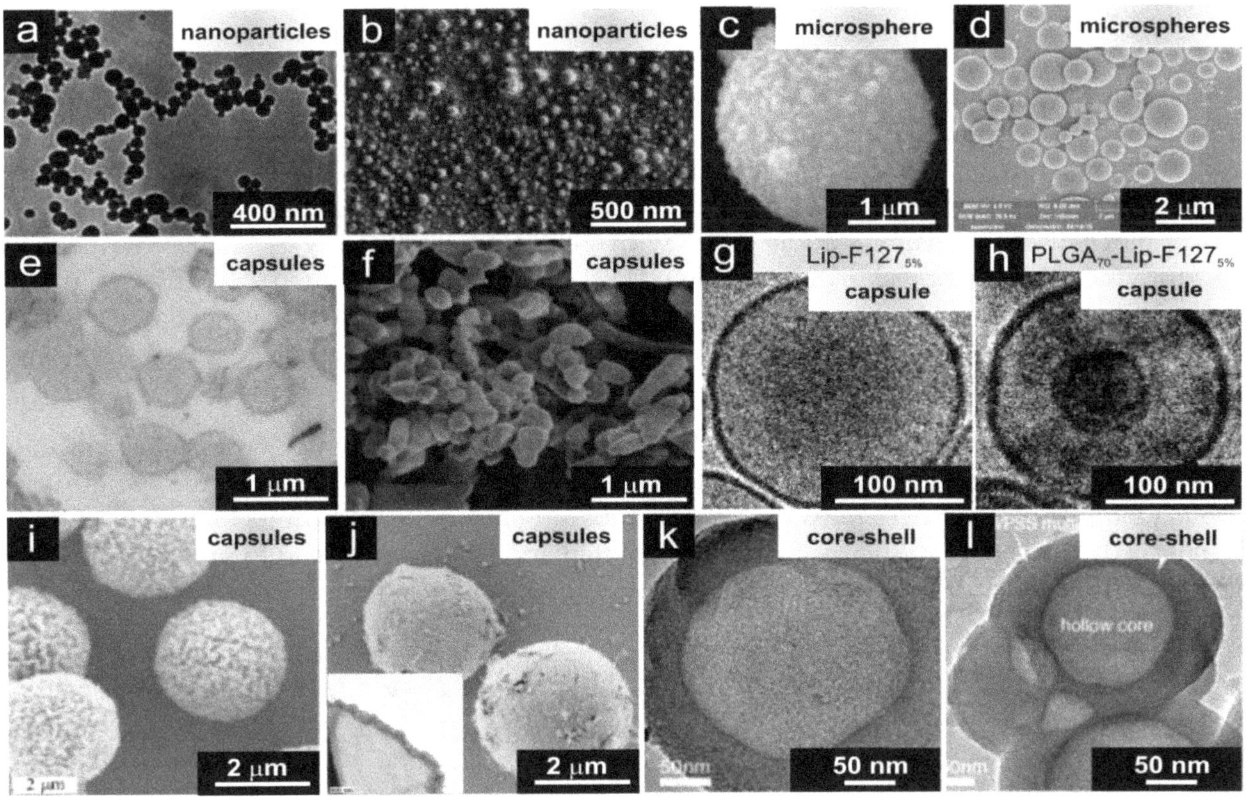

Figure 4. Morphology (structure) of HGs observed by (**a**,**c**,**e**,**g**,**h**) TEM and (**b**,**d**,**f**,**i**,**j**) SEM at different magnifications (the scale bars are marked on the images) obtained by post-loading or in situ loading drugs. (**a**,**b**) Piperlongumine-loaded poly(ethylene glycol)-poly(dehydroabietic ethyl methacrylate) HG nanoparticles [172]. (**c**) Silver alginate HG microspheres [173]. (**d**) Thermosensitive HG microspheres loaded with tenofovir [174]. (**e**,**f**) Polyacrylamide-poly(*N*-isopropylacrylamide) HG capsules loaded with doxorubicin hydrochloride [175]. (**g**) Unloaded lipid capsule (Lip) with F127$_{5\%}$ (5 wt% content of Pluronic F127) [176]. (**h**) Doxorubicin-loaded poly(lactic-co-glycolic acid) (PLGA) core-lipid shell (Lip) with F127$_{5\%}$ structure [176]. Smart organic/inorganic HG polyelectrolyte capsules (poly(allylamine hydrochloride): (**i**) hollow and (**j**) hydroxyapatite [177]. (**k**,**l**) Core-shell mesoporous silica spheres (**l**) loaded with ibuprofen [178].

Drug delivery based on micro- and nanogels are superior when compared with macrosystems (Figure 3b) because: (i) the smaller sizes of these HGs allows for active and passive drug targeting; (ii) controlled drug release leads to improved therapeutic impact and reduced side effects; (iii) drug loading takes place with no chemical reaction (environmental stimuli); (iv) the smaller HGs may infiltrate into tissues via paracellular and transcellular routes; and (v) the smaller HGs are biocompatible and biodegradable [15,179]. Examples of different structures/morphology of HGs are presented in Figure 4. These systems were observed using TEM (transmission electron microscopy) or SEM (scanning electron microscopy). We can distinguish two types of HGs: (i) "core-shell" systems and (ii) homogenously dispersed drugs (Figures 3b and 4). In the core-shell system, a shell is formed by HGs around a central core is drug reservoir (Figure 4e–h,l,k). This structure can be produced in the form of capsules, spheres or slabs, having a high concentration of the drug in the core of the systems, which facilitate the constant release of the drug in the body [126,174,175,180,181]. In the second system, the drug is dispersed homogeneously in a polymer matrix (Figure 4a–d), which in contact with a bio-fluid usually begins swelling, and takes forms of nanoparticles, polymeric micelles, microspheres, etc. [68,172,180,181]. For both types of HGs, releasing of drugs is time-depended process and it is mainly diffusion controlled. Drug releasing from the HG network will be discussed in detail in the next paragraph.

4.2. Immobilization of Drugs

HGs due to their 3D structures may be applied as carriers for drugs, proteins, lipids or cells [15,17,68,182,183]. Additionally, a large amount of water within their structures makes a convenient environment for the immobilization of drugs. However, 3D structures of HG allow the immobilization of drugs in their matrix, in this regard, when immobilization process of active substances is performed, two aspects must be taken into account. The large pore size of HG (large mesh size), as well as the high water content causes that water-soluble drugs with small particles quickly escape from the network, thanks to which they have a short release time [182]. Drug release is much slower when the drug particle size is comparable to the mesh size [17]. When the drug particle size exceeds the mesh size, then the drug is physically trapped in the network [17]. To minimize these problems, the pore size in HG (mesh size) should be "matched" to the size of the immobilized drug.

There are many methods leading to loading of drugs in HG networks/spheres/capsules, and the choice of method depends mainly on the place where the drug should be delivered. Briefly, drugs can be loaded into HG matrices in two ways: post-loading and in situ loading (Table 2 and Figure 5). HGs have proven to be very efficient for local drug delivery, which could lead to prolonged and faster release. Some examples of HG applications are presented in Table 2; different structures are presented in Figure 5.

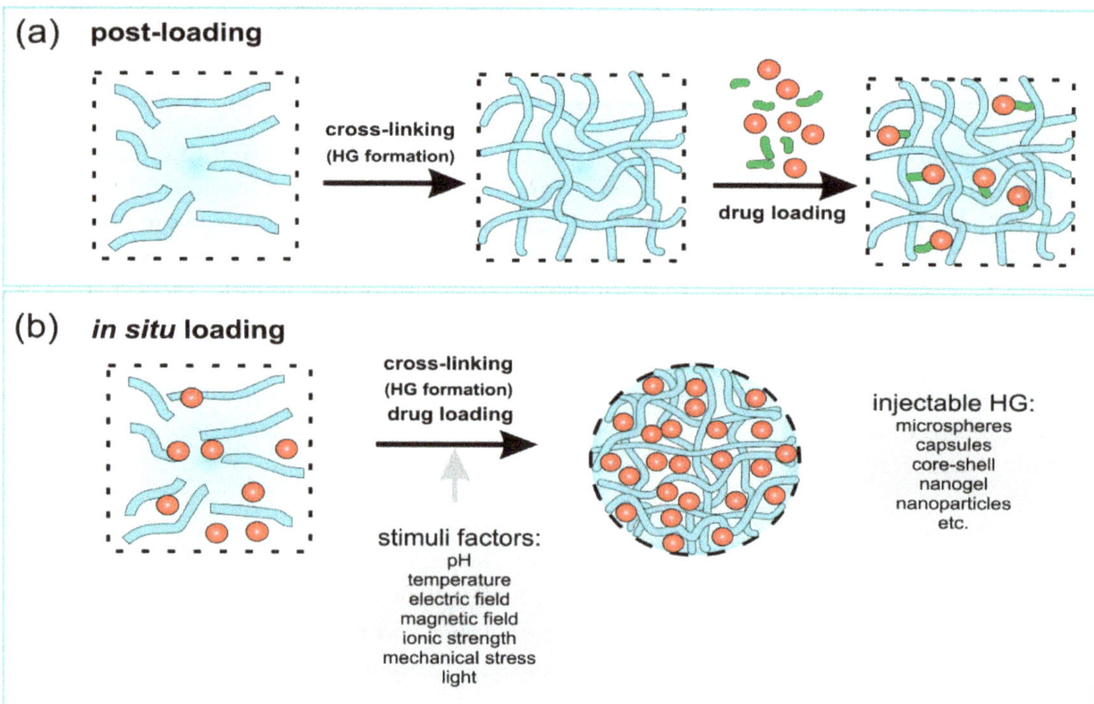

Figure 5. Schematic representation of drug loading in a HG network using (**a**) post-loading and (**b**) in situ loading mechanisms.

Briefly, the post-loading drug process consists of forming a polymer HG matrix (a preformed HG) and immobilizing the drug in the polymeric network (Figure 5a). HGs swell in drug solutions till equilibrium. Depending on the HG macro- or microscopic size, HGs are administered by more or less invasive procedures. Preformed HG gels outside the human body, while being quite simple films or sticky solutions that retain their rheological or mechanical properties after administration [184].

Table 2. Examples of HGs with different routes drug immobilization of and their structures and applications.

Type of Loading Drugs	Hydrogel Precursors	Drug	Structure	Applications	Refs.
Post-loading	AA[17] –BA[18] –DEAP[19]	17-DMAPG [15]	Core-shell [16]	Antitumor activity	[152]
	Carbopol 940 [20]	Vor [11]	Core-shell LPN	Dermal applications	[185]
	Carbopol/stearic acid	Vor	Core-shell	Ophthalmic Application	[186]
	PNIPAAm-*b*-PLA-*b*-PEG-*b*-PLA[7]-*b*-PNIPAAm	Riluzole	-	Neuroprotective drug	[183]
	PAA-PNIPAAm	DOX	Core-shell capsule	Antitumor activity	[175]
	PEG-*b*-PDAEMA [8]	PLGM [9]	Nanoparticle	Antitumor activity	[172]
	Chitosan/Polysaccharide	Tenofovir	Microsphere	Vaginal drug	[174]
	Chitosan/β-GB	DOX-loaded in LTSL [29]	PP[33] HG	Antitumor activity	[187]
	PLGA [30] MicroC PEG derivatives (HG)	DOX-loaded in MicroC [31] Fu [32]-loaded in HG	PP HG	Antitumor activity	[188]
In situ loading	Polysaccharide	Ibuprofen	Core-shell capsule	Oral drug	[126]
	Carbohydrate-NIPAM [22]	Bupivacaine	HG-microgel composite	Anaesthetic drug	[189]
	PNIPAAm-co-AIA [21]	Lopinavir	Microspheres	Antiretroviral drug	[190]
	CmetCel [25] -Dextran	AmB [23]	MacroHG	Antifungal therapy	[191]
	NiPAAm [26]-NtBAAm[27]	Fluvastatin	PP HG	HMG-CoA [25]	[192]
	PPZ [34]	Silibinin	Microspheres	Anticancer and antiangiogenic activity	[193]
	PEG–PCL [35]–PEG	PTX micelles [36]	PP HG	Antitumor activity	[194]

Abbreviations: [1] PNIPAAm: poly(*N*-isopropylacrylamide); [2] PAA: polyacrylamide; [3] PHEMA: poly(hydroxylethyl methacrylate); [4] PVP: poly(vinylpyrrolidone); [5] PEG: poly(ethylene glycol); [6] LPN: lipid nanoparticles; [7] PLA: poly(lactide); [8] PDAEMA: poly(dehydroabietic ethyl methacrylate); [9] PLGM: piperlongumine; [10] DOX: Doxorubicin hydrochloride; [11] Vor: Voriconazole; [12] EGDMA: 2-(2-methyl-acryloyloxy)ethyl 2-methyl-acrylate; [13] HEMA: 2-hydroxethyl 2-methylprop-2-enoate; [14] Indo: Indomethacin; [15] 17-DMAPG: geldanamycin derivative (aminated form, which readily protonates at low pH; [16] core-shell structure of HG-in-LPN; [17] AA: acrylic acid; [18] BA: *N,N′*-methylenebis(acrylamide); [19] DEAP: 2,2-diethoxyacetophenone; [20] Carbopol 940: HG composed of Precirol ATO 5, Labrafil 1944 CS, and Tween 80; [21] AIA: allylamine; [22] NIPAM: poly(*N*-isopropylacrylamide); [23] AmB: Amphotericin B; [24] CmetCel: carboxymethylcellulose-hydrazide; [25] HMG-CoA: reductase inhibitor (statin); [26] NiPAAm: *N*-isopropylacrylamide; [27] NtBAAm: *N-tert*-butylacrylamide; [28] β-GB: β-glycerophosphate; [29] LTSL: lysolipid thermally sensitive liposomes; [30] PLGA: poly(lactide-co-glycolide); [31] MicroC: microcapsule; [32] Fu: 5-fluorouracil; [33] PP: "plum padding"; [34] PPZ: poly(organophosphazene); [35] PCL: poly(ε-caprolactone); [36] PTX: Paclitaxel.

Drugs can be physically or chemically immobilized in HGs and can also be loaded into other species (secondary delivery vehicles) to provide the appropriate environment for targeting. Preformed HGs are solid even when injected [184].

In situ loading of drugs is associated with the simultaneous formation of injectable HGs in the body and the encapsulation of drugs (Figure 5b). Briefly, the whole process shows a sol-to-gel transition in situ that form after injection in vivo.

The resulting HG take the shape of the available space. In situ gel formation usually includes the subsequent steps: (i) gelation as a response to the changes of temperature or pH changes (thermoresponsive or chemical responsive polymers; i.e., "smart" polymers), (ii) ionic or covalent cross-linking, (iii) solvent exchange or crystallization, and/or (iv) thickening upon removal of the injection shear. These external stimuli are shortly summarized in Figure 1a (stimuli factors).

Taking into account the lifetime of HGs, their formation mechanism can be categorized as: (i) pre-gelation (polymer precursor in solution), (ii) therapeutic window (after injection and gelation containing drug), and (iii) degradation (HG degradation products) [18]. These systems may be homopolymeric or multipolymeric or may also be composed of different components, including other systems (e.g., capsule, microgels, and nanoparticles) serving as drug carriers. This latter mentioned gel systems are characterized in the next section.

Immobilization of Drugs in Hydrogel Composites

Some systems containing drugs in matrix/capsules are poorly water-soluble or insoluble. In this sense, soluble therapeutic agents are poorly retained in HGs due to their hydrophilic nature. In this case, there are many problems with loading process of drugs due to their tendency to aggregate resulting in high local concentrations causing toxicity [195]. To overcome these problems, HG composites have been created to exploit the hydrophilic-hydrophobic nature of various components [192,196]. HG composites contain polymeric networks (hydrophilic) swollen with water and nanostructures/microstructures with different physico-chemical properties [192,197–199]. These composites represent a new class of materials with new properties.

The inclusion of nanomaterials in the HG polymer network is an interesting way to adjust the mechanical properties of HG and/or to provide the composite with sensitivity to external stimuli [192,196,197,199]. Different nanomaterials have been immobilized in polymeric networks, including inorganic nanoparticles [200,201], carbon nanomaterials [202], and lipids [99]. Nanoparticle systems have gained considerable attention by being one of the most interesting and promising biomedical materials with the exceptional physicochemical properties, controlled shapes, nano-sized characteristics, comprehensive modification options and well-defined multi-functionality [83]. The preparation of HG composites may be performed using physical and chemical forces.

To overcome the incompatibility of hydrophobic drugs and hydrophilic HG networks, lipid nanoparticles (LPNs) are frequently used to promote good solubility. LPNs have been used for dermal, mucosal, transdermal and intramuscular applications [176,182]. Three types of LPNs have been used in drug delivery systems: (i) lipid nano emulsions (LNEs, where the core is composed of liquid lipids), (ii) solid lipid nanoparticles (SLNs, where the core has lipids in a solid state at room and body temperatures), and (iii) nanostructured lipid carriers (NLCs, where the lipid core is a heterogeneous mixture of solid and liquid lipids) [182]. The lipophilic core of LNPs entraps active ingredients, whereas the surfactant membrane (consisting of phospholipids) ensures the stability of LNPs in hydrophilic environments. In pure lipophilic form, these systems have unsuitable rheological properties and therefore, require structural modifications. These modifications result in the formation of LNP-HG composites [187] as shown in Figure 6.

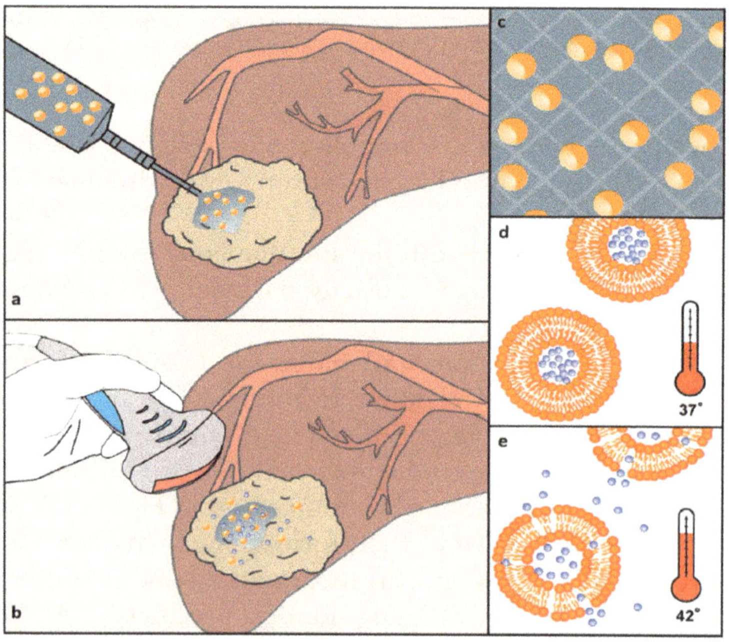

Figure 6. (**a**) Fully syringe-injectable Lipogel consisting of a chitosan/β-GP thermoresponsive gel containing a suspension of DOX-loaded thermosensitive liposomes. (**b**) Release from the gel in situ is controlled using minimally invasive hyperthermia, which is achievable using high intensity-focused ultrasound. A small portion of the drug-loaded liposomes is released from the Lipogel, maximizing the drug delivery distance from the gel implant. (**c**) The majority of liposomes are locked into the gel upon initiation of cross-linking during thermogelation. (**d**,**e**) Liposomes sequester the majority of the drug at body temperature but rapidly become more permeable upon mild hyperthermia and release their drug payload. Reprinted with permission from Ref. [187].

An in situ gelation of chitosan/β-glycerophosphate (GP) and thermoresponsive liposomes was performed [187]. This biocompatible and biodegradable HG was used as a matrix for lysolipid thermally sensitive liposomes (LTSL) loaded with doxorubicin (DOX). LTSLs are bi-layered spherical vesicles that rapidly change structure upon mild hyperthermia (41–43 °C), creating openings in the liposome. DOX was loaded into LTSL by changing solution pH. DOX delivery was also based on the pH-sensitivity of liposomes to acidic pH. A schematic of the controlled-delivery of chitosan/β-GP/DOX-loaded LTSLs and DOX release is presented in Figure 6.

The next very interesting group of composite HGs are "plum pudding gels" (PP gels), which are schematically shown in Figure 7 [179,187,188,192,194]. This type of the composite HG contains microgels or nanogels inside a bulk HG network, which improves the loading and release of drug. In the PP gel structure, the microgels or nanogels act as reservoirs for drugs and can be incorporated into a conventional macroscale HG at the different concentrations to provide two-component gel matrices.

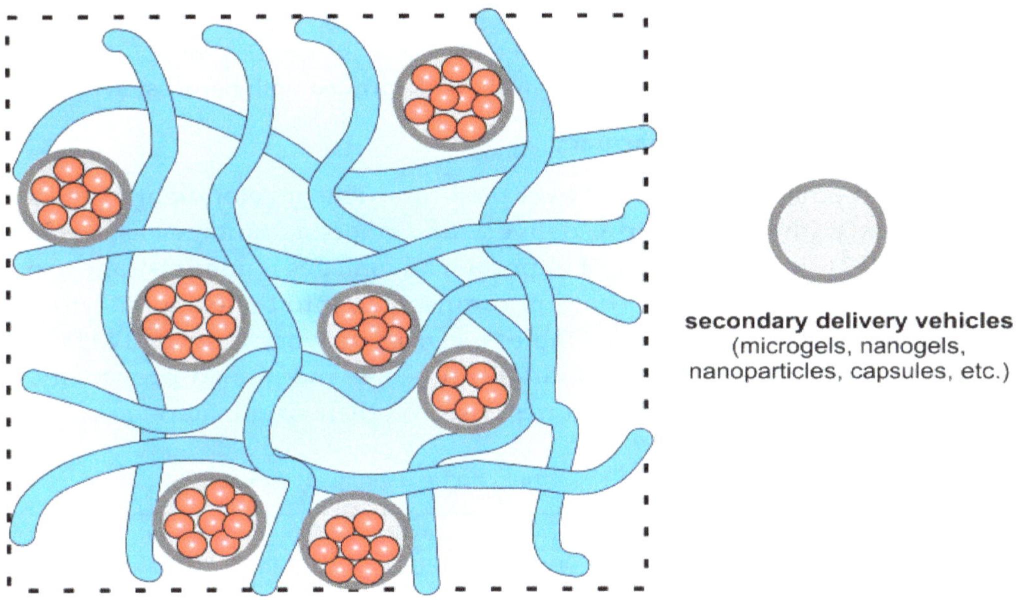

Figure 7. Structure of "plum pudding gels" (PP gels). Composite HG containing a drug embedded in a secondary controlled delivery vehicle (microgels, nanogels, nanoparticles, capsules, etc.).

From a drug delivery perspective, these systems are particularly interesting because the drug delivery limitations of microgels and HGs are minimized, whereas their synergistic effects are observed as soft nanocomposites [179]. The presented chitosan/β-GP/DOX-loaded LTSL system belongs to this group of composites [187]. Other similar systems are listed in Table 2.

4.3. Release Mechanism of Drug from Hydrogel Matrices

The physical and chemical properties of HGs affect their delivery properties, including controlled release. HG structure, diameter, and cross-linking agent density affect the rate of drug diffusion. The kinetics of drug release from HGs is connected to the chemical structure and crosslinking density of the materials, including the HG matrix monomers and coating (Figure 8) [203].

The use of HG networks increases the local concentrations of pharmaceuticals and their slow release at delivery sites. Suitable controlled-release mechanisms include (Figure 8): diffusion [17], swelling [68], chemical and environmental stimuli (degradation or deformation) [67]. Drug release from HGs in response to environmental stimuli may occur due to changes in pH [110,204], temperature [110,205–207], electric field [109,111,208] or ionic strength [209,210]. Some ideas are schematically presented in Figure 8 [17].

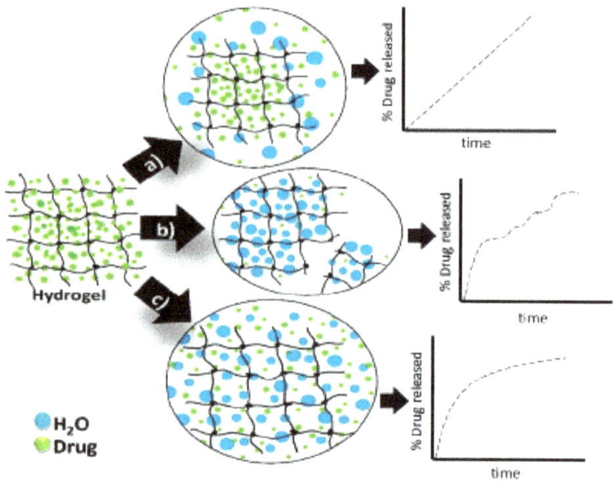

Figure 8. Hydrogels drug release mechanisms and their respective kinetic profiles: (**a**) drug diffusion, (**b**) degradation of the polymeric matrix and (**c**) swelling. Reprinted with permission from Ref. [203].

5. The Use of Hydrogels in Modern Pharmacy

Interest in using HGs has not decreased over the years. The development of specially modified HGs has provided new pathways for drug delivery and offers advantages as a vehicle for active substances [191,192,211–213]. One of the most important advantages is administration route versatility. HGs offer several routes: oral, injection (both intramuscular, into bone and subcutaneous), rectal, vaginal, through wounds, and ophthalmic (Table 3). Drug delivery is strongly connected to drug molecule size and is dependent on administration route. As mentioned previously, HG delivery systems can be classified into three main categories based on their size: macro-, micro- and nanosized.

Table 3. Summary of HGs that can be used as drug carriers.

Hydrogel	Structure/Size	Active Substance	Route of Delivery	Refs.
CTS-g-poly(AA-co-AAm)PVP/MMT	Nanogel	Clarithromycin	Oral	[214]
Salecan/PAMPS	Microgel	Insulin	Oral	[215]
HA	Nanogel	Insulin	Oral	[216]
CTS	Nanogel	Curcumin	Oral	[217]
CTS	-	Camptothecin	Oral	[218]
SS/PVA	Microgel	Gentamycin sulphate	Dermal	[219]
TG/SA/PVA	Microgel	Moxifloxacin	Dermal	[220]
P407/CMCs	Microgel	Cortex Moutan extract	Dermal	[221]
CMCTS/PAD	Macrogel	Voriconazole	Ocular	[12]
HECTS	Macrogel	-	Ocular	[222]
P407	Nanogel	Theaflavin/Nifeviroc	Vaginal	[2]
CTS	Microgel	Tenofovir	Vaginal	[174]
CHC	-	Naringenin	Topical oral	[223]
CTS	Nanogel	Thymol	Topical oral	[224]
GCTS	-	Paclitaxel	Injection	[225]
PF127/HA	Nanogel	Paclitaxel and doxorubicin	Injection	[226]
CTS	-	Curcumin	Injection	[227]
CMCTS	Nanogel	Curcumin	Injection	[228]
CTS/GP	-	Docetaxel	Injection	[229]
Gelatine/laponite (+chitosan or PNIPAM-co-AA)	Nanogel	Rhodamine B	Injection	[230]
Salecan	-	Doxorubicin	Injection	[231]
Agarose	-	Doxorubicin	Injection	[232]
SA	Nanogel	Bevacizumab	Injection	[233]

Abbreviations: CTS: chitosan; AA: acrylic acid; AAm: acrylamide; PVP: polyvinylopyrrolidone; MMT: montmorillonite; PAMPS: poly(2-acryloamido-2-methyl-1-propanesulfonic acid); HA: hyaluronic acid; SS: sericin; PVA: polyvinyl alcohol; TG: tragacanth gum; SA: sodium alginate; P407: poloxamer 407; CMCs: sodium carboxymethyl cellulose; PAD: poly aldehyde dextran; HECTS: hydroxyethylated chitosan; CHC: carboxymethyl-hexanoyl chitosan; GCTS: glycol chitosan; CTS/GP: chitosan/β-glycerophosphate; PNIPAM: poly(*N*-isoproplacrylamide)-co-acrylic acid.

We present some examples of HGs applications in drug delivery. Most informative reports from the last couple of years regarding HGs in health care have been well summarized; however, the literature on HGs is constantly increasing, as well as interest in HG materials. Herein, we highlight only a few studies that only begins to hint at the wide applications of HGs (Table 3).

5.1. Application of Hydrogels for Oral Administration

Oral administrative routes are classic and accepted means for delivering drugs. The vast majority of medicines available on the market are taken through oral routes. Several pills are often taken daily at appropriate intervals to achieve effective therapy. This reduces associated risks of skipping or missing doses and thereby lowering the effectiveness of the therapy. The development of delayed release capsules that prolong the delivery of active substances has been a breakthrough and has allowed for increased compliance. With these delayed release capsules, the amount of tablets consumed is reduced, usually to only one per day. Acid-sensitive drugs require protection against harmful effects of gastric juice typically encountered when delivering drugs vial oral routes. Protection can be offered by using special tablets coated with polymers soluble only at basic pH, such as in the intestines. As a result, drugs survive transit through the stomach and are released only in the intestines thereby promoting higher absorption into the bloodstream.

HGs have also been explored for oral delivery applications. The appropriate selection of gel or the addition of pH-dependent coatings enable the controlled release of active substances from HGs.

The first modification was presented by Panahi et al. [214] (Table 3). Chitosan (CTS)-based gels with acrylic acid (AA), acrylamide (AAm) and polyvinylpyrrolidone (PVP) were prepared [214]. During HG formation, a mineral (montmorillonite, MMT), which has ability to absorb water, was used. Clarithromycin (CAM), a macrolide antibiotic, was used to eradicate *H. Pylori* from the gastrointestinal tract was immobilized in the HG network. It was important to achieve a prolonged release of the antibiotic to increase the chances of an effective therapy. MMT increased the pore diameter in the gel structure, which increased the immobilization of the active substance. However, this also prevented solvent from readily reaching CAM through more intricate pathways in the network, which complicated drug release.

The dependence of the release of the drug on the pH level was explored by Qi et al. [215] (Table 3). An HG system was prepared based on salecan (beta glucan) with pH-sensitive poly(2-acrylamido-2-methyl-1-propanesulfonic acid) (PAMPS). The system had the ability to take or donate protons depending on the pH of the environment, while reducing or increasing the network volume. The authors showed that salecan in combination with PAMPS had the ability to release the active substance depending on the pH of the environment. Using insulin as an exemplary drug, at acidic pH insulin was released at a lower level than at neutral or slightly alkaline pH.

Insulin release from HGs was more extensively studied [216]. Special nanocarriers based on methacrylic acid were synthesized. In a neutral environment, the methacrylic polymer chains started to repel each other, thereby loosening the nanocarrier network and allowing the release of insulin. This property was exploited in preparing HA-doped HG. In the intestines, where the pH is above 7, insulin release increased dramatically compared with release in the stomach. By using HGs as a drug carrier, the release of insulin was extended over time.

In another study, a unique biodegradable, super porous, swellable and pH-sensitive nanocellulose reinforced CTS HG was prepared for the oral administration of curcumin [217]. The in vitro degradation of HG was dependent on the swelling ratio and the number of cellulose nanocrystals (CNCs) in the HG. All HGs showed maximum swelling ratios greater than 300%. The drug release occurred in simulated gastric media; the drug maintained its chemical activity after in vitro release. According to this study, CNC-reinforced CTS HGs can be used to improve the bioavailability of curcumin for absorption from the stomach and upper intestinal tract.

Finally, tetrakis(hydroxymethyl)phosphonium chloride was used as a crosslinking agent in a Mannich reaction to obtain chitosan-based HGs [218]. These pH-sensitive HGs showed low toxicity, high biocompatibility, and allowed for the modified release of encapsulated drugs, namely camptothecin, for 48 h. According to the obtained results, the oral administration of camptothecin through HGs provided low concentrations of the drug at the absorption site, avoiding carrier saturation and reducing intestinal toxicity [218].

5.2. Hydrogels for Dermal Applications

Due to their fairly compact consistency, HGs can also be applied to wounds or other skin issues. Commercially available HG-based dressings used for exudative wounds, pressure sores or burns, exploit the adhesive properties and ability of HGs to absorb liquids. The addition of antibacterial substances may further improve the applications of HG dressings.

Researchers from Southwest University in China developed a sericin (SS) and polyvinyl alcohol (PVA)-based HG (Table 3) [219]. This gel showed good biocompatibility, humidity and self-healing properties, i.e., ideal for dressings. Gentamycin sulphate, a known antibiotic substance and aminoglycoside, was added to this HG. To determine the properties of the obtained antibacterial HG, a number of in vitro tests were carried out, which measured wettability, swelling, microbiological activity, drug substance release, cytotoxicity, and immunotoxicity. The studies showed that the antibacterial HG ensured a prolonged release. For a deeper analysis of the HG properties, a model infected tissue was prepared. Tests confirmed that the HG was cytocompatible with mammalian cells and did not affect the growth of healthy cells.

The material used in wound dressing should fulfil many requirements [220], including isolation from harmful external factors, such as secondary wound infection, but should also provide sufficient water vapour permeability and oxygen availability. HGs based on tragacanth gum (TG), sodium alginate (SA) and PVA meet these properties and have potential applications [220]. In addition to good permeability for water vapour and oxygen, these HGs also provide barriers against secondary wound infection. These properties were confirmed by in vitro studies. Additionally, the HGs had haemolytic and mucoadhesive properties. Dressings based on these HGs were able to release antimicrobial active substances (moxifloxacin, an antibiotic from the fluoroquinolone group used to treat a wide spectrum of microorganisms). The results showed prolonged release of up to 24 h without an initial burst release.

Patients struggling with atopic skin changes very often use strong steroid drugs to alleviate emerging inflammation. Unfortunately, topical steroid therapy also leads to skin dryness and irritation, which patients with atopic dermatitis should avoid. Therefore, adequate skin hydration in atopic dermatitis therapy is maintained through the systematic and frequent use of appropriate emollients. Wang et al. combined the administration of an anti-inflammatory substance and maintenance of proper skin hydration (Figure 9) [221].

A HG prepared from a mixture of poloxamer 407 (P407) and sodium carboxymethyl cellulose (CMC) was used to achieve this goal (Table 3) [221]. A special nonwoven fabric was covered with the HG mixture. The addition of CMCs resulted in an increase in hydrophilicity of the resulting gel structure and also significantly reduced the sol-gel transition temperature, which advantageously promoted the fabrication of the coated nonwoven fabric. The HG exhibited moisture retaining properties, and the nonwoven fabric material prevented excessive water transpiration. The anti-inflammatory effect was provided by the addition of a Cortex Moutan extract, a well-known plant popular in Chinese medicine, during HG preparation. To determine the drug release profile, in vitro and ex vivo studies were performed. The in vitro studies showed that the release of the anti-inflammatory substance occurred in a prolonged manner up to several dozen hours, ensuring prolonged and elevated levels of the anti-inflammatory substance. Ex vivo tests on pork ear confirmed the results of the in vitro tests. The nonwoven fabric coated with a mixture of HGs composed of P407 and CMCs and Cortex Moutan extract showed potential for treating and caring for atopic lesions in patients with active skin inflammation.

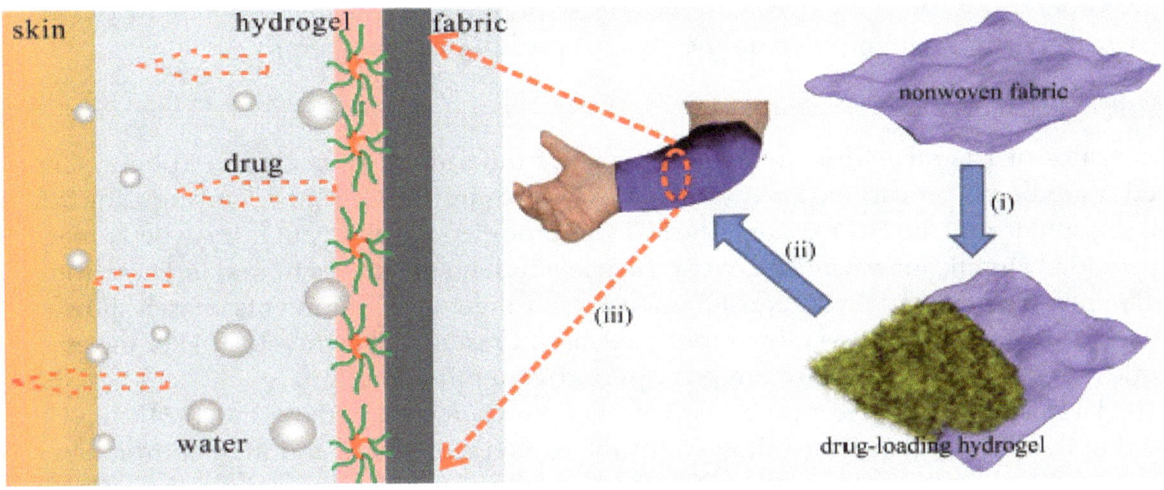

Figure 9. Diagram of a dual-functional fabric; (i) representation showing how the fabric is covered with HG, (ii) representation showing how the HG-coated fabric is applied to the patient's skin, and (iii) representation showing how the drug diffuses across the skin. Reprinted with permission from Ref. [221].

5.3. *Hydrogels for Ocular Applications*

The administration of a slightly soluble substance in the eye can be quite challenging [12,222]. Chitosan-based HGs showed promise as polymeric carriers for both hydrophilic and lyophilic drugs for ocular applications [234]. HGs based on carboxymethyl chitosan (CMCTS) and polyaldehyde dextran (PAD) were prepared [12]. The poor water solubility of the active substance (voriconazole), was addressed by encapsulating in cyclodextrin, which significantly increased the bioavailability of voriconazole and facilitated its application. The HG has the ability to gel in situ, allowing for easier intraocular injection. However, the prolonged release of voriconazole from the gel remained an issue.

Scientists from the Ocean University of China focused on the gelling process [222]. HGs based on hydroxyethylated chitosan (HECTS) with a special azide group showed the ability to polymerize under UV radiation. The polymerization lasted up to 30 s and was carried out in vivo. While the experiments, which were performed on New Zealand rabbits, should be confirmed on the human body, they already gave promising results and were thriving to recognize this HG as a good carrier for the intraocular administration of anti-glaucoma medications.

5.4. *Hydrogels for Vaginal Applications*

A HG made of P407 with nanosized layered double hydroxides allowed to include both hydrophilic and hydrophobic substances in the gel structure, which significantly widens the spectrum of administered drugs to patients [2]. Additionally, the HG has an important ability to gel transition at body temperature, so that during application it is a solution and in contact with the human body temperature it solidifies and stays on the tissues. As sample drugs, water-soluble theaflavin and Nile red dye were used to determine release profiles from the HG in rabbit vagina in independent and simultaneous states [2]. The antiviral properties of theaflavin were preserved and was able to limit the entry of HIV into the immune system. These tests were repeated against nifeviroc as a hydrophobic active and the effect was amplified. Thus, this HG acts as a potential carrier for the delivery of a broad spectrum of antiviral drugs to the human body.

HGs have also been applied in the vaginal administration of antiviral drug in the treatment of HIV [174]. HGs based on CTS with glycerol phosphate gelled upon contact with the human body, at a temperature of approximately 37 °C. Additionally, by enclosing active substances (e.g., tenofovir) in microspheres and immobilizing them in the HG structure (PP gels, Figure 7), a much longer release profile was obtained when compared with the release profile from the microspheres or HG alone. This provides an opportunity to improve on the effectiveness of immunotherapy.

5.5. Hydrogels for Topical Oral Applications

In the use of HG structures in the treatment of inflammatory periodontal bent, Chang et al. prepared a gel based on carboxymethyl-hexanoyl chitosan (CHC) [223]. Through the addition of glycerol phosphate into the HG network, the HG was modified to solidify at human body temperatures, which provided significant advantages over the use of other substances in oral inflammation therapy. Anti-inflammatory properties were carried out using naringenin. Experiments on rats showed that the anti-inflammatory substance was more rapidly released from the HG when the pH of the environment was acidic (~5.5), thereby rapidly treating the periodontal inflammation.

CTS HG can also be used to treat oral inflammation when used with thymol [224]. In vitro studies showed that the resulting structure allowed for the prolonged release and high antimicrobial activity of thymol against microorganisms up to 72 h. Furthermore, in the first two days, the active substance was increasingly released. This dual action HG demonstrated anti-inflammatory properties and the treatment of bacterial biofilms in the oral cavity.

5.6. Injection of Hydrogels

Therapeutic injections are usually least favoured by the patient and requires specialized HGs. The key challenge is to prepare a structure that will be fluid enough to squeeze through the needle but also sufficiently rigid that when applied does not spread and remains at the injection site [17,135,136]. Therefore, an important property of these structures is shear thinning, i.e., the ability to decrease viscosity of fluid under shear strain.

CTS-based in situ HGs are frequently adopted in the treatment for age-related macular degeneration (AMD), glaucoma and mucosal allergic diseases [234]. The HGs offer a convenient matrix for in situ gelling systems containing other nanoparticles, such as micelles. Injectable CTS-based in situ gels have been applied as in situ forming implants and as drug carriers in nasal and ocular delivery due to good biocompatibility, simple manufacture and sustained-release properties. These systems have been utilized to deliver several chemotherapeutic agents, including camptothecin [218,235], paclitaxel (PTX) [225,226], DOX [226], curcumin [217,227,228], and docetaxel (DTX) [229,236].

An injectable drug delivery system based on a visible light-cured glycol chitosan (GCS) HG containing PTX-complexed beta-cyclodextrin (β-CD) (GCS/CD/PTX) was tested for ovarian cancer therapy using a tumour-bearing mouse model [225]. The swollen GCS HG affected the release of PTX and CD/PTX. These systems exhibited a controlled release of PTX for 7 days. Additionally, GC/CD/PTX resulted in a superior antitumor effect against ovarian cancer.

An interesting application of HGs as dual carriers for PTX and DOX was proposed by Rezazadeh et al. [226]. An injectable thermosensitive HG for simultaneous intra-tumoral administration of PTX and DOX was prepared using mixed micelles composed of Pluronic F127 and α-tocopheryl polyethylene glycol 1000 succinate (TPGS) and a thermosensitive Pluronic F127/hyaluronic acid (PF127/HA) HG containing fixed amount of DOX [226]. PP gel formation temperature, rheological properties, injectability, degradation rates of the HG, and the release rate of DOX and PTX from the HG were examined. The HG containing PTX-loaded micelles and DOX converted to a semisolid with increasing temperature to 35 °C. DOX and PTX were released from the HG at different rates within 12 h and 3 days, respectively. This novel thermosensitive HG could be used for the co-delivery of PTX and DOX in solid tumours.

A series of injectable in situ-forming chitosan-based HGs were prepared by the chemical cross-linking of CTS and genipin in the presence of different inorganic salts [227]. In situ HG formation, with curcumin as an active substance, was detected after subcutaneous injections in rats. In vitro curcumin release profiles exhibited sustained release properties with an initial burst release with approximately three to six times higher cumulative release than other gel controls.

CTS-based HGs may also show magnetic properties, when magnetic Fe_3O_4 and $MnFe_2O_4$ nanoparticles are incorporated into their networks [228]. The Fe_3O_4 and $MnFe_2O_4$ on CMCTS HGs indicated a pH-sensitive behaviour; their release performances were investigated by curcumin as a model drug. The effects of applied magnetic fields on drug release for composites containing Fe_3O_4 were higher compared with $MnFe_2O_4$. The results showed that HGs containing Fe_3O_4 and $MnFe_2O_4$ can be applied for novel drug delivery systems.

DTX is an anticancer drug used for treatment of various solid tumours [229]. But it's low water solubility and a lack of specification has limited its clinical use. Therefore, new solutions have been explored to use this drug in targeted therapy. A thermosensitive chitosan/β-glycerophosphate (CTS/GP) DTX-loaded HG for intratumoral delivery was studied. The results of an in vitro release study demonstrated that DTX-C/GP was released over a period of 3 weeks. The tumour volume was minimized by the intratumoral injection of DTX-CTS/GP (at 20 mg/kg in H22 tumour-bearing mice). Further, the in vivo pharmacokinetic characteristics of DTX-CTS/GP correlated well with the in vitro release. DTX-CTS/GP significantly prolonged DTX retention, supported a high DTX concentration in tumours, and toxicity was effectively reduced.

Carbon nanostructures were also successfully applied in hydrophilic, porous materials as a component of HGs for DTX carriers [236]. A functionalized graphene oxide (GO)-based thermosensitive HG loaded with DTX for intratumoral delivery was designed. First, GO was functionalized by using chitosan to achieve high stability in physiological solutions. Next, HGs containing few components were formed: GO-chitosan, Poloxamer 407 and Poloxamer 188 and DTX. GO/chitosan HG was stable in physiological solution; DTX released much more slowly from this gel compared with free DTX with a pH-responsive feature. The DTX–GO/chitosan gel released higher concentrations and longer resident times in the tumour tissues of mice in vivo giving nontoxic effects to normal organs. Additionally, the combination of near-infrared laser irradiation at 808 nm significantly enhanced tumour inhibition in vitro and in vivo.

Other composite-based HGs were also evaluated. Gharaie et al. used gelatin and laponite in various proportions to obtain appropriate shear thinning properties (Figure 10) [230]. Additionally, by loading with CTS or poly(*N*-isopropylacrylamide)-co-acrylic acid (PNIPAM-co-AA) to the gel structure, pH-responsive abilities were gained, resulting in a different release profiles. As a model substance, rhodamine B was used to test the release. The results of these experiments showed that the gel could be easily and accessibly applied, whereas the release of the active substance was dependent on the pH level (in acidic and neutral environments, the release was negligible, whereas release increased at basic pH.

The key point of interest of many scientists is the fight against cancer. Also in this case HG can also be used to treat cancer [36]. Hu et al. combined salecan, a beta-glucan polysaccharide, with Fe_3O_4 nanoparticles and agarose [231]. The resulting HG gained magnetic properties and was used as a carrier for DOX (an anthracycline cytostatic used in anti-cancer therapy). The salecan-based HG with iron oxide nanoparticles had a pH-dependent drug release profile. In an acidic environment, unlike alkaline environments, a larger amount of DOX was released. Due to the acidic pH of cancer cells, this result indicated significant promise. Additionally, due to the presence of Fe_3O_4 nanoparticles, the amount of active drug released was also manipulated. With an external electromagnetic field, inorganic particles can be vibrated, thereby loosening the gel structure enabling easier release of DOX.

The technical aspects of DOX release from HGs were examined by a group from Drexel University [232]. In this study, an agarose-based HG was used wherein DOX-dextran sulphate complexes were provided. The structure was doped with divalent metallic ions, Ca^{2+} from $CaCl_2$ and Mg^{2+} from $MgCl_2$, at different concentrations. The divalent ions interfered with the binding between DOX and dextran sulphate, promoting prolonged release of the active substance from the HG and thereby providing a sustained chemotherapeutic effect for destroying cancer cells. Alginate (sodium alginate, SA)-based HGs with immobilized bevacizumab were also examined [233]. Anti-angiogenic active ingredients were released at prolonged and elevated levels to cancerous and neighbouring cells. As a result, tumour growth was inhibited.

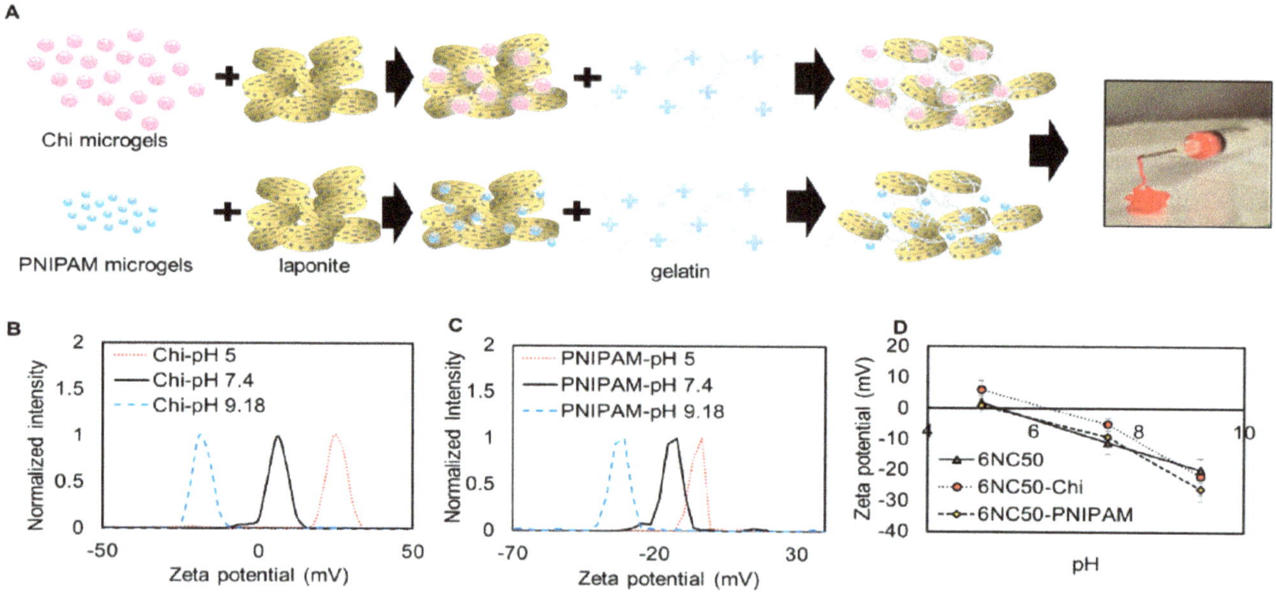

Figure 10. Electrostatic interactions between gelatin and laponite resulted in formation of pH responsive nanocomposite. (**A**) Schematic preparation of shear-thinning HG with laponite. Zeta potential at different pH of (**B**) CTS particles, (**C**) PNIPAM-*co*-Acrylic acid particles and (**D**) PNIPAM-*co*-Acrylic acid and laponite particles. Reprinted with permission from Ref. [230].

6. Future Outlook

Recent developments of HGs as drug delivery carriers for biological and biomedical applications were reviewed. Major synthetic strategies for the preparation of HGs, their classification, the physicochemical properties and their applications were described in detail. The wide variety of recently reported work has demonstrated the application of HG materials as drug delivery systems with different dimensions (macro, micro and nano) in various administration routes.

There are advantages in using HGs as vehicles for active substances. First, HGs can be modified for prolonged or rapid release. This feature is very important in planning therapies for patients and improves compliance with drug regimens. Additionally, by using modified HG materials, drug release can be tailored on demand. Therefore, greater control over health and treatment process can be achieved. Another advantage of functional modifications of HGs is the ability to adjust the controlled release of drugs. By adding specific enzymes or ionisable groups, the entire HG network structure acquires the ability to react to pH changes or to the presence of specific ions.

Technological challenges and problems in the production of HGs are primarily observed in maintaining a balance between chemical structure, composition, drug release and biocompatibility. HGs appear to be very promising materials and forward-looking and have yet to be fully realized. Due to a relatively simple manufacturing process, HGs can be readily modified and functionalized for use in targeted therapy. By using HG structures in medicine, it is easier to achieve better compliance, which is desirable in therapy.

However, the studies reviewed herein are mostly proof-of-concept. There remains limited information on HG in vivo experiments and HG biocompatibility. Most of these studies have focused on in vitro studies to show the non-cytotoxicity of the materials studied. Research on the biocompatibility and biodegradability of these materials, combined with in vivo research, remains a niche topic and has many unresolved questions. The future design and development of effective HG-based drug carriers requires a high degree of control over their properties in vitro and in vivo. These properties include controlled stability for prolonged circulation and biodegradability for facile removal after drug release. One future goal should be the improved design of HG with specific targeting residues to enable highly selective uptake in particular cells or organs. In this way, careful control over size, biodegradability, stability, functionality, and bioconjugation will guide the development of next generation HGs.

Author Contributions: Conceptualization, M.E.P.-B.; writing—original draft preparation, M.E.P.-B.; M.T.; A.C.; writing—review and editing, M.E.P.-B., M.T.; visualization, supervision and project administration, M.E.P.-B.; funding acquisition, M.E.P.-B. All authors have read and agreed to the published version of the manuscript.

References

1. Korde, J.M.; Kandasubramanian, B. Naturally biomimicked smart shape memory hydrogels for biomedical functions. *Chem. Eng. J.* **2020**, *379*, 122430. [CrossRef]
2. Tian, W.; Han, S.; Huang, X.; Han, M.; Cao, J.; Liang, Y.; Sun, Y. LDH hybrid thermosensitive hydrogel for intravaginal delivery of anti-HIV drugs. *Artif. Cells Nanomed. Biotechnol.* **2019**, *47*, 1234–1240. [CrossRef] [PubMed]
3. Tibbitt, M.W.; Dahlman, J.E.; Langer, R. Emerging frontiers in drug delivery. *J. Am. Chem. Soc.* **2016**, *138*, 704–717. [CrossRef] [PubMed]
4. Fujiyabu, T.; Yoshikawa, Y.; Chung, U.; Sakai, T. Structure-property relationship of a model network containing solvent. *Sci. Technol. Adv. Mater.* **2019**, *20*, 608–621. [CrossRef] [PubMed]
5. Kirschner, C.M.; Anseth, K.S. Hydrogels in healthcare: From static to dynamic material microenvironments. *Acta Mater.* **2013**, *61*, 931–944. [CrossRef] [PubMed]
6. Chatterjee, S.; Chi-leung Hui, P. Stimuli-responsive hydrogels: An interdisciplinary overview. In *Hydrogels—Smart Materials for Biomedical Applications*; Popa, L., Violeta Ghica, M., Dinu-Pîrvu, C.-E., Eds.; IntechOpen: London, UK, 2019; ISBN 978-1-78985-875-4.
7. Shafiee, S.; Ahangar, H.A.; Saffar, A. Taguchi method optimization for synthesis of Fe_3O_4 @chitosan/Tragacanth Gum nanocomposite as a drug delivery system. *Carbohydr. Polym.* **2019**, *222*, 114982. [CrossRef] [PubMed]
8. Ullah, K.; Sohail, M.; Buabeid, M.A.; Murtaza, G.; Ullah, A.; Rashid, H.; Khan, M.A.; Khan, S.A. Pectin-based (LA-co-MAA) semi-IPNS as a potential biomaterial for colonic delivery of oxaliplatin. *Int. J. Pharm.* **2019**, *569*, 118557. [CrossRef]
9. Nazlı, A.B.; Açıkel, Y.S. Loading of cancer drug resveratrol to pH-Sensitive, smart, alginate-chitosan hydrogels and investigation of controlled release kinetics. *J. Drug Deliv. Sci. Technol.* **2019**, *53*, 101199. [CrossRef]
10. Kim, C.; Jeong, D.; Kim, S.; Kim, Y.; Jung, S. Cyclodextrin functionalized agarose gel with low gelling temperature for controlled drug delivery systems. *Carbohydr. Polym.* **2019**, *222*, 115011. [CrossRef]
11. Cocarta, A.-I.; Hobzova, R.; Sirc, J.; Cerna, T.; Hrabeta, J.; Svojgr, K.; Pochop, P.; Kodetova, M.; Jedelska, J.; Bakowsky, U.; et al. Hydrogel implants for transscleral drug delivery for retinoblastoma treatment. *Mater. Sci. Eng. C* **2019**, *103*, 109799. [CrossRef]
12. Yang, C.; Gao, L.; Liu, X.; Yang, T.; Yin, G.; Chen, J.; Guo, H.; Yu, B.; Cong, H. Injectable Schiff base polysaccharide hydrogels for intraocular drug loading and release. *J. Biomed. Mater. Res.* **2019**, *107*. [CrossRef] [PubMed]
13. Alvarez-Rivera, F.; Serro, A.P.; Silva, D.; Concheiro, A.; Alvarez-Lorenzo, C. Hydrogels for diabetic eyes: Naltrexone loading, release profiles and cornea penetration. *Mater. Sci. Eng. C* **2019**, *105*, 110092. [CrossRef] [PubMed]
14. Dragan, E.S.; Dinu, M.V. Polysaccharides constructed hydrogels as vehicles for proteins and peptides. A review. *Carbohydr. Polym.* **2019**, *225*, 115210. [CrossRef] [PubMed]
15. Duwa, R.; Emami, F.; Lee, S.; Jeong, J.-H.; Yook, S. Polymeric and lipid-based drug delivery systems for treatment of glioblastoma multiforme. *J. Ind. Eng. Chem.* **2019**, *79*, 261–273. [CrossRef]
16. Riley, L.; Schirmer, L.; Segura, T. Granular hydrogels: Emergent properties of jammed hydrogel microparticles and their applications in tissue repair and regeneration. *Curr. Opin. Biotechnol.* **2019**, *60*, 1–8. [CrossRef]
17. Li, J.; Mooney, D.J. Designing hydrogels for controlled drug delivery. *Nat. Rev. Mater.* **2016**, *1*, 10671. [CrossRef]
18. Bakaic, E.; Smeets, N.M.B.; Hoare, T. Injectable hydrogels based on poly (ethylene glycol) and derivatives as functional biomaterials. *RSC Adv.* **2015**, *5*, 35469–35486. [CrossRef]

19. Norouzi, M.; Nazari, B.; Miller, D.W. Injectable hydrogel-based drug delivery systems for local cancer therapy. *Drug Dis. Today* **2016**, *21*, 1835–1849. [CrossRef]
20. Nguyen, Q.V.; Huynh, D.P.; Park, J.H.; Lee, D.S. Injectable polymeric hydrogels for the delivery of therapeutic agents: A review. *Eur. Polym. J.* **2015**, *72*, 602–619. [CrossRef]
21. Soni, K.S.; Desale, S.S.; Bronich, T.K. Nanogels: An overview of properties, biomedical applications and obstacles to clinical translation. *J. Control. Release* **2016**, *240*, 109–126. [CrossRef]
22. Nita, L.E.; Chiriac, A.P.; Rusu, A.G.; Bercea, M.; Ghilan, A.; Dumitriu, R.P.; Mititelu-Tartau, L. New self-healing hydrogels based on reversible physical interactions and their potential applications. *Eur. Polym. J.* **2019**, *118*, 176–185. [CrossRef]
23. Wang, J.; Liu, L.; Chen, J.; Deng, M.; Feng, X.; Chen, L. Supramolecular nanoplatforms via cyclodextrin host-guest recognition for synergistic gene-photodynamic therapy. *Eur. Polym. J.* **2019**, *118*, 222–230. [CrossRef]
24. Marafon, P.; Fachel, F.N.S.; Dal Prá, M.; Bassani, V.L.; Koester, L.S.; Henriques, A.T.; Braganhol, E.; Teixeira, H.F. Development, physico-chemical characterization and in-vitro studies of hydrogels containing rosmarinic acid-loaded nanoemulsion for topical application. *J. Pharm. Pharmacol.* **2019**, *71*, 1199–1208. [CrossRef] [PubMed]
25. Miranda, M.; Cruz, M.T.; Vitorino, C.; Cabral, C. Nanostructuring lipid carriers using *Ridolfia segetum* (L.) Moris essential oil. *Mater. Sci. Eng. C* **2019**, *103*, 109804. [CrossRef] [PubMed]
26. Sharaf, S.; El-Naggar, M.E. Wound dressing properties of cationized cotton fabric treated with carrageenan/cyclodextrin hydrogel loaded with honey bee propolis extract. *Int. J. Biol. Macromol.* **2019**, *133*, 583–591. [CrossRef]
27. Liu, Z.; Zheng, Y.; Dang, J.; Zhang, J.; Dong, F.; Wang, K.; Zhang, J. A novel antifungal plasma-activated hydrogel. *ACS Appl. Mater. Interfaces* **2019**, *11*, 22941–22949. [CrossRef]
28. Wang, K.; Wang, J.; Li, L.; Xu, L.; Feng, N.; Wang, Y.; Fei, X.; Tian, J.; Li, Y. Synthesis of a novel anti-freezing, non-drying antibacterial hydrogel dressing by one-pot method. *Chem. Eng. J.* **2019**, *372*, 216–225. [CrossRef]
29. Chen, W.; Zhu, Y.; Zhang, Z.; Gao, Y.; Liu, W.; Borjihan, Q.; Qu, H.; Zhang, Y.; Zhang, Y.; Wang, Y.-J.; et al. Engineering a multifunctional N-halamine-based antibacterial hydrogel using a super-convenient strategy for infected skin defect therapy. *Chem. Eng. J.* **2020**, *379*, 122238. [CrossRef]
30. Xue, H.; Hu, L.; Xiong, Y.; Zhu, X.; Wei, C.; Cao, F.; Zhou, W.; Sun, Y.; Endo, Y.; Liu, M.; et al. Quaternized chitosan-Matrigel-polyacrylamide hydrogels as wound dressing for wound repair and regeneration. *Carbohydr. Polym.* **2019**, *226*, 115302. [CrossRef]
31. Huang, L.; Zhu, Z.; Wu, D.; Gan, W.; Zhu, S.; Li, W.; Tian, J.; Li, L.; Zhou, C.; Lu, L. Antibacterial poly (ethylene glycol) diacrylate/chitosan hydrogels enhance mechanical adhesiveness and promote skin regeneration. *Carbohydr. Polym.* **2019**, *225*, 115110. [CrossRef]
32. Liang, Y.; Zhao, X.; Hu, T.; Han, Y.; Guo, B. Mussel-inspired, antibacterial, conductive, antioxidant, injectable composite hydrogel wound dressing to promote the regeneration of infected skin. *J. Coll. Interface Sci.* **2019**, *556*, 514–528. [CrossRef] [PubMed]
33. Solomevich, S.O.; Bychkovsky, P.M.; Yurkshtovich, T.L.; Golub, N.V.; Mirchuk, P.Y.; Revtovich, M.Y.; Shmak, A.I. Biodegradable pH-sensitive prospidine-loaded dextran phosphate based hydrogels for local tumor therapy. *Carbohydr. Polym.* **2019**, *226*, 115308. [CrossRef] [PubMed]
34. Chen, H.; Wei, X.; Chen, H.; Wei, H.; Wang, Y.; Nan, W.; Zhang, Q.; Wen, X. The study of establishment of an in vivo tumor model by three-dimensional cells culture systems methods and evaluation of antitumor effect of biotin-conjugated pullulan acetate nanoparticles. *Artif. Cells Nanomed. Biotechnol.* **2019**, *47*, 123–131. [CrossRef] [PubMed]
35. Cao, D.; Zhang, X.; Akabar, M.D.; Luo, Y.; Wu, H.; Ke, X.; Ci, T. Liposomal doxorubicin loaded PLGA-PEG-PLGA based thermogel for sustained local drug delivery for the treatment of breast cancer. *Artif. Cells Nanomed. Biotechnol.* **2019**, *47*, 181–191. [CrossRef]
36. Wu, Q.; He, Z.; Wang, X.; Zhang, Q.; Wei, Q.; Ma, S.; Ma, C.; Li, J.; Wang, Q. Cascade enzymes within self-assembled hybrid nanogel mimicked neutrophil lysosomes for singlet oxygen elevated cancer therapy. *Nat. Commun.* **2019**, *10*, 240. [CrossRef]
37. Puertas-Bartolomé, M.; Benito-Garzón, L.; Fung, S.; Kohn, J.; Vázquez-Lasa, B.; San Román, J. Bioadhesive functional hydrogels: Controlled release of catechol species with antioxidant and antiinflammatory behavior. *Mater. Sci. Eng. C* **2019**, *105*, 110040. [CrossRef]

38. Zheng, J.; Fan, R.; Wu, H.; Yao, H.; Yan, Y.; Liu, J.; Ran, L.; Sun, Z.; Yi, L.; Dang, L.; et al. Directed self-assembly of herbal small molecules into sustained release hydrogels for treating neural inflammation. *Nat. Commun.* **2019**, *10*, 1604. [CrossRef]
39. Uehara, M.; Li, X.; Sheikhi, A.; Zandi, N.; Walker, B.; Saleh, B.; Banouni, N.; Jiang, L.; Ordikhani, F.; Dai, L.; et al. Anti-IL-6 eluting immunomodulatory biomaterials prolong skin allograft survival. *Sci. Rep.* **2019**, *9*, 6535. [CrossRef]
40. García, J.R.; Quirós, M.; Han, W.M.; O'Leary, M.N.; Cox, G.N.; Nusrat, A.; García, A.J. IFN-γ-tethered hydrogels enhance mesenchymal stem cell-based immunomodulation and promote tissue repair. *Biomaterials* **2019**, *220*, 119403. [CrossRef]
41. Hertegård, S.; Nagubothu, S.R.; Malmström, E.; Ström, C.E.; Tolf, A.; Davies, L.C.; Le Blanc, K. Hyaluronan hydrogels for the local delivery of mesenchymal stromal cells to the injured vocal fold. *Stem Cells Dev.* **2019**, *28*, 1177–1190. [CrossRef]
42. Grigoras, A.G. Drug delivery systems using pullulan, a biocompatible polysaccharide produced by fungal fermentation of starch. *Environ. Chem. Lett.* **2019**, *17*, 1209–1223. [CrossRef]
43. Ge, W.; Cao, S.; Shen, F.; Wang, Y.; Ren, J.; Wang, X. Rapid self-healing, stretchable, moldable, antioxidant and antibacterial tannic acid-cellulose nanofibril composite hydrogels. *Carbohydr. Polym.* **2019**, *224*, 115147. [CrossRef] [PubMed]
44. Clegg, J.R.; Wagner, A.M.; Shin, S.R.; Hassan, S.; Khademhosseini, A.; Peppas, N.A. Modular fabrication of intelligent material-tissue interfaces for bioinspired and biomimetic devices. *Prog. Mater. Sci.* **2019**, *106*, 100589. [CrossRef]
45. Bezerra, U.T.; Ferreira, H.S.; Barbosa, N.P. Hydrogels: Types, structure, properties, and applications. In *Frontiers in Biomaterials*; Razavi, M., Ed.; Bentham Science Publishers Ltd.: Sharjah, UAE, 2017; Volume 4, pp. 143–169. ISBN 978-1-68108-536-4.
46. Chatterjee, S.; Hui, P.; Kan, C. Thermoresponsive hydrogels and their biomedical applications: Special insight into their applications in textile based transdermal therapy. *Polymers* **2018**, *10*, 480. [CrossRef]
47. Akhtar, M.F.; Hanif, M.; Ranjha, N.M. Methods of synthesis of hydrogels ... A review. *Saudi Pharm. J.* **2016**, *24*, 554–559. [CrossRef]
48. Buwalda, S.J.; Boere, K.W.M.; Dijkstra, P.J.; Feijen, J.; Vermonden, T.; Hennink, W.E. Hydrogels in a historical perspective: From simple networks to smart materials. *J. Control. Release* **2014**, *190*, 254–273. [CrossRef]
49. Zhang, Y.S.; Khademhosseini, A. Advances in engineering hydrogels. *Science* **2017**, *356*, eaaf3627. [CrossRef]
50. Chai, Q.; Jiao, Y.; Yu, X. Hydrogels for biomedical applications: Their characteristics and the mechanisms behind them. *Gels* **2017**, *3*, 6. [CrossRef]
51. Ahmed, E.M. Hydrogel: Preparation, characterization, and applications: A review. *J. Adv. Res.* **2015**, *6*, 105–121. [CrossRef]
52. Straccia, M.; d'Ayala, G.; Romano, I.; Oliva, A.; Laurienzo, P. Alginate hydrogels coated with chitosan for wound dressing. *Mar. Drugs* **2015**, *13*, 2890–2908. [CrossRef]
53. Yuan, L.; Wu, Y.; Fang, J.; Wei, X.; Gu, Q.; El-Hamshary, H.; Al-Deyab, S.S.; Morsi, Y.; Mo, X. Modified alginate and gelatin cross-linked hydrogels for soft tissue adhesive. *Artif. Cells Nanomed. Biotechnol.* **2017**, *45*, 76–83. [CrossRef] [PubMed]
54. Kaczmarek-Pawelska, A. Alginate-based hydrogels in regenerative medicine. In *Alginates*; IntechOpen: London, UK, 2019.
55. Hu, Y.; Zheng, M.; Dong, X.; Zhao, D.; Cheng, H.; Xiao, X. Preparation and characterization of alginate-hyaluronic acid-chitosan based composite gel beads. *J. Wuhan Univ. Technol.-Mater. Sci. Ed.* **2015**, *30*, 1297–1303. [CrossRef]
56. Parlato, M.; Reichert, S.; Barney, N.; Murphy, W.L. Poly(ethylene glycol) hydrogels with adaptable mechanical and degradation properties for use in biomedical applications. *Macromol. Biosci.* **2014**, *14*, 687–698. [CrossRef] [PubMed]
57. Zustiak, S.P.; Leach, J.B. Hydrolytically degradable poly(ethylene glycol) hydrogel scaffolds with tunable degradation and mechanical properties. *Biomacromolecules* **2010**, *11*, 1348–1357. [CrossRef]
58. Basu, A.; Kunduru, K.R.; Doppalapudi, S.; Domb, A.J.; Khan, W. Poly(lactic acid) based hydrogels. *Adv. Drug Deliv. Rev.* **2016**, *107*, 192–205. [CrossRef]
59. Korzhikov-Vlakh, V.; Krylova, M.; Sinitsyna, E.; Ivankova, E.; Averianov, I.; Tennikova, T. Hydrogel layers on the surface of polyester-based materials for improvement of their biointeractions and controlled release of proteins. *Polymers* **2016**, *8*, 418. [CrossRef]

60. Palmese, L.L.; Thapa, R.K.; Sullivan, M.O.; Kiick, K.L. Hybrid hydrogels for biomedical applications. *Curr. Opin. Chem. Eng.* **2019**, *24*, 143–157. [CrossRef]
61. Stagnaro, P.; Schizzi, I.; Utzeri, R.; Marsano, E.; Castellano, M. Alginate-polymethacrylate hybrid hydrogels for potential osteochondral tissue regeneration. *Carbohydr. Polym.* **2018**, *185*, 56–62. [CrossRef]
62. Jia, X.; Kiick, K.L. Hybrid multicomponent hydrogels for tissue engineering. *Macromol. Biosci.* **2009**, *9*, 140–156. [CrossRef]
63. Vieira, V.M.P.; Hay, L.L.; Smith, D.K. Multi-component hybrid hydrogels—Understanding the extent of orthogonal assembly and its impact on controlled release. *Chem. Sci.* **2017**, *8*, 6981–6990. [CrossRef]
64. Hu, S.; Zhou, L.; Tu, L.; Dai, C.; Fan, L.; Zhang, K.; Yao, T.; Chen, J.; Wang, Z.; Xing, J.; et al. Elastomeric conductive hybrid hydrogels with continuous conductive networks. *J. Mater. Chem. B* **2019**, *7*, 2389–2397. [CrossRef]
65. Radvar, E.; Azevedo, H.S. Supramolecular peptide/polymer hybrid hydrogels for biomedical applications. *Macromol. Biosci.* **2019**, *19*, 1800221. [CrossRef] [PubMed]
66. Li, J.; Illeperuma, W.R.K.; Suo, Z.; Vlassak, J.J. Hybrid hydrogels with extremely high stiffness and toughness. *ACS Macro Lett.* **2014**, *3*, 520–523. [CrossRef]
67. Narayanaswamy, R.; Torchilin, V.P. Hydrogels and their applications in targeted drug delivery. *Molecules* **2019**, *24*, 603. [CrossRef] [PubMed]
68. Caccavo, D.; Cascone, S.; Lamberti, G.; Barba, A.A.; Larsson, A. Swellable hydrogel-based systems for controlled drug delivery. In *Smart Drug Delivery System*; Sezer, A.D., Ed.; InTech: London, UK, 2016; ISBN 978-953-51-2247-0.
69. Parhi, R. Cross-linked hydrogel for pharmaceutical applications: A review. *Adv. Pharm. Bull.* **2017**, *7*, 515–530. [CrossRef] [PubMed]
70. Tonda-Turo, C.; Gnavi, S.; Ruini, F.; Gambarotta, G.; Gioffredi, E.; Chiono, V.; Perroteau, I.; Ciardelli, G. Development and characterization of novel agar and gelatin injectable hydrogel as filler for peripheral nerve guidance channels: Novel agar and gelatin injectable hydrogel for peripheral nerve guidance channels. *J. Tissue Eng. Regen. Med.* **2017**, *11*, 197–208. [CrossRef]
71. Wakhet, S.; Singh, V.K.; Sahoo, S.; Sagiri, S.S.; Kulanthaivel, S.; Bhattacharya, M.K.; Kumar, N.; Banerjee, I.; Pal, K. Characterization of gelatin–agar based phase separated hydrogel, emulgel and bigel: A comparative study. *J. Mater. Sci. Mater. Med.* **2015**, *26*, 118. [CrossRef]
72. Sadeghi, M.; Heidari, B. Crosslinked graft copolymer of methacrylic acid and gelatin as a novel hydrogel with pH-responsiveness properties. *Materials* **2011**, *4*, 543–552. [CrossRef]
73. Lanzalaco, S.; Turon, P.; Weis, C.; Alemán, C.; Armelin, E. The mechanism of adhesion and graft polymerization of a PNIPAAm thermoresponsive hydrogel to polypropylene meshes. *Soft Matter* **2019**, *15*, 3432–3442. [CrossRef]
74. Singh, R.; Mahto, V. Synthesis, characterization and evaluation of polyacrylamide graft starch/clay nanocomposite hydrogel system for enhanced oil recovery. *Pet. Sci.* **2017**, *14*, 765–779. [CrossRef]
75. Varaprasad, K.; Raghavendra, G.M.; Jayaramudu, T.; Yallapu, M.M.; Sadiku, R. A mini review on hydrogels classification and recent developments in miscellaneous applications. *Mater. Sci. Eng. C* **2017**, *79*, 958–971. [CrossRef] [PubMed]
76. Mohammadi, S.; Vafaie Sefti, M.; Baghban Salehi, M.; Mousavi Moghadam, A.; Rajaee, S.; Naderi, H. Hydrogel swelling properties: Comparison between conventional and nanocomposite hydrogels for water shutoff treatment: Comparing Conventional hydrogels with Nanocomposite. *Asia Pac. J. Chem. Eng.* **2015**, *10*, 743–753. [CrossRef]
77. Monir, T.S.B.; Afroz, S.; Khan, R.A.; Miah, M.Y.; Takafuji, M.; Alam, M.A. pH-sensitive hydrogel from polyethylene oxide and acrylic acid by gamma radiation. *J. Compos. Sci.* **2019**, *3*, 58. [CrossRef]
78. Hennink, W.E.; van Nostrum, C.F. Novel crosslinking methods to design hydrogels. *Adv. Drug Deliv. Rev.* **2012**, *64*, 223–236. [CrossRef]
79. Bauri, K.; Nandi, M.; De, P. Amino acid-derived stimuli-responsive polymers and their applications. *Polym. Chem.* **2018**, *9*, 1257–1287. [CrossRef]
80. Kahn, J.S.; Hu, Y.; Willner, I. Stimuli-responsive dna-based hydrogels: From basic principles to applications. *Acc. Chem. Res.* **2017**, *50*, 680–690. [CrossRef] [PubMed]
81. Alexander, A.; Ajazuddin; Khan, J.; Saraf, S.; Saraf, S. Poly(ethylene glycol)–poly(lactic-co-glycolic acid) based thermosensitive injectable hydrogels for biomedical applications. *J. Control. Release* **2013**, *172*, 715–729. [CrossRef]

82. Larrañeta, E.; Stewart, S.; Ervine, M.; Al-Kasasbeh, R.; Donnelly, R. Hydrogels for hydrophobic drug delivery. Classification, synthesis and applications. *J. Funct. Biomater.* **2018**, *9*, 13. [CrossRef]
83. Zhao, F.; Yao, D.; Guo, R.; Deng, L.; Dong, A.; Zhang, J. Composites of polymer hydrogels and nanoparticulate systems for biomedical and pharmaceutical applications. *Nanomaterials* **2015**, *5*, 2054–2130. [CrossRef]
84. Laftah, W.A.; Hashim, S.; Ibrahim, A.N. Polymer hydrogels: A review. *Polym. Plast. Technol. Eng.* **2011**, *50*, 1475–1486. [CrossRef]
85. Purushotham, S.; Ramanujan, R.V. Thermoresponsive magnetic composite nanomaterials for multimodal cancer therapy. *Acta Biomater.* **2010**, *6*, 502–510. [CrossRef] [PubMed]
86. Qiu, Y.; Park, K. Environment-sensitive hydrogels for drug delivery. *Adv. Drug Deliv. Rev.* **2012**, *64*, 49–60. [CrossRef]
87. Gong, C.; Qi, T.; Wei, X.; Qu, Y.; Wu, Q.; Luo, F.; Qian, Z. Thermosensitive polymeric hydrogels as drug delivery systems. *Curr. Med. Chem.* **2012**, *20*, 79–94. [CrossRef]
88. Ferreira, N.N.; Ferreira, L.M.B.; Cardoso, V.M.O.; Boni, F.I.; Souza, A.L.R.; Gremião, M.P.D. Recent advances in smart hydrogels for biomedical applications: From self-assembly to functional approaches. *Eur. Polym. J.* **2018**, *99*, 117–133. [CrossRef]
89. Cochis, A.; Bonetti, L.; Sorrentino, R.; Contessi Negrini, N.; Grassi, F.; Leigheb, M.; Rimondini, L.; Farè, S. 3D printing of thermo-responsive methylcellulose hydrogels for cell-sheet engineering. *Materials* **2018**, *11*, 579. [CrossRef]
90. Contessi Negrini, N.; Bonetti, L.; Contili, L.; Farè, S. 3D printing of methylcellulose-based hydrogels. *Bioprinting* **2018**, *10*, e00024. [CrossRef]
91. Larrañeta, E.; Barturen, L.; Ervine, M.; Donnelly, R.F. Hydrogels based on poly(methyl vinyl ether-co-maleic acid) and Tween 85 for sustained delivery of hydrophobic drugs. *Int. J. Pharm.* **2018**, *538*, 147–158. [CrossRef]
92. Hwang, T.; Frank, Z.; Neubauer, J.; Kim, K.J. High-performance polyvinyl chloride gel artificial muscle actuator with graphene oxide and plasticizer. *Sci. Rep.* **2019**, *9*, 1–9. [CrossRef]
93. Bae, J.W.; Shin, E.-J.; Jeong, J.; Choi, D.-S.; Lee, J.E.; Nam, B.U.; Lin, L.; Kim, S.-Y. High-performance PVC gel for adaptive micro-lenses with variable focal length. *Sci. Rep.* **2017**, *7*, 2068. [CrossRef]
94. Kim, M.H.; Kim, B.S.; Park, H.; Lee, J.; Park, W.H. Injectable methylcellulose hydrogel containing calcium phosphate nanoparticles for bone regeneration. *Int. J. Biol. Macromol.* **2018**, *109*, 57–64. [CrossRef]
95. Contessi, N.; Altomare, L.; Filipponi, A.; Farè, S. Thermo-responsive properties of methylcellulose hydrogels for cell sheet engineering. *Mater. Lett.* **2017**, *207*, 157–160. [CrossRef]
96. Safronov, A.P.; Terziyan, T.V. Formation of chemical networks of acrylamide and acrylic acid hydrogels initiated by ammonium persulfate. *Polym. Sci. Ser. B* **2015**, *57*, 481–487. [CrossRef]
97. Jalani, G.; Naccache, R.; Rosenzweig, D.H.; Haglund, L.; Vetrone, F.; Cerruti, M. Photocleavable hydrogel-coated upconverting nanoparticles: A multifunctional theranostic platform for nir imaging and on-demand macromolecular delivery. *J. Am. Chem. Soc.* **2016**, *138*, 1078–1083. [CrossRef]
98. Li, L.; Scheiger, J.M.; Levkin, P.A. Design and applications of photoresponsive hydrogels. *Adv. Mater.* **2019**, *31*, 1807333. [CrossRef]
99. Makhlouf, A.S.H.; Abu-Thabit, N.Y. (Eds.) *Stimuli Responsive Polymeric Nanocarriers for Drug Delivery Applications*; Elsevierz: Amsterdam, The Netherlands, 2018; Volume 1, ISBN 978-0-08-101997-9.
100. Tomatsu, I.; Peng, K.; Kros, A. Photoresponsive hydrogels for biomedical applications. *Adv. Drug Deliv. Rev.* **2011**, *63*, 1257–1266. [CrossRef]
101. Truong, V.X.; Li, F.; Ercole, F.; Forsythe, J.S. Wavelength-selective coupling and decoupling of polymer chains via reversible [2 + 2] photocycloaddition of styrylpyrene for construction of cytocompatible photodynamic hydrogels. *ACS Macro Lett.* **2018**, *7*, 464–469. [CrossRef]
102. Rosales, A.M.; Vega, S.L.; DelRio, F.W.; Burdick, J.A.; Anseth, K.S. Hydrogels with reversible mechanics to probe dynamic cell microenvironments. *Angew. Chem. Int. Ed.* **2017**, *56*, 12132–12136. [CrossRef]
103. Yan, B.; Boyer, J.-C.; Habault, D.; Branda, N.R.; Zhao, Y. near infrared light triggered release of biomacromolecules from hydrogels loaded with upconversion nanoparticles. *J. Am. Chem. Soc.* **2012**, *134*, 16558–16561. [CrossRef]
104. Ariffin, A.; Musa, M.S.; Othman, M.B.H.; Razali, M.A.A.; Yunus, F. Effects of various fillers on anionic polyacrylamide systems for treating kaolin suspensions. *Coll. Surf. A Physicochem. Eng. Asp.* **2014**, *441*, 306–311. [CrossRef]
105. Ullah, F.; Othman, M.B.H.; Javed, F.; Ahmad, Z.; Akil, H.M. Classification, processing and application of hydrogels: A review. *Mater. Sci. Eng. C* **2015**, *57*, 414–433. [CrossRef]

106. Steichen, S.D.; Caldorera-Moore, M.; Peppas, N.A. A review of current nanoparticle and targeting moieties for the delivery of cancer therapeutics. *Eur. J. Pharm. Sci.* **2013**, *48*, 416–427. [CrossRef] [PubMed]
107. Sharpe, L.A.; Daily, A.M.; Horava, S.D.; Peppas, N.A. Therapeutic applications of hydrogels in oral drug delivery. *Exp. Opin. Drug Deliv.* **2014**, *11*, 901–915. [CrossRef] [PubMed]
108. Liu, L.; Yao, W.; Rao, Y.; Lu, X.; Gao, J. pH-Responsive carriers for oral drug delivery: Challenges and opportunities of current platforms. *Drug Deliv.* **2017**, *24*, 569–581. [CrossRef] [PubMed]
109. Qu, J.; Zhao, X.; Ma, P.X.; Guo, B. Injectable antibacterial conductive hydrogels with dual response to an electric field and pH for localized "smart" drug release. *Acta Biomater.* **2018**, *72*, 55–69. [CrossRef] [PubMed]
110. Chen, Y.; Cheng, G.; Hu, R.; Chen, S.; Lu, W.; Gao, S.; Xia, H.; Wang, B.; Sun, C.; Nie, X.; et al. A nasal temperature and pH dual-responsive in situ gel delivery system based on microemulsion of huperzine A: Formulation, evaluation, and in vivo pharmacokinetic study. *AAPS PharmSciTech* **2019**, *20*, 301. [CrossRef] [PubMed]
111. Kiaee, G.; Mostafalu, P.; Samandari, M.; Sonkusale, S. A pH-mediated electronic wound dressing for controlled drug delivery. *Adv. Healthcare Mater.* **2018**, *7*, 1800396. [CrossRef]
112. Anirudhan, T.S.; Mohan, A.M. Novel pH switchable gelatin based hydrogel for the controlled delivery of the anti cancer drug 5-fluorouracil. *RSC Adv.* **2014**, *4*, 12109. [CrossRef]
113. Indermun, S.; Choonara, Y.E.; Kumar, P.; du Toit, L.C.; Modi, G.; Luttge, R.; Pillay, V. An interfacially plasticized electro-responsive hydrogel for transdermal electro-activated and modulated (TEAM) drug delivery. *Int. J. Pharm.* **2014**, *462*, 52–65. [CrossRef]
114. Reddy, N.N.; Mohan, Y.M.; Varaprasad, K.; Ravindra, S.; Joy, P.A.; Raju, K.M. Magnetic and electric responsive hydrogel-magnetic nanocomposites for drug-delivery application. *J. Appl. Polym. Sci.* **2011**, *122*, 1364–1375. [CrossRef]
115. Siangsanoh, C.; Ummartyotin, S.; Sathirakul, K.; Rojanapanthu, P.; Treesuppharat, W. Fabrication and characterization of triple-responsive composite hydrogel for targeted and controlled drug delivery system. *J. Mol. Liq.* **2018**, *256*, 90–99. [CrossRef]
116. Uva, M.; Pasqui, D.; Mencuccini, L.; Fedi, S.; Barbucci, R. Influence of alternating and static magnetic fields on drug release from hybrid hydrogels containing magnetic nanoparticles. *J. Biomater. Nanobiotechnol.* **2014**, *5*, 116–127. [CrossRef]
117. Crippa, F.; Moore, T.L.; Mortato, M.; Geers, C.; Haeni, L.; Hirt, A.M.; Rothen-Rutishauser, B.; Petri-Fink, A. Dynamic and biocompatible thermo-responsive magnetic hydrogels that respond to an alternating magnetic field. *J. Magn. Magn. Mater.* **2017**, *427*, 212–219. [CrossRef]
118. Jain, E.; Hill, L.; Canning, E.; Sell, S.A.; Zustiak, S.P. Control of gelation, degradation and physical properties of polyethylene glycol hydrogels through the chemical and physical identity of the crosslinker. *J. Mater. Chem. B* **2017**, *5*, 2679–2691. [CrossRef]
119. Deng, Y.; Yang, L. Preparation and characterization of polyethylene glycol (PEG) hydrogel as shape-stabilized phase change material. *Appl. Therm. Eng.* **2017**, *114*, 1014–1017. [CrossRef]
120. Fukasawa, M.; Sakai, T.; Chung, U.; Haraguchi, K. Synthesis and mechanical properties of a nanocomposite gel consisting of a tetra-PEG/clay network. *Macromolecules* **2010**, *43*, 4370–4378. [CrossRef]
121. Matsunaga, T.; Sakai, T.; Akagi, Y.; Chung, U.; Shibayama, M. SANS and SLS studies on tetra-arm PEG gels in as-prepared and swollen states. *Macromolecules* **2009**, *42*, 6245–6252. [CrossRef]
122. Matsunaga, T.; Sakai, T.; Akagi, Y.; Chung, U.; Shibayama, M. Structure characterization of tetra-PEG gel by small-angle neutron scattering. *Macromolecules* **2009**, *42*, 1344–1351. [CrossRef]
123. Fujii, K.; Asai, H.; Ueki, T.; Sakai, T.; Imaizumi, S.; Chung, U.; Watanabe, M.; Shibayama, M. High-performance ion gel with tetra-PEG network. *Soft Matter* **2012**, *8*, 1756–1759. [CrossRef]
124. Asai, H.; Fujii, K.; Ueki, T.; Sakai, T.; Chung, U.; Watanabe, M.; Han, Y.-S.; Kim, T.-H.; Shibayama, M. Structural analysis of high performance ion-gel comprising tetra-PEG network. *Macromolecules* **2012**, *45*, 3902–3909. [CrossRef]
125. Oveissi, F.; Naficy, S.; Le, T.Y.L.; Fletcher, D.F.; Dehghani, F. Tough hydrophilic polyurethane-based hydrogels with mechanical properties similar to human soft tissues. *J. Mater. Chem. B* **2019**, *7*, 3512–3519. [CrossRef]
126. Chen, Z.; Wang, T.; Yan, Q. Building a polysaccharide hydrogel capsule delivery system for control release of ibuprofen. *J. Biomater. Sci. Polym. Ed.* **2018**, *29*, 309–324. [CrossRef] [PubMed]
127. Jana, S.; Saha, A.; Nayak, A.K.; Sen, K.K.; Basu, S.K. Aceclofenac-loaded chitosan-tamarind seed polysaccharide interpenetrating polymeric network microparticles. *Coll. Surf. B Biointerfaces* **2013**, *105*, 303–309. [CrossRef] [PubMed]

128. Liou, G.-S.; Lin, P.-H.; Yen, H.-J.; Yu, Y.-Y.; Tsai, T.-W.; Chen, W.-C. Highly flexible and optical transparent 6F-PI/TiO2 optical hybrid films with tunable refractive index and excellent thermal stability. *J. Mater. Chem.* **2010**, *20*, 531–536. [CrossRef]
129. Koetting, M.C.; Peters, J.T.; Steichen, S.D.; Peppas, N.A. Stimulus-responsive hydrogels: Theory, modern advances, and applications. *Mater. Sci. Eng. R Rep.* **2015**, *93*, 1–49. [CrossRef]
130. Jayaramudu, T.; Raghavendra, G.M.; Varaprasad, K.; Sadiku, R.; Raju, K.M. Development of novel biodegradable Au nanocomposite hydrogels based on wheat: For inactivation of bacteria. *Carbohydr. Polym.* **2013**, *92*, 2193–2200. [CrossRef]
131. Gaharwar, A.K.; Peppas, N.A.; Khademhosseini, A. Nanocomposite hydrogels for biomedical applications: Nanocomposite hydrogels. *Biotechnol. Bioeng.* **2014**, *111*, 441–453. [CrossRef]
132. Chen, M.H.; Wang, L.L.; Chung, J.J.; Kim, Y.-H.; Atluri, P.; Burdick, J.A. Methods to assess shear-thinning hydrogels for application as injectable biomaterials. *ACS Biomater. Sci. Eng.* **2017**, *3*, 3146–3160. [CrossRef]
133. Rodell, C.B.; Lee, M.E.; Wang, H.; Takebayashi, S.; Takayama, T.; Kawamura, T.; Arkles, J.S.; Dusaj, N.N.; Dorsey, S.M.; Witschey, W.R.T.; et al. Injectable shear-thinning hydrogels for minimally invasive delivery to infarcted myocardium to limit left ventricular remodeling. *Circ. Cardiovasc. Interv.* **2016**, *9*, e004058. [CrossRef]
134. Nep, E.I.; Conway, B. Grewia gum 2: Mucoadhesive properties of compacts and gels. *Trop. J. Pharm. Res.* **2011**, *10*, 393–401. [CrossRef]
135. Tsintou, M.; Dalamagkas, K.; Seifalian, A. Injectable hydrogel versus plastically compressed collagen scaffold for central nervous system applications. *Int. J. Biomater.* **2018**, *2018*, 1–10. [CrossRef]
136. Bae, K.H.; Wang, L.-S.; Kurisawa, M. Injectable biodegradable hydrogels: Progress and challenges. *J. Mater. Chem. B* **2013**, *1*, 5371. [CrossRef]
137. Mathew, A.P.; Uthaman, S.; Cho, K.-H.; Cho, C.-S.; Park, I.-K. Injectable hydrogels for delivering biotherapeutic molecules. *Int. J. Biol. Macromol.* **2018**, *110*, 17–29. [CrossRef] [PubMed]
138. Tong, R.; Chen, G.; Pan, D.; Qi, H.; Li, R.; Tian, J.; Lu, F.; He, M. Highly stretchable and compressible cellulose ionic hydrogels for flexible strain sensors. *Biomacromolecules* **2019**, *20*, 2096–2104. [CrossRef]
139. Zhou, Y.; Wan, C.; Yang, Y.; Yang, H.; Wang, S.; Dai, Z.; Ji, K.; Jiang, H.; Chen, X.; Long, Y. Highly Stretchable, Elastic, and Ionic Conductive Hydrogel for Artificial Soft Electronics. *Adv. Funct. Mater.* **2019**, *29*, 1806220. [CrossRef]
140. Zhang, X.; Sheng, N.; Wang, L.; Tan, Y.; Liu, C.; Xia, Y.; Nie, Z.; Sui, K. Supramolecular nanofibrillar hydrogels as highly stretchable, elastic and sensitive ionic sensors. *Mater. Horiz.* **2019**, *6*, 326–333. [CrossRef]
141. Liu, S.; Oderinde, O.; Hussain, I.; Yao, F.; Fu, G. Dual ionic cross-linked double network hydrogel with self-healing, conductive, and force sensitive properties. *Polymer* **2018**, *144*, 111–120. [CrossRef]
142. Franzén, H.; Draget, K.; Langebäck, J.; Nilsen-Nygaard, J. Characterization and properties of hydrogels made from neutral soluble chitosans. *Polymers* **2015**, *7*, 373–389. [CrossRef]
143. Shams Es-haghi, S.; Weiss, R.A. Fabrication of tough hydrogels from chemically cross-linked multiple neutral networks. *Macromolecules* **2016**, *49*, 8980–8987. [CrossRef]
144. Weller, C.; Weller, C.; Team, V. Interactive dressings and their role in moist wound management. In *Advanced Textiles for Wound Care*; Elsevier: Amsterdam, The Netherlands, 2019; pp. 105–134. ISBN 978-0-08-102192-7.
145. Seliktar, D. Designing cell-compatible hydrogels for biomedical applications. *Science* **2012**, *336*, 1124–1128. [CrossRef]
146. Kumar, A.; Kumar, A. Antimicrobial polymeric gels. In *Polymeric Gels*; Elsevier: Amsterdam, The Netherlands, 2018; pp. 357–371. ISBN 978-0-08-102179-8.
147. McKenzie, M.; Betts, D.; Suh, A.; Bui, K.; Kim, L.; Cho, H. Hydrogel-based drug delivery systems for poorly water-soluble drugs. *Molecules* **2015**, *20*, 20397–20408. [CrossRef]
148. Gu, D.; O'Connor, A.J.; Qiao, G.G.H.; Ladewig, K. Hydrogels with smart systems for delivery of hydrophobic drugs. *Exp. Opin. Drug Deliv.* **2017**, *14*, 879–895. [CrossRef] [PubMed]
149. Jiang, Y.; Chen, J.; Deng, C.; Suuronen, E.J.; Zhong, Z. Click hydrogels, microgels and nanogels: Emerging platforms for drug delivery and tissue engineering. *Biomaterials* **2014**, *35*, 4969–4985. [CrossRef] [PubMed]
150. Barthelat, F.; Yin, Z.; Buehler, M.J. Structure and mechanics of interfaces in biological materials. *Nat. Rev. Mater.* **2016**, *1*, 16007. [CrossRef]
151. Thorne, J.B.; Vine, G.J.; Snowden, M.J. Microgel applications and commercial considerations. *Coll. Polym. Sci.* **2011**, *289*, 625–646. [CrossRef]

152. Wang, Y.; Tu, S.; Pinchuk, A.N.; Xiong, M.P. Active drug encapsulation and release kinetics from hydrogel-in-liposome nanoparticles. *J. Coll. Interface Sci.* **2013**, *406*, 247–255. [CrossRef]
153. Nayak, A.K.; Das, B. Introduction to polymeric gels. In *Polymeric Gels*; Elsevier: Amsterdam, The Netherlands, 2018; pp. 3–27. ISBN 978-0-08-102179-8.
154. Kawaguchi, H. Micro hydrogels: Preparation, properties, and applications. *J. Oleo Sci.* **2013**, *62*, 865–871. [CrossRef]
155. Vinogradov, S. Colloidal microgels in drug delivery applications. *Curr. Pharm. Des.* **2006**, *12*, 4703–4712. [CrossRef]
156. Panda, J.J.; Mishra, A.; Basu, A.; Chauhan, V.S. Stimuli responsive self-assembled hydrogel of a low molecular weight free dipeptide with potential for tunable drug delivery. *Biomacromolecules* **2008**, *9*, 2244–2250. [CrossRef]
157. Kim, B.; Peppas, N.A. In vitro release behavior and stability of insulin in complexation hydrogels as oral drug delivery carriers. *Int. J. Pharm.* **2003**, *266*, 29–37. [CrossRef]
158. Na, K.; Lee, K.H.; Bae, Y.H. pH-sensitivity and pH-dependent interior structural change of self-assembled hydrogel nanoparticles of pullulan acetate/oligo-sulfonamide conjugate. *J. Control. Release* **2004**, *97*, 513–525. [CrossRef]
159. Fleige, E.; Quadir, M.A.; Haag, R. Stimuli-responsive polymeric nanocarriers for the controlled transport of active compounds: Concepts and applications. *Adv. Drug Deliv. Rev.* **2012**, *64*, 866–884. [CrossRef] [PubMed]
160. Setia, A.; Ahuja, P. Nanohydrogels. In *Organic Materials as Smart Nanocarriers for Drug Delivery*; Elsevier: Amsterdam, The Netherlands, 2018; pp. 293–368. ISBN 978-0-12-813663-8.
161. Kim, S.H.; Kim, S.-H.; Nair, S.; Moore, E. Reactive electrospinning of cross-linked poly(2-hydroxyethyl methacrylate) nanofibers and elastic properties of individual hydrogel nanofibers in aqueous solutions. *Macromolecules* **2005**, *38*, 3719–3723. [CrossRef]
162. Gil, E.; Hudson, S. Stimuli-reponsive polymers and their bioconjugates. *Prog. Polym. Sci.* **2004**, *29*, 1173–1222. [CrossRef]
163. Konwar, R.; Ahmed, A.B. Nanoparticle: An overview of preparation, characterization and application. *Int. Res. J. Pharm.* **2016**, *4*, 47–57. [CrossRef]
164. Kumari, A.; Yadav, S.K.; Yadav, S.C. Biodegradable polymeric nanoparticles based drug delivery systems. *Coll. Surf. B Biointerfaces* **2010**, *75*, 1–18. [CrossRef]
165. Guvendiren, M.; Lu, H.D.; Burdick, J.A. Shear-thinning hydrogels for biomedical applications. *Soft Matter* **2012**, *8*, 260–272. [CrossRef]
166. Metters, A.T.; Bowman, C.N.; Anseth, K.S. Verification of scaling laws for degrading PLA-*b*-PEG-*b*-PLA hydrogels. *AIChE J.* **2001**, *47*, 1432–1437. [CrossRef]
167. Mason, M.N.; Metters, A.T.; Bowman, C.N.; Anseth, K.S. Predicting controlled-release behavior of degradable PLA-*b*-PEG-*b*-PLA hydrogels. *Macromolecules* **2001**, *34*, 4630–4635. [CrossRef]
168. Lustig, S.R.; Peppas, N.A. Solute diffusion in swollen membranes. IX. Scaling laws for solute diffusion in gels. *J. Appl. Polym. Sci.* **1988**, *36*, 735–747. [CrossRef]
169. Metters, A.T.; Anseth, K.S.; Bowman, C.N. A statistical kinetic model for the bulk degradation of PLA-*b*-PEG-*b*-PLA hydrogel networks: Incorporating network non-idealities. *J. Phys. Chem. B* **2001**, *105*, 8069–8076. [CrossRef]
170. Tan, H.; Marra, K.G. Injectable, biodegradable hydrogels for tissue engineering applications. *Materials* **2010**, *3*, 1746–1767. [CrossRef]
171. Lee, J.H. Injectable hydrogels delivering therapeutic agents for disease treatment and tissue engineering. *Biomater. Res.* **2018**, *22*, 1–14. [CrossRef] [PubMed]
172. Wang, J.; Yao, K.; Wang, C.; Tang, C.; Jiang, X. Synthesis and drug delivery of novel amphiphilic block copolymers containing hydrophobic dehydroabietic moiety. *J. Mater. Chem. B* **2013**, *1*, 2324. [CrossRef]
173. Lengert, E.; Yashchenok, A.M.; Atkin, V.; Lapanje, A.; Gorin, D.A.; Sukhorukov, G.B.; Parakhonskiy, B.V. Hollow silver alginate microspheres for drug delivery and surface enhanced Raman scattering detection. *RSC Adv.* **2016**, *6*, 20447–20452. [CrossRef]
174. Yang, T.-T.; Cheng, Y.-Z.; Qin, M.; Wang, Y.-H.; Yu, H.-L.; Wang, A.-L.; Zhang, W.-F. Thermosensitive chitosan hydrogels containing polymeric microspheres for vaginal drug delivery. *BioMed Res. Int.* **2017**, *2017*, 1–12. [CrossRef]

175. Nan, J.; Chen, Y.; Li, R.; Wang, J.; Liu, M.; Wang, C.; Chu, F. Polymeric hydrogel nanocapsules: A thermo and pH dual-responsive carrier for sustained drug release. *Nano-Micro Lett.* **2014**, *6*, 200–208. [CrossRef]
176. Yu, M.; Xu, L.; Tian, F.; Su, Q.; Zheng, N.; Yang, Y.; Wang, J.; Wang, A.; Zhu, C.; Guo, S.; et al. Rapid transport of deformation-tuned nanoparticles across biological hydrogels and cellular barriers. *Nat. Commun.* **2018**, *9*, 2607. [CrossRef]
177. Shchukin, D.G.; Sukhorukov, G.B.; Möhwald, H. Smart inorganic/organic nanocomposite hollow microcapsules. *Angew. Chem. Int. Ed.* **2003**, *42*, 4472–4475. [CrossRef]
178. Zhu, Y.; Shi, J.; Shen, W.; Dong, X.; Feng, J.; Ruan, M.; Li, Y. Stimuli-responsive controlled drug release from a hollow mesoporous silica sphere/polyelectrolyte multilayer core-shell structure. *Angew. Chem. Int. Ed.* **2005**, *44*, 5083–5087. [CrossRef]
179. Bayat, M.; Nasri, S. Injectable microgel–hydrogel composites "plum pudding gels": New system for prolonged drug delivery. In *Nanomaterials for Drug Delivery and Therapy*; Elsevier: Amsterdam, The Netherlands, 2019; pp. 343–372. ISBN 978-0-12-816505-8.
180. Basso, J.; Miranda, A.; Nunes, S.; Cova, T.; Sousa, J.; Vitorino, C.; Pais, A. Hydrogel-based drug delivery nanosystems for the treatment of brain tumors. *Gels* **2018**, *4*, 62. [CrossRef]
181. Motornov, M.; Roiter, Y.; Tokarev, I.; Minko, S. Stimuli-responsive nanoparticles, nanogels and capsules for integrated multifunctional intelligent systems. *Prog. Polym. Sci.* **2010**, *35*, 174–211. [CrossRef]
182. Desfrançois, C.; Auzély, R.; Texier, I. Lipid nanoparticles and their hydrogel composites for drug delivery: A review. *Pharmaceuticals* **2018**, *11*, 118. [CrossRef] [PubMed]
183. Pertici, V.; Pin-Barre, C.; Rivera, C.; Pellegrino, C.; Laurin, J.; Gigmes, D.; Trimaille, T. Degradable and injectable hydrogel for drug delivery in soft tissues. *Biomacromolecules* **2019**, *20*, 149–163. [CrossRef] [PubMed]
184. Sosnik, A.; Seremeta, K. Polymeric hydrogels as technology platform for drug delivery applications. *Gels* **2017**, *3*, 25. [CrossRef]
185. Song, S.H.; Lee, K.M.; Kang, J.B.; Lee, S.G.; Kang, M.J.; Choi, Y.W. Improved skin delivery of voriconazole with a nanostructured lipid carrier-based hydrogel formulation. *Chem. Pharm. Bull.* **2014**, *62*, 793–798. [CrossRef]
186. Khare, A.; Singh, I.; Pawar, P.; Grover, K. Design and evaluation of voriconazole loaded solid lipid nanoparticles for ophthalmic application. *J. Drug Deliv.* **2016**, *2016*, 1–11. [CrossRef]
187. López-Noriega, A.; Hastings, C.L.; Ozbakir, B.; O'Donnell, K.E.; O'Brien, F.J.; Storm, G.; Hennink, W.E.; Duffy, G.P.; Ruiz-Hernández, E. Hyperthermia-induced drug delivery from thermosensitive liposomes encapsulated in an injectable hydrogel for local chemotherapy. *Adv. Healthcare Mater.* **2014**, *3*, 854–859. [CrossRef]
188. Kim, D.Y.; Kwon, D.Y.; Kwon, J.S.; Park, J.H.; Park, S.H.; Oh, H.J.; Kim, J.H.; Min, B.H.; Park, K.; Kim, M.S. Synergistic anti-tumor activity through combinational intratumoral injection of an in-situ injectable drug depot. *Biomaterials* **2016**, *85*, 232–245. [CrossRef]
189. Sivakumaran, D.; Maitland, D.; Hoare, T. Injectable microgel-hydrogel composites for prolonged small-molecule drug delivery. *Biomacromolecules* **2011**, *12*, 4112–4120. [CrossRef]
190. Town, A.R.; Giardiello, M.; Gurjar, R.; Siccardi, M.; Briggs, M.E.; Akhtar, R.; McDonald, T.O. Dual-stimuli responsive injectable microgel/solid drug nanoparticle nanocomposites for release of poorly soluble drugs. *Nanoscale* **2017**, *9*, 6302–6314. [CrossRef]
191. Hudson, S.P.; Langer, R.; Fink, G.R.; Kohane, D.S. Injectable in situ cross-linking hydrogels for local antifungal therapy. *Biomaterials* **2010**, *31*, 1444–1452. [CrossRef] [PubMed]
192. McGillicuddy, F.C.; Lynch, I.; Rochev, Y.A.; Burke, M.; Dawson, K.A.; Gallagher, W.M.; Keenan, A.K. Novel "plum pudding" gels as potential drug-eluting stent coatings: Controlled release of fluvastatin. *J. Biomed. Mater. Res. Part A* **2006**, *79*, 923–933. [CrossRef] [PubMed]
193. Cho, J.-K.; Park, J.W.; Song, S.-C. Injectable and biodegradable poly(organophosphazene) gel containing silibinin: Its physicochemical properties and anticancer activity. *J. Pharm. Sci.* **2012**, *101*, 2382–2391. [CrossRef]
194. Lei, N.; Gong, C.; Qian, Z.; Luo, F.; Wang, C.; Wang, H.; Wei, Y. Therapeutic application of injectable thermosensitive hydrogel in preventing local breast cancer recurrence and improving incision wound healing in a mouse model. *Nanoscale* **2012**, *4*, 5686. [CrossRef]
195. Chen, M.-C.; Tsai, H.-W.; Liu, C.-T.; Peng, S.-F.; Lai, W.-Y.; Chen, S.-J.; Chang, Y.; Sung, H.-W. A nanoscale drug-entrapment strategy for hydrogel-based systems for the delivery of poorly soluble drugs. *Biomaterials* **2009**, *30*, 2102–2111. [CrossRef]

196. Biondi, M.; Borzacchiello, A.; Mayol, L.; Ambrosio, L. Nanoparticle-integrated hydrogels as multifunctional composite materials for biomedical applications. *Gels* **2015**, *1*, 162–178. [CrossRef]
197. Li, Y.; Huang, G.; Zhang, X.; Li, B.; Chen, Y.; Lu, T.; Lu, T.J.; Xu, F. Magnetic hydrogels and their potential biomedical applications. *Adv. Funct. Mater.* **2013**, *23*, 660–672. [CrossRef]
198. Meid, J.; Friedrich, T.; Tieke, B.; Lindner, P.; Richtering, W. Composite hydrogels with temperature sensitive heterogeneities: Influence of gel matrix on the volume phase transition of embedded poly-(N-isopropylacrylamide) microgels. *Phys. Chem. Chem. Phys.* **2011**, *13*, 3039–3047. [CrossRef]
199. Salvati, A.; Söderman, O.; Lynch, I. Plum-pudding gels as a platform for drug delivery: Understanding the effects of the different components on the diffusion behavior of solutes. *J. Phys. Chem. B* **2007**, *111*, 7367–7376. [CrossRef]
200. Li, X.; Rombouts, W.; van der Gucht, J.; de Vries, R.; Dijksman, J.A. Mechanics of composite hydrogels approaching phase separation. *PLoS ONE* **2019**, *14*, e0211059. [CrossRef]
201. Tan, H.-L.; Teow, S.-Y.; Pushpamalar, J. Application of metal nanoparticle–hydrogel composites in tissue regeneration. *Bioengineering* **2019**, *6*, 17. [CrossRef] [PubMed]
202. Alam, A.; Zhang, Y.; Kuan, H.-C.; Lee, S.-H.; Ma, J. Polymer composite hydrogels containing carbon nanomaterials—Morphology and mechanical and functional performance. *Prog. Polym. Sci.* **2018**, *77*, 1–18. [CrossRef]
203. Rocha-García, D.; Guerra-Contreras, A.; Rosales-Mendoza, S.; Palestino, G. Role of porous silicon/hydrogel composites on drug delivery. *Open Mater. Sci.* **2016**, *3*, 93–101. [CrossRef]
204. Ayub, A.D.; Chiu, H.I.; Mat Yusuf, S.N.A.; Abd Kadir, E.; Ngalim, S.H.; Lim, V. Biocompatible disulphide cross-linked sodium alginate derivative nanoparticles for oral colon-targeted drug delivery. *Artif. Cells Nanomed. Biotechnol.* **2019**, *47*, 353–369. [CrossRef] [PubMed]
205. Havanur, S.; Batish, I.; Cheruku, S.P.; Gourishetti, K.; JagadeeshBabu, P.E.; Kumar, N. Poly(N,N-diethyl acrylamide)/functionalized graphene quantum dots hydrogels loaded with doxorubicin as a nano-drug carrier for metastatic lung cancer in mice. *Mater. Sci. Eng. C* **2019**, *105*, 110094. [CrossRef]
206. Hou, F.; Xi, B.; Wang, X.; Yang, Y.; Zhao, H.; Li, W.; Qin, J.; He, Y. Self-healing hydrogel with cross-linking induced thermo-response regulated light emission property. *Coll. Surf. B Biointerfaces* **2019**, *183*, 110441. [CrossRef]
207. Zarrintaj, P.; Jouyandeh, M.; Ganjali, M.R.; Hadavand, B.S.; Mozafari, M.; Sheiko, S.S.; Vatankhah-Varnoosfaderani, M.; Gutiérrez, T.J.; Saeb, M.R. Thermo-sensitive polymers in medicine: A review. *Eur. Polym. J.* **2019**, *117*, 402–423. [CrossRef]
208. Zhang, Y.; An, Q.; Tong, W.; Li, H.; Ma, Z.; Zhou, Y.; Huang, T.; Zhang, Y. A new way to promote molecular drug release during medical treatment: A polyelectrolyte matrix on a piezoelectric-dielectric energy conversion substrate. *Small* **2018**, *14*, 1802136. [CrossRef]
209. Dadou, S.M.; El-Barghouthi, M.I.; Antonijevic, M.D.; Chowdhry, B.Z.; Badwan, A.A. Elucidation of the controlled-release behavior of metoprolol succinate from directly compressed xanthan gum/chitosan polymers: Computational and experimental studies. *ACS Biomater. Sci. Eng.* **2019**. [CrossRef]
210. Gu, S.; Yang, L.; Li, S.; Yang, J.; Zhang, B.; Yang, J. Thermo- and glucose-sensitive microgels with improved salt tolerance for controlled insulin release in a physiological environment: Thermo- and glucose-sensitive microgels with improved salt tolerance. *Polym. Int.* **2018**, *67*, 1256–1265. [CrossRef]
211. Wang, X.; Wang, C.; Zhang, Q.; Cheng, Y. Near infrared light-responsive and injectable supramolecular hydrogels for on-demand drug delivery. *Chem. Commun.* **2016**, *52*, 978–981. [CrossRef] [PubMed]
212. Sattari, S.; Dadkhah Tehrani, A.; Adeli, M. pH-responsive hybrid hydrogels as antibacterial and drug delivery systems. *Polymers* **2018**, *10*, 660. [CrossRef] [PubMed]
213. Li, X.; Fu, M.; Wu, J.; Zhang, C.; Deng, X.; Dhinakar, A.; Huang, W.; Qian, H.; Ge, L. pH-sensitive peptide hydrogel for glucose-responsive insulin delivery. *Acta Biomater.* **2017**, *51*, 294–303. [CrossRef]
214. Panahi, Y.; Gharekhani, A.; Hamishehkar, H.; Zakeri-Milani, P.; Gharekhani, H. Stomach-specific drug delivery of clarithromycin using asemi interpenetrating polymeric network hydrogel made ofmontmorillonite and chitosan: Synthesis, characterization and in vitro drug release study. *Adv. Pharm. Bull.* **2019**, *9*, 159–173. [CrossRef]
215. Qi, X.; Wei, W.; Li, J.; Zuo, G.; Pan, X.; Su, T.; Zhang, J.; Dong, W. Salecan-based pH-sensitive hydrogels for insulin delivery. *Mol. Pharm.* **2017**, *14*, 431–440. [CrossRef]

216. Li, L.; Jiang, G.; Yu, W.; Liu, D.; Chen, H.; Liu, Y.; Huang, Q.; Tong, Z.; Yao, J.; Kong, X. A composite hydrogel system containing glucose-responsive nanocarriers for oral delivery of insulin. *Mater. Sci. Eng. C* **2016**, *69*, 37–45. [CrossRef]
217. Udeni Gunathilake, T.; Ching, Y.; Chuah, C. Enhancement of curcumin bioavailability using nanocellulose reinforced chitosan hydrogel. *Polymers* **2017**, *9*, 64. [CrossRef]
218. Martínez-Martínez, M.; Rodríguez-Berna, G.; Bermejo, M.; Gonzalez-Alvarez, I.; Gonzalez-Alvarez, M.; Merino, V. Covalently crosslinked organophosphorous derivatives-chitosan hydrogel as a drug delivery system for oral administration of camptothecin. *Eur. J. Pharm. Biopharm.* **2019**, *136*, 174–183. [CrossRef]
219. Tao, G.; Wang, Y.; Cai, R.; Chang, H.; Song, K.; Zuo, H.; Zhao, P.; Xia, Q.; He, H. Design and performance of sericin/poly(vinyl alcohol) hydrogel as a drug delivery carrier for potential wound dressing application. *Mater. Sci. Eng. C* **2019**, *101*, 341–351. [CrossRef]
220. Singh, B.; Varshney, L.; Francis, S.; Rajneesh. Designing tragacanth gum based sterile hydrogel by radiation method for use in drug delivery and wound dressing applications. *Int. J. Biol. Macromol.* **2016**, *88*, 586–602. [CrossRef]
221. Wang, W.; Wat, E.; Hui, P.C.L.; Chan, B.; Ng, F.S.F.; Kan, C.-W.; Wang, X.; Hu, H.; Wong, E.C.W.; Lau, C.B.S.; et al. Dual-functional transdermal drug delivery system with controllable drug loading based on thermosensitive poloxamer hydrogel for atopic dermatitis treatment. *Sci. Rep.* **2016**, *6*, 24112. [CrossRef] [PubMed]
222. Qiao, X.; Peng, X.; Qiao, J.; Jiang, Z.; Han, B.; Yang, C.; Liu, W. Evaluation of a photocrosslinkable hydroxyethyl chitosan hydrogel as a potential drug release system for glaucoma surgery. *J. Mater. Sci. Mater. Med.* **2017**, *28*, 149. [CrossRef] [PubMed]
223. Chang, P.-C.; Chao, Y.-C.; Hsiao, M.-H.; Chou, H.-S.; Jheng, Y.-H.; Yu, X.-H.; Lee, N.; Yang, C.; Liu, D.-M. Inhibition of periodontitis induction using a stimuli-responsive hydrogel carrying naringin. *J. Periodontol.* **2017**, *88*, 190–196. [CrossRef] [PubMed]
224. Alvarez Echazú, M.I.; Olivetti, C.E.; Anesini, C.; Perez, C.J.; Alvarez, G.S.; Desimone, M.F. Development and evaluation of thymol-chitosan hydrogels with antimicrobial-antioxidant activity for oral local delivery. *Mater. Sci. Eng. C* **2017**, *81*, 588–596. [CrossRef] [PubMed]
225. Hyun, H.; Park, M.; Jo, G.; Kim, S.; Chun, H.; Yang, D. Photo-cured glycol chitosan hydrogel for ovarian cancer drug delivery. *Mar. Drugs* **2019**, *17*, 41. [CrossRef]
226. Rezazadeh, M.; Akbari, V.; Amuaghae, E.; Emami, J. Preparation and characterization of an injectable thermosensitive hydrogel for simultaneous delivery of paclitaxel and doxorubicin. *Res. Pharm. Sci.* **2018**, *13*, 181.
227. Songkroh, T.; Xie, H.; Yu, W.; Liu, X.; Sun, G.; Xu, X.; Ma, X. Injectable in situ forming chitosan-based hydrogels for curcumin delivery. *Macromol. Res.* **2015**, *23*, 53–59. [CrossRef]
228. Naderi, Z.; Azizian, J. Synthesis and characterization of carboxymethyl chitosan/Fe3O4 and MnFe2O4 nanocomposites hydrogels for loading and release of curcumin. *J. Photochem. Photobiol. B Biol.* **2018**, *185*, 206–214. [CrossRef]
229. Li, C.; Ren, S.; Dai, Y.; Tian, F.; Wang, X.; Zhou, S.; Deng, S.; Liu, Q.; Zhao, J.; Chen, X. Efficacy, pharmacokinetics, and biodistribution of thermosensitive chitosan/β-glycerophosphate hydrogel loaded with docetaxel. *AAPS PharmSciTech* **2014**, *15*, 417–424. [CrossRef]
230. Samimi Gharaie, S.; Dabiri, S.; Akbari, M. Smart shear-thinning hydrogels as injectable drug delivery systems. *Polymers* **2018**, *10*, 1317. [CrossRef]
231. Hu, X.; Wang, Y.; Zhang, L.; Xu, M.; Zhang, J.; Dong, W. Magnetic field-driven drug release from modified iron oxide-integrated polysaccharide hydrogel. *Int. J. Biol. Macromol.* **2018**, *108*, 558–567. [CrossRef] [PubMed]
232. Niu, X.; Zhang, Z.; Zhong, Y. Hydrogel loaded with self-assembled dextran sulfate-doxorubicin complexes as a delivery system for chemotherapy. *Mater. Sci. Eng. C* **2017**, *77*, 888–894. [CrossRef] [PubMed]
233. Ferreira, N.N.; Ferreira, L.M.; Miranda-Gonçalves, V.; Reis, R.M.; Seraphim, T.V.; Borges, J.C.; Baltazar, F.; Gremião, M.P.D. Alginate hydrogel improves anti-angiogenic bevacizumab activity in cancer therapy. *Eur. J. Pharm. Biopharm.* **2017**, *119*, 271–282. [CrossRef]
234. Liu, L.; Gao, Q.; Lu, X.; Zhou, H. In situ forming hydrogels based on chitosan for drug delivery and tissue regeneration. *Asian J. Pharm. Sci.* **2016**, *11*, 673–683. [CrossRef]

235. Li, X.; Kong, X.; Zhang, J.; Wang, Y.; Wang, Y.; Shi, S.; Guo, G.; Luo, F.; Zhao, X.; Wei, Y.; et al. Pharmaceutical nanotechnology: A novel composite hydrogel based on chitosan and inorganic phosphate for local drug delivery of camptothecin nanocolloids. *J. Pharm. Sci.* **2011**, *100*, 232–241. [CrossRef]
236. Zhu, X.; Zhang, Y.; Huang, H.; Zhang, H.; Hou, L.; Zhang, Z. Functionalized graphene oxide-based thermosensitive hydrogel for near-infrared chemo-photothermal therapy on tumor. *J. Biomater. Appl.* **2016**, *30*, 1230–1241. [CrossRef]

10

Injectable Thermosensitive Formulation Based on Polyurethane Hydrogel/Mesoporous Glasses for Sustained Co-Delivery of Functional Ions and Drugs

Monica Boffito [1,†], Carlotta Pontremoli [2,†], Sonia Fiorilli [2,*], Rossella Laurano [1], Gianluca Ciardelli [1,‡] and Chiara Vitale-Brovarone [2,‡]

1 Department of Mechanical and Aerospace Engineering, Politecnico di Torino, Corso Duca degli Abruzzi 24, 10129 Torino, Italy; monica.boffito@polito.it (M.B.); rossella.laurano@polito.it (R.L.); gianluca.ciardelli@polito.it (G.C.)
2 Department of Applied Science and Technology, Politecnico di Torino, Corso Duca degli Abruzzi 24, 10129 Torino, Italy; carlotta.pontremoli@polito.it (C.P.); chiara.vitale@polito.it (C.V.-B.)
* Correspondence: sonia.fiorilli@polito.it
† These authors contributed equally.
‡ Joint last authorship.

Abstract: Mini-invasively injectable hydrogels are widely attracting interest as smart tools for the co-delivery of therapeutic agents targeting different aspects of tissue/organ healing (e.g., neo-angiogenesis, inflammation). In this work, copper-substituted bioactive mesoporous glasses (Cu-MBGs) were prepared as nano- and micro-particles and successfully loaded with ibuprofen through an incipient wetness method (loaded ibuprofen approx. 10% *w/w*). Injectable hybrid formulations were then developed by dispersing ibuprofen-loaded Cu-MBGs within thermosensitive hydrogels based on a custom-made amphiphilic polyurethane. This procedure showed almost no effects on the gelation potential (gelation at 37 °C within 3–5 min). Cu^{2+} and ibuprofen were co-released over time in a sustained manner with a significantly lower burst release compared to MBG particles alone (burst release reduction approx. 85% and 65% for ibuprofen and Cu^{2+}, respectively). Additionally, released Cu^{2+} species triggered polyurethane chemical degradation, thus enabling a possible tuning of gel residence time at the pathological site. The overall results suggest that hybrid injectable thermosensitive gels could be successfully designed for the simultaneous localized co-delivery of multiple therapeutics.

Keywords: polyurethane; injectable hydrogels; ion/drug delivery; mesoporous bioactive glasses; tissue regeneration

1. Introduction

Tissue regeneration is the result of a complex process, which involves the synergistic contributes of cells, biomaterials, and bioactive factors (e.g., drugs, ions, growth factors). In most cases the complete regeneration of tissues fails due to a lack of vascularization; hence insufficient angiogenesis is one of the major current pathological concerns. In addition, the occurrence of drug-resistant infections may lead to several complications and greatly enhance the number of non-healing cases [1]. In order to overcome these issues, much attention has focused on the design of multifunctional systems which are able to simultaneously promote all the processes involved in the tissue/organ healing cascade. The incorporation of drugs, growth factors or inorganic nanomaterials into hydrogels has been extensively investigated [2,3], with the aim of combining in a single formulation several therapeutic abilities (such as pro-angiogenesis, anti-bacterial, anti-inflammatory). Among the approaches already explored, the combination of hydrogels with inorganic nanocarriers, which are able to incorporate and release several agents, represents a promising therapeutic strategy with a high potential for clinical translation. With this perspective, Zhu et al. prepared chitosan/mesoporous silica nanoparticle (MSN) composite hydrogels for localized co-delivery of drugs and macromolecules [4]. Similar hydrogel embedding ibuprofen-loaded MSN was proposed for surface coating of titanium implants [5] and poly(vinyl alcohol) hydrogels carrying oil-loaded MSNs containing curcumin were studied for dermal application [6]. More recently, a similar strategy has been explored to design thermosensitive hydrogels based on a poly(N-isopropylacrylamide) (PNIPAM) copolymer carrying mesoporous silica for dual-responsive (i.e., temperature and light) drug release [7] and for bone tissue regeneration [8].

More recently, in the field of tissue regeneration, considerable attention has been addressed towards the use of mesoporous bioactive glasses (MBGs) enriched with specific metallic ions (i.e., Sr^{2+}, Cu^{2+}, Ag^{+}, Ce^{3+}), as multifunctional therapeutic platforms for advanced medical devices [9,10]. Among the elements which can exert therapeutic properties, copper has been extensively investigated, due to the well documented pro-angiogenic effect alongside its antibacterial potential [11,12]. Several works have evidenced the antibacterial potential of Cu-containing MBGs against both planktonic bacteria and biofilms. In particular, Wu et al. [11] tested the successful antibacterial potential of Cu-containing MBG scaffolds against *Escherichia coli bacteria* and, accordingly with this, the authors recently demonstrated that Cu-containing MBG nanoparticles and their ionic extracts exert promising antibacterial activity against both Gram positive and Gram negative bacteria (*Staphylococcus aureus*, *Staphylococcus epidermidis* and *E. coli*) and are effective in inhibiting and preventing biofilm produced by *S. epidermidis* [13]. In addition to antibacterial abilities, Cu-substituted bioactive glasses were also demonstrated to stimulate angiogenesis and promote revascularization of soft and hard tissues [14,15].

Based on these promising results, we have recently reported the development of hybrid formulations able to combine the injectability of thermosensitive poly(ether urethane)-based (PEU) hydrogels and the capability of MBG particles to release functional copper ions [16]. This system was developed for a prolonged and sustained release of copper ions, with the final aim to promote simultaneously angiogenesis and anti-microbial effect [13,17–19]. However, no effects against persistent inflammation could be achieved with the formulated system. Hence, in order to expand the potentialities of the previously developed hybrid platform, Cu-substituted MBGs, in the form of micro- and nano-particles, were loaded with ibuprofen (Ibu), chosen as an anti-inflammatory agent, and embedded into PEU hydrogels. The resulting hybrid formulations were evaluated in terms of ion/drug co-delivery kinetics, gelation behavior and stability in an aqueous environment.

Since the main goal of this contribution was the definition and the characterization of a novel and adaptable drug/ion release platform, our investigation mainly focused to identify the maximum amount of particles which could be incorporated within the hydrogel and to assess the related effect on the gelation behavior as well as the ion/drug co-release capacity that the final combined formulation could provide. The high potentiality of the proposed strategy lies in its wide versatility, as by tailoring the composition and cargo of MBGs, different ions and bioactive factors can be co-released according to the therapeutic effects required by the final targeted application. Moreover, their release timing and dosages can be finally optimized according to the requirements of each specific application, to make the released payload effective (i.e., releasing kinetics within the therapeutic window), while avoiding cytotoxic concentrations. In addition, the use of a custom-made PEU hydrogel as the vehicle phase of the MBGs provides the final system with a further degree of freedom. The characteristic LEGO-like chemical structure of PEUs allows polymer properties to be finely tuned by changing their constituting building blocks. This versatility opens the way to the design of stimuli-responsive hydrogels with an enhanced control over payload release and/or hydrogel dissolution/degradation, thus improving the release properties compared to those observed for MBGs alone. To the best of our knowledge, this is the first attempt to design a hybrid injectable formulation based on a thermo-sensitive hydrogel embedding MBGs able to co-release therapeutic ions and drugs.

2. Materials and Methods

2.1. Synthesis of Cu-Substituted MBGs

2.1.1. Materials

Cetyltrimethylammonium bromide (CTAB ≥ 98%), ammonium hydroxide solution (NH_4OH), double distilled water (ddH_2O), tetraethyl orthosilicate (TEOS), calcium nitrate tetrahydrate ($Ca(NO_3)_2 \cdot 4H_2O$, 99%), copper chloride ($CuCl_2$, 99%), Pluronic P123 ($EO_{20}PO_{70}EO_{20}$, M_n ~5800 Da), ibuprofen (>98% GC), Trizma® base, primary standard and buffer, ≥99.9% (titration) were purchased from Sigma Aldrich, Milan, Italy and used as received. All solvents were purchased from Sigma Aldrich (Milan, Italy) in analytical grade.

2.1.2. Cu-Substituted MBG Nanoparticles

Cu-substituted MBGs nanoparticles (nominal molar ratio Cu/Ca/Si = 2/13/85, hereafter named as MBG_Cu2%_SG) were prepared using a base-catalyzed template sol-gel synthesis, following an already optimized protocol [16]. In brief, 6.6 g of CTAB, acting as template, and 12 mL of NH_4OH were dissolved in 600 mL of ddH_2O under magnetic stirring (350 rpm) for 30 min. Then, 30 mL of TEOS, 4.888 g of $Ca(NO_3)_2 \cdot 4H_2O$ and 0.428 g of $CuCl_2$ were added, and the obtained solution was vigorously stirred for 3 h at room temperature (RT). The powder was collected by centrifugation (Hermle Labortechnik Z326, Hermle LaborTechnik GmbH, Wehingen, Germany) at 10,000 rpm for 5 min, washed twice with ddH_2O and once with absolute ethanol. The final precipitate was dried at 70 °C for 12 h and calcined at 600 °C in air for 5 h at a heating rate of 1 °C min^{-1} using a Carbolite 1300 CWF 15/5 (Carbolite Ltd., Hope Valley, UK), in order to completely remove CTAB.

2.1.3. Cu-Substituted MBG Microspheres

Cu-substituted MBG microspheres (nominal molar ratio Cu/Ca/Si=2/13/85, hereafter named as MBG_Cu2%_SD) were synthesized following the aerosol-assisted spray-drying method reported by Pontremoli, Boffito et al. [16]. Briefly, 2.030 g of Pluronic P123, acting as template, were dissolved in 85 g of ddH_2O. Simultaneously, in a separate batch, a solution of 10.73 g of TEOS was pre-hydrolyzed under acidic conditions using 5 g of an aqueous HCl solution at pH 2. The solution with TEOS was then added drop-wise into the template solution and kept stirring for half an hour. Then, 0.163 g of $CuCl_2$ and 1.86 g of $Ca(NO_3)_2 \cdot 4H_2O$ were added. The final solution was stirred for 15 min and then sprayed with a Büchi, Mini Spray-Dryer B-290 (Büchi Labortechnik AG, Flawil, Switzerland), using N_2 as atomizing gas (inlet temperature 220 °C, N_2 pressure 60 mm Hg, feed rate 5 mL min^{-1}). The obtained powder was finally calcined at 600 °C in air for 5 h at a heating rate of 1 °C min^{-1} using a Carbolite 1300 CWF 15/5 (Carbolite Ltd., Hope Valley, UK).

2.1.4. Ibuprofen Loading Procedure

Ibuprofen was loaded into MBG_Cu2%_SG and MBG_Cu2%_SD through the incipient wetness method [20]. In brief, 0.1 g of both Cu-substituted MBGs were impregnated several times by dropping consecutive small aliquots of an ibuprofen solution in ethanol (at the final concentration of 30 mg/mL) onto the powders at RT. After each impregnation, ethanol was evaporated at 50 °C for 10 min and the dried powder mixed with a spatula. In order to completely fill the mesopores with ibuprofen the impregnation procedure was carried out with four 100 μL aliquots. Lastly, the obtained powders were dried at 50 °C overnight and named as follows: MBG_Cu2%_SG_Ibu and MBG_Cu2%_SD_Ibu.

2.2. Characterization of Cu-Substituted MBGs Loaded with Ibu

The morphology and particle size of the prepared powders were analyzed by field-emission scanning electron microscopy (FE-SEM) using a ZEISS MERLIN instrument (Oberkochen, Germany). For FE-SEM observations, 10 mg of MBG_Cu2%_SG_Ibu were dispersed in 10 mL of isopropanol using an ultrasonic bath (Digitec DT 103H, Bandelin, Berlin, Germany) for 5 min to obtain a stable suspension. A drop of the resulting suspension was put on a copper grid (3.05 mm Diam. 200 MESH, TAAB), allowed to dry and successively chromium-plated prior to imaging (Cr layer 7 nm). MBG_Cu2%_SD_Ibu sample was dispersed directly onto the double face carbon tape placed on a sample stub and then coated with a Cr layer. Compositional analysis of the powders was performed by energy dispersive spectroscopy (EDS; AZtec EDS, Oxford instruments, Abingdon-on-Thames, UK). EDS spectra were acquired on powder dispersed on carbon tape by analyzing an area of $75 \times 50\ \mu m^2$. Nitrogen adsorption–desorption isotherms were measured by using an adsorption analyzer ASAP2020 Micromeritics (ASAP 2020 Plus Physisorption, Norcross, GA, USA) at a temperature of −196 °C. Before nitrogen adsorption–desorption measurements, loaded samples were outgassed at 37 °C for 5 h, in order to avoid the degradation of the drug. The Brunauer–Emmett–Teller (BET) equation was used to calculate the specific surface area (SSA_{BET}) from the adsorption data (relative pressures 0.04–0.2). The pore size distribution was calculated through the DFT method (density functional theory) using the NLDFT kernel of equilibrium isotherms (desorption branch). The mesopore structure was investigated by transmission electron microscopy (TEM, Fei Company, Hillsboro, OR, USA) using a FEI Tecnai G2 operated at 200 kV. The samples were prepared by suspending the powders in ethanol and drop-wise placed on carbon coated copper grids. Thermo-gravimetric analysis (TGA) of the samples was performed on a TG 209 F1 Libra instrument from Netzsch (Selb, Germany) over a temperature range of 25–600 °C under air flux at a heating rate of 10 °C min^{-1}. The drug content was determined from the weight loss between 200 and 600 °C, by applying a correction for the weight loss in the same range of temperature due to the surface silanol condensation as recorded on Cu-substituted MBGs before Ibu loading. Fourier transformed infrared (FT-IR) spectra of the drug-loaded samples were collected on a Bruker Equinox 55 spectrometer (Bruker, Billerica, MA, USA) over a range of wavenumbers from 4000 to 400 cm^{-1} (resolution 2 cm^{-1}). In order to assess the amorphous state of incorporated Ibu, X-ray patterns were collected using an X'Pert PRO, PANalytical instrument (X'Pert PRO, PANalytical, Almelo, The Netherlands) (CuKα radiation at 40 kV and 40 mA). Data were obtained from 10° to 80° (diffraction angle 2ϑ) at a step size of 0.0130° and a scan step time of 60 s. Differential scanning calorimetry (DSC) analysis of Ibu-loaded samples was carried out with a DSC 204 F1 Phoenix (Netzsch) instrument ((Selb, Germany). The samples were heated from 37 °C to 200 °C at a heating rate of 10 °C min^{-1} under N_2 flux.

2.3. Synthesis of Amphiphilic Poly(ether urethane)

2.3.1. Materials

Amphiphilic water-soluble PEU was synthesized starting from Poloxamer®407 (P407, poly(ethylene oxide)-poly(propylene oxide)-poly(ethylene oxide) PEO-PPO-PEO triblock copolymer, 70% PEO, M_n 12,600 g/mol), 1,6-hexamethylene diisocyanate (HDI) and 1,4-cyclohexanedimethanol (CDM), purchased from Sigma Aldrich, Milan, Italy. Before the synthesis, all the reagents were anhydrified according to the following protocols: P407 was dried for 8 h at 100 °C and then cooled down at 40 °C at a pressure lower than 200 mbar; HDI was distilled under reduced pressure; CDM was vacuum-dried in a dessicator at RT. Dibutyiltin dilaurate (DBTDL) was also purchased from Sigma Aldrich, Milan, Italy and used as received to catalyze the polymerization reaction. Anhydrous 1,2-dichoroethane (DCE, Carlo Erba Reagents, Cornaredo, Italy) was prepared by pouring the solvent over activated (at 120 °C, overnight) molecular sieves (4Å, Sigma Aldrich, Milano, Italy) under N_2 atmosphere for 8 h. All other solvents were purchased from Carlo Erba Reagents, Cornaredo, Italy in the analytical grade and used as received.

2.3.2. Poly(ether urethane) Synthesis

PEU synthesis was carried out according to Boffito et al. [21]. P407, HDI and CDM were reacted at 1:2:1 molar ratio and the synthesis was conducted under N_2 atmosphere following a prepolymerization method with a first reaction between P407 and HDI to form an N=C=O-terminated prepolymer which was then chain extended through the addition of CDM. In detail, the required amount of HDI was added to a 20% *w/v* concentrated P407 solution previously prepared in DCE and equilibrated at 80 °C. DBTDL was also added at 0.1% *w/w* concentration with respect to P407 and the reagents reacted for 150 min. Then, the reaction mixture was cooled down at 60 °C and a 3% *w/v* concentrated CDM solution previously prepared in DCE was added to start the chain extension reaction which lasted 90 min and was finally terminated through the addition of MeOH. The synthesized PEU was collected by precipitation in an excess of petroleum ether (petroleum ether: DCE = 4:1 *v/v*) and further purified by solubilization in DCE (20% *w/v*) and precipitation in a diethyl ether/MeOH mixture (98:2 *v/v*, 5:1 volume ratio with respect to DCE). PEU was collected by centrifugation (MIKRO 220R, Hettich, Tuttlingen, Germany), dried overnight, grinded and stored under vacuum at 4 °C until use. Hereafter, the synthesized PEU will be referred to with the acronym CHP407, where C, H and P407 refer to CDM, HDI and Poloxamer®407, respectively.

2.4. Chemical Characterization of the As-Synthesized PEU

The successful synthesis of CHP407 poly(ether urethane) was assessed by attenuated total reflectance Fourier transformed infrared (ATR-FTIR) spectroscopy and size exclusion chromatography (SEC). CHP407 and P407 ATR-FTIR spectra were registered using a Perkin Elmer (Waltham, MA, USA) Spectrum 100 instrument equipped with an ATR diamond crystal (UATR KRS5). Spectra were obtained as an average of 16 scans registered at RT within the spectral range 4000–600 cm^{-1} (resolution 4 cm^{-1}). CHP407 molecular weight distribution was assessed by SEC using an Agilent Technologies 1200 Series (Agilent Technologies, Inc., Santa Clara, CA, USA) instrument equipped with a refractive index detector (RID) and two columns (Waters Styragel HR1 and HR4, Waters Corporation, Sesto San Giovanni, Italy). Analyses were conducted at 55 °C using N,N-dimethylformammide (DMF, CHROMASOLV Plus, inhibitor-free, for HPLC, Carlo Erba Reagents, Cornaredo, Italy), added with 0.1% *w/v* LiBr (Sigma Aldrich, Milano, Italy) as eluent at a flow rate of 0.5 mL/min. Samples were prepared at 2 mg/mL concentration in the mobile phase and filtered through a 0.45 µm syringe filter (Macherey-Nagel, Düren, Germany poly(tetrafluoro ethylene) membrane) before analysis. The Agilent ChemStation software was finally used to estimate CHP407 Number Average Molecular Weight (M_n) and polydispersity index (Đ) based on a calibration curve previously constructed starting from 10 poly(methyl methacrylate) standards with M_n ranging between 940 and 214,600 g/mol.

2.5. Preparation of CHP407-Based Hydrogels Carrying Cu-MBGs Loaded with Ibu

CHP407 thermosensitive hydrogels were prepared at a final PEU concentration of 15% *w/v* [16,21]. Cu-MBGs loaded with Ibu were encapsulated into CHP407-based hydrogels with final particle concentration of 20 mg/mL. In detail, hybrid hydrogels were prepared by adding an aliquot of particle suspension in ddH_2O (100 mg/mL), previously sonicated for 3 min at 20% amplitude, to a CHP407-based solution prepared in physiological saline solution (0.9% NaCl). The starting concentration of CHP407 solution was determined in order to reach the desired PEU and particle contents in the final system. Both CHP407 solubilization and particle addition were carried out at 4 °C to avoid undesired gelation during sample preparation. Sample mixing was conducted using a Vortex mixer for 30 s to ensure homogeneous particle dispersion within the sol-gel systems. Particles were added to CHP407 aqueous solutions immediately before use to avoid premature payload release before characterization tests. Pure CHP407 sol-gel systems and CHP407 hydrogels loaded with Ibu were also prepared as control samples. Loading of Ibu in CHP407 sol-gel systems was carried out by adding CHP407 aqueous solutions prepared at higher concentration with a predefined volume of an Ibu stock solution (at 40 mg/mL in ethanol) to reach an average content equal to the Ibu amount incorporated into MBG_Cu2%_SG_Ibu and MBG_Cu2%_SD_Ibu, as assessed through TGA analysis. Based on this calculation, CHP407 sol-gel systems were loaded with Ibu at a final concentration of 2.5 mg/mL. Hereafter, the developed sol-gel systems will be referred to with the acronyms reported in Table 1. For all the conducted tests, hydrogels were prepared in Bijou sample containers (inner diameter 17 mm, Carlo Erba Reagents, Cornaredo, Italy) at a final volume of 1 mL, to avoid geometry and volume influence on the performed characterizations.

Table 1. Compositional information and acronyms of the designed sol-gel systems.

Acronym	Composition
CHP407	CHP407 poly(ether urethane) (PEU) at 15% *w/v*
CHP407_Ibu	CHP407 PEU at 15% *w/v* + ibuprofen at a concentration equal to the mean drug amount assessed in MBG_Cu2%_SG_Ibu and MBG_Cu2%_SD_Ibu (i.e., 2.5 mg/mL)
CHP407_MBG_Cu2%_SG_Ibu	CHP407 PEU at 15% *w/v* + MBG_Cu2%_SG_Ibu (20 mg/mL MBG concentration and the corresponding amount of ibuprofen)
CHP407_MBG_Cu2%_SD_Ibu	CHP407 PEU at 15% *w/v* + MBG_Cu2%_SD_Ibu (20 mg/mL MBG concentration and the corresponding amount of ibuprofen)

2.6. *Characterization of Hybrid Sol-Gel Systems*

The thermosensitive behavior of pure CHP407 (i.e., without particle) and hybrid hydrogels (i.e., containing MBG_Cu2%_SG_Ibu, MBG_Cu2%_SD_Ibu or Ibu) was studied through tube inverting test in temperature ramp mode and isothermal conditions (i.e., at 37 °C) to assess the effects of drug/particle incorporation on hydrogel sol-to-gel transition. In view of their potential clinical application as injectable depots for the prolonged and sustained payload release, the delivery profile of ibuprofen and copper ion was investigated in physiological mimicking conditions. Furthermore, gel swelling potential and residence time in watery environment at physiological temperature were also assessed.

2.6.1. Thermosensitive Behavior of CHP407-Based Sol-Gel Systems

Tube inverting test in temperature ramp conditions was carried out to estimate hydrogel Lower Critical Gelation Temperature (LCGT). In detail, samples were subjected to a step-by-step temperature increase within the range 5–40 °C at a rate of 1 °C/step. In each step, temperature was kept constant for 5 min and the samples were finally inverted for 30 s to visually inspect their sol, biphasic or gel state (in the gel state no flow was observed within the set inversion time). The same test was carried out in isothermal conditions at 37 °C to assess hydrogel gelation time. In this test, instead of temperature, incubation time at 37 °C was varied from 1 to 10 min with a rate of 1 min/step. Each step consisted in sample equilibration in the sol state for 10 min, incubation at 37 °C for the required time, inversion for 30 s and visual inspection.

2.6.2. Gel Swelling and Stability in Aqueous Media

Gel swelling and stability in physiological mimicking conditions, that is, in aqueous media and 37 °C, were investigated on the designed sol-gel systems up to 14 days incubation time [16]. Samples (1 mL) were first incubated at 37 °C (Memmert IF75, Schwabach, Germany) for 15 min to allow a complete gelation and then added with 1 mL of Trizma® (0.1 M, pH 7.4) previously equilibrated at 37 °C. Complete medium refresh was performed every two days. On predefined time points of 6h, 1d, 3d, 7d and 14d three samples were collected, weighted upon removal of the residual buffer, lyophilized (Martin Christ ALPHA 2–4 LSC, Osterode am Harz, Germany) and weighted again. The collected data were finally used to estimate sample percentage of swelling (weight change in wet state %) and polymer weight loss (weight loss in dry state %) [16]. Samples collected on day 14 were also analyzed by SEC to assess changes in polymer molecular weight distribution during incubation in aqueous media at 37 °C.

2.6.3. Payload Release Studies

Payload release studies were carried out on hydrogels incorporating MBG_Cu2%_SG_Ibu, MBG_Cu2%_SD_Ibu and simply dispersed Ibu. Tests were conducted at 37 °C up to 14 days using

Trizma® as release medium. Complete gelation of the samples was ensured through incubation at 37 °C for 15 min; then, 1 mL of release medium (previously equilibrated at 37 °C) was added to each sample and the release test started. Release media were collected and completely refreshed at 1h, 3h, 5h, 1d, 2d, 3d, 4d, 8d, 10d, and 14d incubation time. Released Ibu was quantified through a high performance liquid chromatography (HPLC, Thermo Scientific, Dionex Ultimate 3000, Waltham, MA, USA) instrument equipped with a C18 column (5 μm, 120 Å) according to the protocol described by Alsirawan et al. [22]. A mixture of acetonitrile (ACN, Carlo Erba Reagents, Cornaredo, Italy, HPLC grade) and phosphoric acid solution at 0.03% *w/v* concentration (pH 2.25) at 60/40 *v/v* was used as mobile phase at 1.7 mL/min. Analysis were conducted with an injection volume of 20 μL, at RT and 214 nm for 5 min. In order to prepare the samples, the collected extracts were mixed with ACN at 40/60 volume ratio and filtered through a 0.45 μm syringe filter (Macherey-Nagel, Düren, Germany, poly(tetrafluoro ethylene) membrane). Ibu content was finally quantified with respect to a calibration curve based on ibuprofen standards with concentration ranging between 0 and 2.5 mg/mL. The collected extracts were also characterized by inductively coupled plasma atomic emission spectrometry technique (ICP-AES) (ICP-MS, Thermo Scientific, Waltham, MA, USA) to measure the concentration of released copper ions. In order to express the results in terms of released percentage, the amount of copper initially incorporated into the MBG framework was measured by dissolving MBG_Cu2%_SG_Ibu and MBG_Cu2%_SD_Ibu in a mixture of nitric and hydrofluoric acids (0.5 mL of HNO_3 and 2 mL of HF for 10 mg of powder) and quantifying copper concentration through ICP-AES. To compare the ion/drug release kinetics from MBGs as such and embedded within the hydrogel, release tests from particle alone were also conducted as follows: drug-loaded powders were dispersed in physiological saline solution at 20 mg/mL MBG concentration and Trizma® was added as release medium at 37 °C (1:1 volume ratio), as previously performed with the hydrogel systems. Release tests from free MBG particles were conducted up to 24 h observation time. In order to better characterize copper ion and ibuprofen release mechanism from the hydrogels incorporating MBG_Cu2%_SG_Ibu, MBG_Cu2%_SD_Ibu and Ibu as such, the Korsmeyer-Peppas equation was used in the form recently reported by Boffito et al. [23] to estimate the release exponent n, whose value classifies the type of release. Specifically, an n value of 0.45 or 0.89 is typical of a diffusion- or swelling/relaxation-controlled release, respectively. An n value within the range 0.45–0.89 characterizes an anomalous release, meanwhile when n shows a value higher than 0.89 other processes are ongoing in addition to diffusion and swelling/relaxation.

2.7. *Statistical Analysis*

Statistical analysis was performed on the data collected from swelling, stability, and payload release tests. All tests were performed in triplicate and results have been reported as mean ± standard deviation. Comparison among results was performed through GraphPad Prism (GraphPad Software, Inc., La Jolla, CA, USA, version 5.03, 2009; http://www.graphpad.com) using a Two-way ANOVA analysis followed by Bofferoni's multiple comparison tests. The degree of statistical difference among the results was defined in accordance to Boffito et al. [21].

3. Results and Discussion

3.1. *Cu-MBGs Loaded with Ibu*

Morphological and Structural Characterization

FE-SEM images of MBG_Cu2%_SG_Ibu (Figure 1A) and MBG_Cu2%_SD_Ibu (Figure 1C) showed nanoparticles with a monodispersed spherical shape (size range: 150–200 nm) and microspheres in the range of 1–5 μm, respectively. EDS spectra (Figure 1B,D) of both powders confirmed the presence of copper inside the framework, with a Cu/Si molar ratio in good agreement with the nominal ratio for both MBGs.

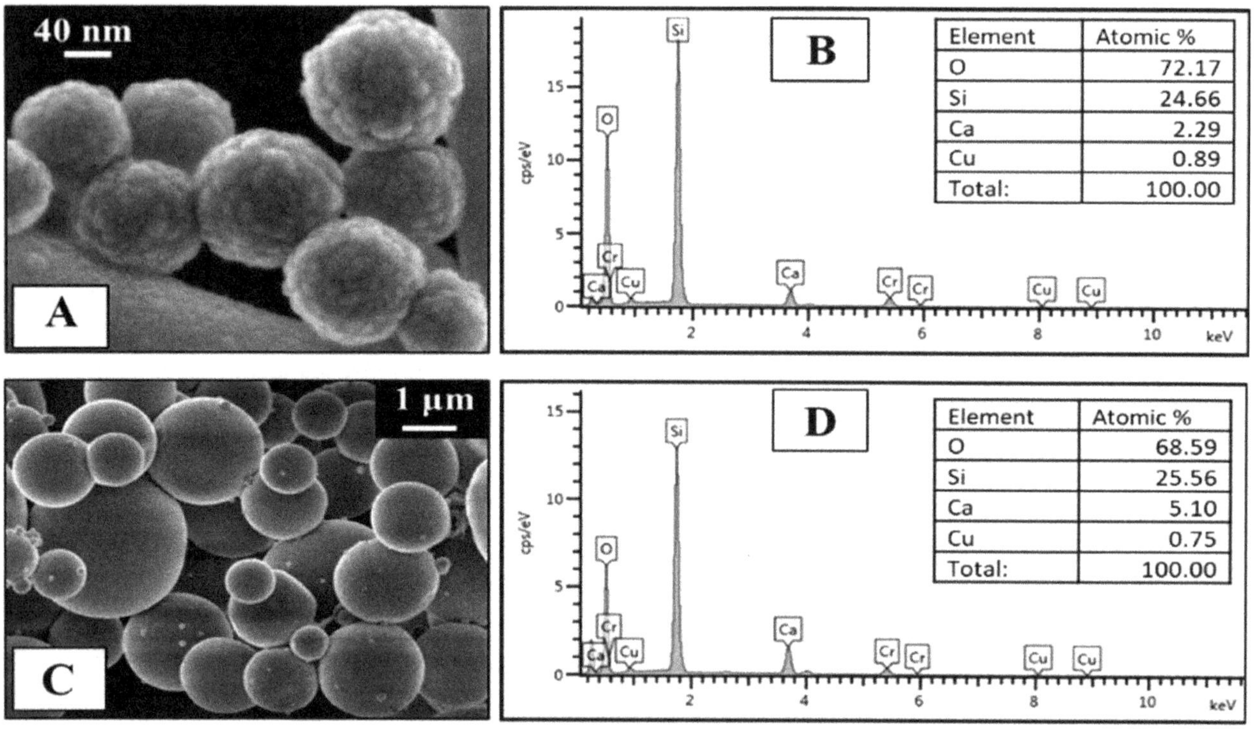

Figure 1. Field-emission scanning electron microscopy (FE-SEM) image of MBG_Cu2%_SG_Ibu (**A**) and MBG_Cu2%_SD_Ibu (**C**). Energy dispersive spectroscopy (EDS) spectrum of MBG_Cu2%_SG_Ibu (**B**) and MBG_Cu2%_SD_Ibu (**D**).

FESEM observations and EDS analysis evidenced that ibuprofen incorporation did not significantly alter the morphological features and the chemical composition of Cu-substituted MBGs, which resulted very similar to those reported for not-loaded samples [16]. In particular, the amount of copper revealed by EDS before and after the drug loading resulted unaffected, evidencing that the loading procedure did not induce any copper release (data not shown).

Figure 2 shows the nitrogen adsorption–desorption isotherms and the pore size distribution of the sample before and after drug loading. As expected, before loading, MBG_Cu2%_SG showed a type IV sorption isotherm, according to the IUPAC classification, with a well-defined step around 0.4 (P/P_0), indicative of uniform mesopores. The specific surface area and pore volume values reported in Table 2 are characteristic of mesoporous materials with uniform pores and remarkable value of specific surface area (SSA_{BET}) [24]. The mesopore size distribution was centered at around 4.2 nm, thus allowing the incorporation of ibuprofen whose molecular size is about 1 nm [25–27]. As expected, drug up-loading induced a significant modification of the adsorption-desorption isotherm (reduction of the adsorbed volume and presence of hysteresis loop) and a drastic reduction of the pore volume, as shown in Figure 2. In particular, the modification of the isotherm curve upon drug incorporation suggested that most of the mesopores were completely filled with Ibu. On the other hand, the remaining population underwent size reduction and shape modification from cylinder to ink-bottle pores, in analogy to the results reported by Hong et al. [28] for similar systems. In addition, the drastic reduction of pore volume as a consequence of drug incorporation was confirmed by the disappearance of the component centered at 4.2 nm (Figure 2B). The isotherm of MBG_Cu2%_SD was a type IV curve (Figure 2C), with H1 hysteresis loop, typical of mesoporous material with pores larger than 4 nm. Although the specific surface area was lower compared to that of MBG_Cu2%_SG, it resulted much higher compared to not-templated sol-gel glasses (few m^2/g), conferring increased surface reactivity to MBGs in the biological environment [29]. The worm-like mesoporous structure was further confirmed by TEM images, reported in Figure S1. The pore size distribution evidenced multisized pores in the range between 8 and 11 nm (Figure 2D), which easily allows the diffusion and incorporation of ibuprofen molecules. A drastic reduction in SSA_{BET} was observed in MBG_Cu2%_SD_Ibu sample, while the pore volume reduction was lower compared to MBG_Cu2%_SG_Ibu sample (Table 2). Hence, in MBG_Cu2%_SD the incorporation of drug molecules occurred without a full occlusion of the available pore volume. The total amount of loaded drug was quantified by TGA analysis on both samples after drug incorporation. As reference, TGA analysis was also conducted on not-loaded MBG samples, proving the complete absence of residual organic species at 600 °C. TGA thermograms of MBG_Cu2%_SG_Ibu and MBG_Cu2%_SD_Ibu exhibited a significant weight decrease between 300 and 400 °C, which can be ascribed to ibuprofen loss [30], due to the rupture of the multiple H-bonding interactions between the drug and the hydroxyl groups of the inner MBG surface, in accordance with Mellaerts and co-workers [26]. The weight percentage of loaded ibuprofen, based on TGA analysis, turned out to be 12% in MBG_Cu2%_SG and 10% in MBG_Cu2%_SD. These results confirmed that the drug loading capacity increases with the increase of MGB surface area and pore volume, according to data reported in the literature for mesoporous silicas [31].

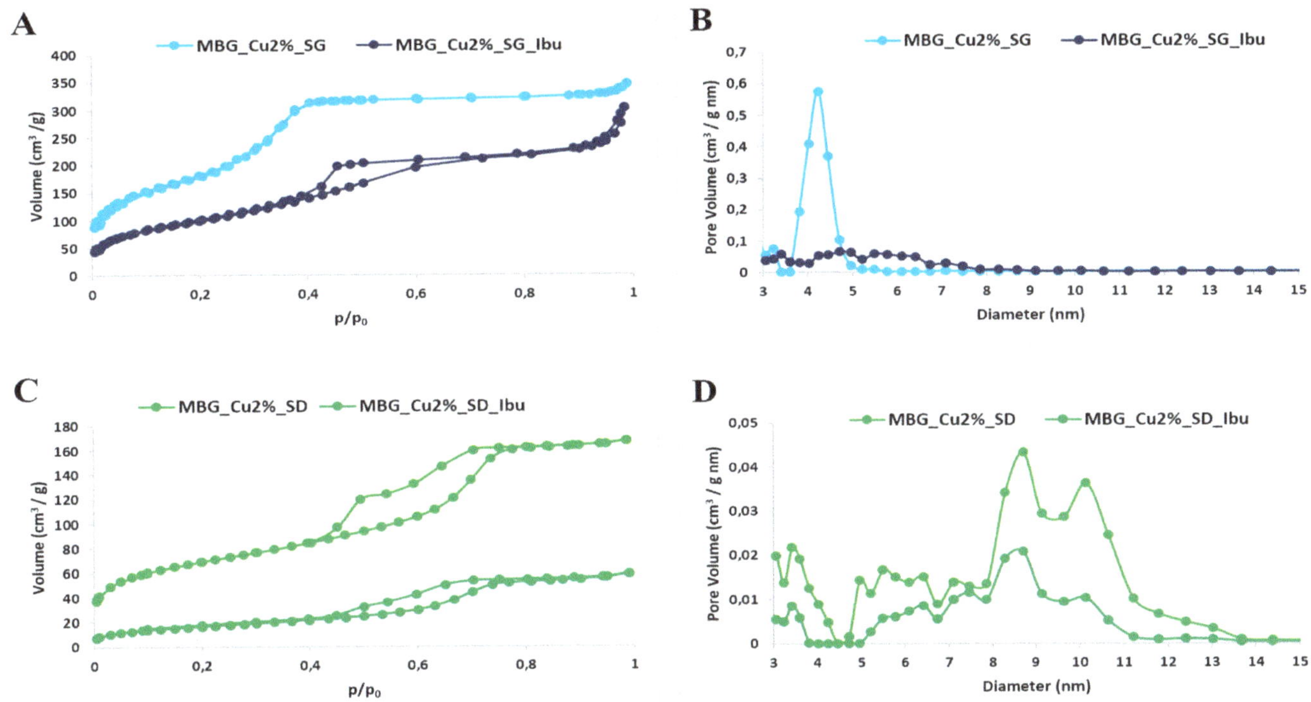

Figure 2. N_2 adsorption–desorption isotherm of MBG_Cu2%_SG and MBG_Cu2%_SG_Ibu (**A**), MBG_Cu2%_SD and MBG_Cu2%_SD_Ibu (**C**). DFT (density functional theory) pore size distribution of MBG_Cu2%_SG and MBG_Cu2%_SG_Ibu (**B**), MBG_Cu2%_SD and MBG_Cu2%_SD_Ibu (**D**).

Table 2. Structural properties (i.e., specific surface area -SSA_{BET}-, pore volume, pore size) of MBG_Cu2%_SG, MBG_Cu2%_SD, MBG_Cu2%_SG_Ibu and MBG_Cu2%_SD_Ibu.

Acronym	SSA_{BET} ($m^2\ g^{-1}$)	Pore Volume ($cm^3\ g^{-1}$)	Pore Size (nm)
MBG_Cu2%_SG	740	0.65	4.2
MBG_Cu2%_SG_Ibu	330	0.35	4–6
MBG_Cu2%_SD	226	0.24	8–11
MBG_Cu2%_SD_Ibu	54	0.081	8–9

The FTIR spectra of Cu-substituted MBGs before (curves b–d) and after ibuprofen loading (curves c–e) are reported in Figure 3A and compared to the FTIR spectrum of ibuprofen alone (curve a). MBG samples showed the typical adsorption bands of H-bonded hydroxyls (stretching vibration) in the range of 3750–3000 cm^{-1}. For what concerns drug-loaded samples, spectra showed the typical bands of ibuprofen molecule: the absorption bands at 2933 and 2871 cm^{-1} ascribed to C–H stretching modes and the signals at 1475 and 1421 cm^{-1} attributed to C–H bending vibrations. At variance with the spectrum of the drug alone which showed a clear adsorption band at 1706 cm^{-1}, due to the C=O stretching vibration in –COOH groups, for ibuprofen-loaded samples two bands appeared at 1550 and 1407 cm^{-1}, due to the asymmetric (ν_{as}) and symmetric (ν_s) stretching vibration of the carboxylate group COO^-, respectively [32], resulting from proton-transfer reactions from carboxylic moieties to hydroxyl groups at MBG surface [33]. As widely reported in the literature [34,35], drug loading in their amorphous form results in an increased dissolution rates and solubility. Hence, DSC and X-ray powder diffraction (XRD) analyses of ibuprofen-loaded samples were conducted to assess the amorphous state of the drug and exclude the presence of large crystalline aggregates. Figure 3 compares the DSC thermograms of Ibu as such, MBG_Cu2%_SG_Ibu and MBG_Cu2%_SD_Ibu samples. A single endothermic melting peak at 76 °C, ascribed to crystal phase melting, was observed only for ibuprofen as such, confirming the non-crystalline state of ibuprofen loaded into the mesopores. The amorphous state of the drug was also confirmed by XRD analysis (Figure 3D). XRD pattern of ibuprofen powder showed several characteristic X-ray diffraction peaks, which completely disappeared upon drug loading into the pores of Cu-substituted MBGs, which, in accordance with DSC data, strongly suggested that re-crystallization did not occur inside the pores upon solvent evaporation during the incorporation process. This behavior has been previously reported by Bràs et al. [30], who confirmed the amorphous state of ibuprofen confined inside SBA-15 silicas with similar pore size. The proposed attribution is also supported by several authors [36,37] who reported that re-crystallization of the entrapped drug molecules is suppressed below a critical pore diameter, showing that crystallization can occur only when pore size is significantly larger (about 20 times) compared to the drug size [36].

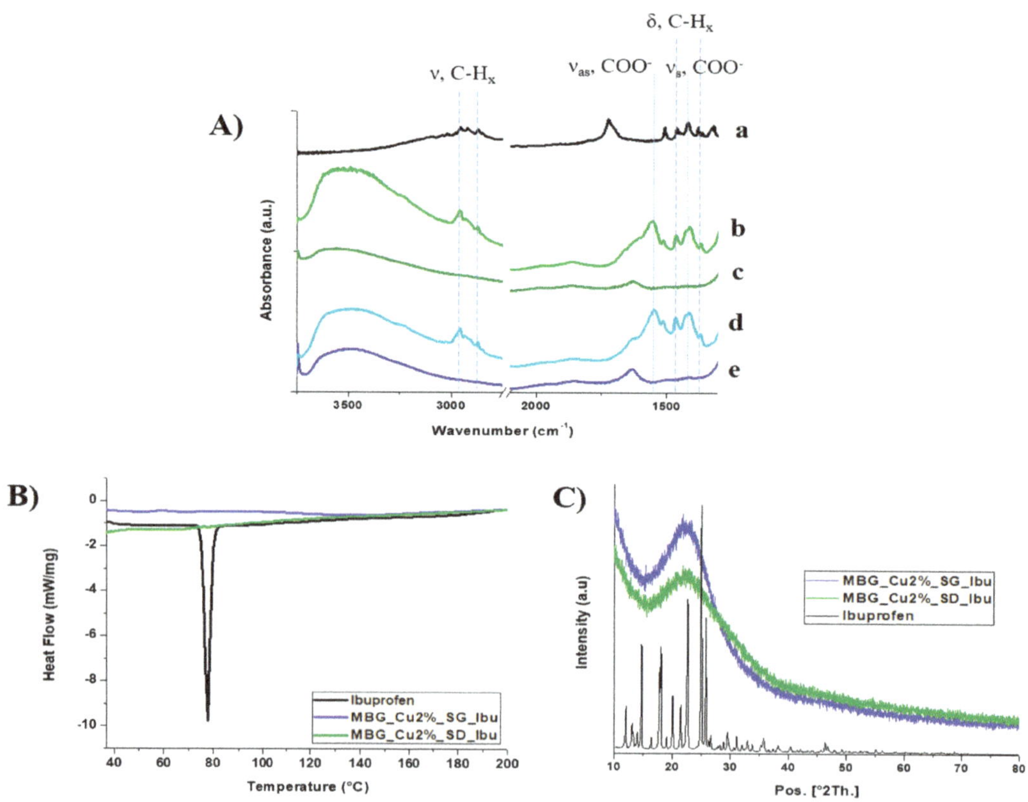

Figure 3. (**A**) Fourier transformed infrared (FTIR) spectra of ibuprofen (**a**), MBG_Cu 2%_SG_Ibu (**b**), MBG_Cu2%_SG (**c**), MBG_Cu 2%_SD_Ibu (**d**) and MBG_Cu2%_SD (**e**). (**B**) Differential scanning calorimetry (DSC) thermograms of ibuprofen, MBG_Cu2%_SG_Ibu and MBG_Cu2%_SD_Ibu samples. (**C**) X-ray powder diffraction (XRD) patterns of ibuprofen, MBG_Cu2%_SG_Ibu and MBG_Cu2%_SD_Ibu samples.

3.2. Poly(ether urethane) Chemical Characterization

The successful synthesis of a PEU carrying P407 blocks in its backbone was confirmed by attenuated total reflectance Fourier transformed infrared (ATR-FTIR) spectroscopy (Figure 4). The appearance of new transmission peaks in CHP407 spectrum, compared to P407 one, clearly proved the formation of urethane bonds among PEU building blocks [16,21]. In detail, the formation of N-H bonds was proved by the appearance of a new peak at 3342 cm^{-1} (stretching vibration), while the signals at 1720 and 1642 cm^{-1} could be ascribed to the stretching vibration of urethane free and bound carbonyl groups (C=O), respectively. N-H bonds also showed a bending vibration at 1540 cm^{-1} concurrent with C-N bond stretching. CHP407 showed M_n of 71,670 Da and a polydispersity index of 1.7, further confirming the success of the polymerization reaction.

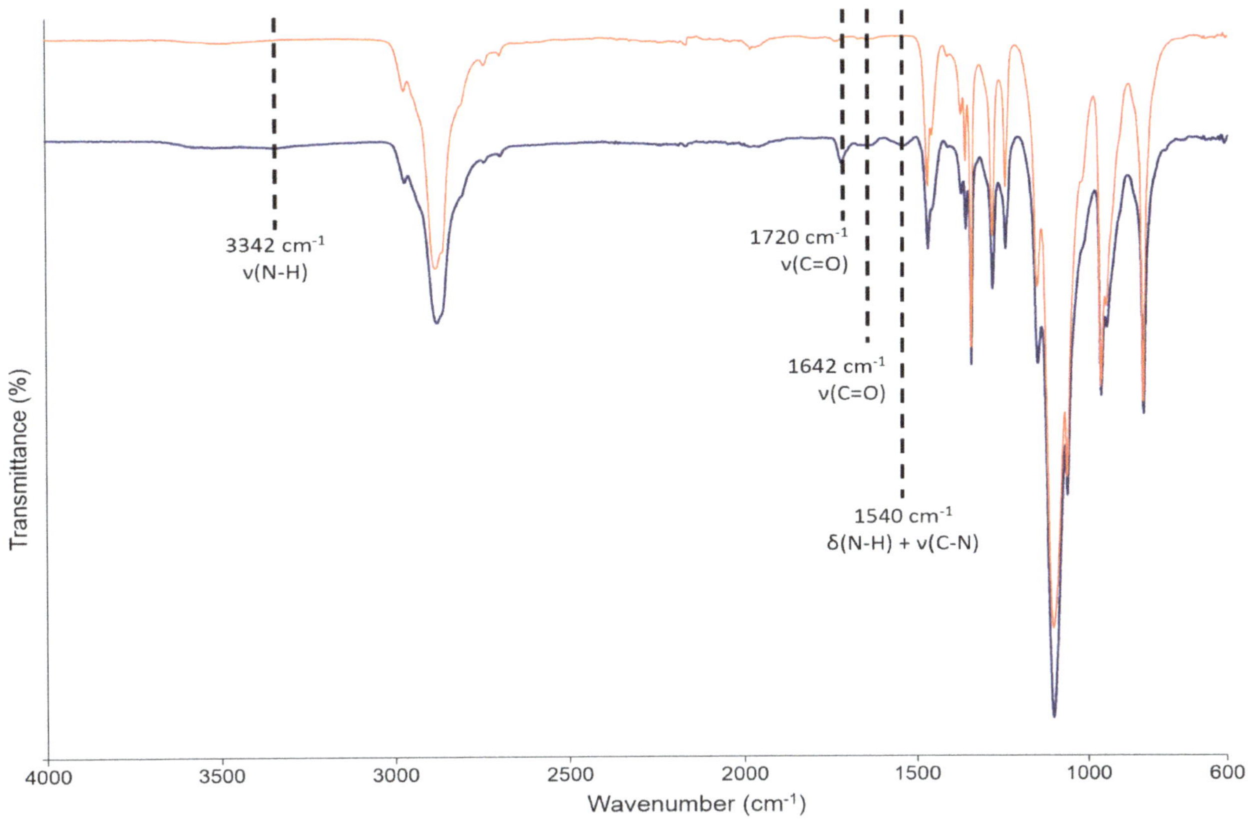

Figure 4. Attenuated total reflectance Fourier transformed infrared (ATR-FTIR) spectra of P407 (red) and CHP407 (blue). Dashed lines identify the characteristic signals of newly formed urethane bonds in CHP407.

3.3. Characterization of Hybrid Sol-Gel Systems

3.3.1. Thermosensitive Behavior of CHP407-Based Hydrogels

The temperature-dependent sol-to-gel transition of the developed systems was characterized through tube inverting tests carried out in temperature ramp mode and in isothermal conditions at 37 °C. The former test allowed the estimation of hydrogel LCGT, while the latter was conducted to evaluate the time required for a complete gelation in physiological conditions. Table 3 reports LCGT values and gelation time in physiological conditions of pure CHP407 hydrogel and CHP407 hybrid hydrogels.

Table 3. Lower critical gelation temperature (LGCT) and gelation time at 37 °C of CHP407, CHP407_Ibu, CHP407_ MBG_Cu2%_SG_Ibu and CHP407_ MBG_Cu2%_SD_Ibu.

Acronym	LCGT (°C) [1]	Gelation Time @ 37 °C (min) [2]
CHP407	28	5
CHP407_Ibu	27	5
CHP407_MBG_Cu2%_SG_Ibu	29	4
CHP407_MBG_Cu2%_SD_Ibu	30	6

[1] Error: ± 0.5 °C. [2] Error: ± 0.5 min.

The incorporation of MBG_Cu2%_SG_Ibu, MBG_Cu2%_SD_Ibu or ibuprofen as such was found to slightly influence the transition kinetics of the designed sol-gel systems, in accordance with our previous work [16]. Particle incorporation marginally increased hydrogel gelation temperature, suggesting that MBG particles act as defects in the gel network, initially hindering and then slowing down the kinetics of the sol-to-gel transition [16]. On the other hand, the slight decrease of gelation time in physiological conditions observed for CHP407 gels containing MBG_Cu2%_SG_Ibu particles could also result from the criterion adopted to define the "sol" and the "gel" states, that is, presence or absence of sample flow within 30 s of vial inversion. Indeed, particle addition to the hydrogels induced an increase in viscosity that, as a consequence, inevitably accounted for the shorter incubation time at 37 °C requested for not observing any flow within the observation time. Similarly, the slightly lower gelation temperature of CHP407_MBG_Cu2%_SG_Ibu compared to CHP407_MBG_Cu2%_SD_Ibu could be correlated to their dimensional differences, which result in different hydrogel viscosity. Indeed, at a fixed MBG concentration of 20 mg/mL, the number of MBG_Cu2%_SG_Ibu contained throughout the gel is expected to be higher compared to MBG_Cu2%_SD_Ibu, due to the lower size of SG particles. Regarding the addition of ibuprofen as such, no effects were observed in gelation time in physiological conditions, while LCGT value slightly decreased. This behavior did not result from the addition of a small volume of EtOH (used to solubilize Ibu) to the sol-gel systems (data not reported), but rather to the intrinsic nature of the drug. In fact, being hydrophobic, ibuprofen is expected to be partly loaded within the core of the forming CHP407 micelles, thus inducing an increase of micelle volume, which then achieves the critical value required for the onset of thermal gelation [8] at a lower temperature. Despite the commented slight changes in LCGT and gelation time at 37 °C, neither the addition of MBG particles of different size nor the incorporation of a hydrophobic drug significantly affected the gelation potential of CHP407-based hydrogels upon temperature increase.

3.3.2. Gel Characterization through Swelling and Stability to Dissolution Tests

CHP407-based gels, both virgin and hybrid formulations, were characterized in terms of aqueous medium absorption (Figure 5A) and dissolution/degradation (Figure 5B) over time in a physiological mimicking environment, that is, at 37 °C in the presence of a physiological-like buffer at pH 7.4. The incorporation of ibuprofen as such within CHP407 gels did not significantly affect gel behavior in aqueous media. Indeed, the percentage of swelling increased overtime up to 7d, followed by a drastic decrease on day 14 for both CHP407 and CHP407_Ibu samples. This change in medium absorption trend can be correlated to two concurrent phenomena occurring in the samples and their balance, namely swelling and dissolution/degradation resulting from the progressive absorption of aqueous media within the gels. The decrease in the swelling percentage observed on day 14 in CHP407 and CHP407_Ibu is thus due to the increasing gel instability in aqueous media over time. This hypothesis was demonstrated by the progressive increase in the percentage of weight loss (statistically significant increase at each time point, with the exception of day 1), that reached a value of 46.9 ± 0.6% and 45.8 ± 1.9% for CHP407 and CHP407_Ibu, respectively, after 14 days incubation in aqueous environment. Differently from ibuprofen, the embedding of MBGs in CHP407 hydrogels significantly affected gel long-term stability in aqueous environment (statistical differences between particle-loaded and not-loaded gels observed from day 3 in terms of swelling and day 1 in terms of weight loss percentage). In fact, both CHP407_MBG_Cu2%_SG_Ibu and CHP407_MBG_Cu2%_SD_Ibu showed negative swelling percentages starting from day 7 of incubation time suggesting that dissolution/degradation had completely prevailed on absorption phenomena. This observation was further proved by weight loss data, with CHP407_MBG_Cu2%_SG_Ibu and CHP407_MBG_Cu2%_SD_Ibu being almost completely dissolved/degraded after 14 days incubation in aqueous medium (weight loss percentage of 83.9 ± 2.2% and 68.9 ± 4.7% for CHP407_MBG_Cu2%_SG_Ibu and CHP407_MBG_Cu2%_SD_Ibu, respectively). The collected data confirmed the behavior previously observed for similar systems [16], with slight differences due to the different sample geometry, that is, gel thickness and extension of the surface in contact with the aqueous medium. More in detail, since day 1, CHP407_MBG_Cu2%_SG_Ibu and CHP407_MBG_Cu2%_SD_Ibu showed statistically different dissolution/degradation, while swelling percentage became significantly different from day 3 on, with hydrogel containing MBG_Cu2%_SG_Ibu exhibiting higher destabilization induced by the progressive absorption of aqueous medium.

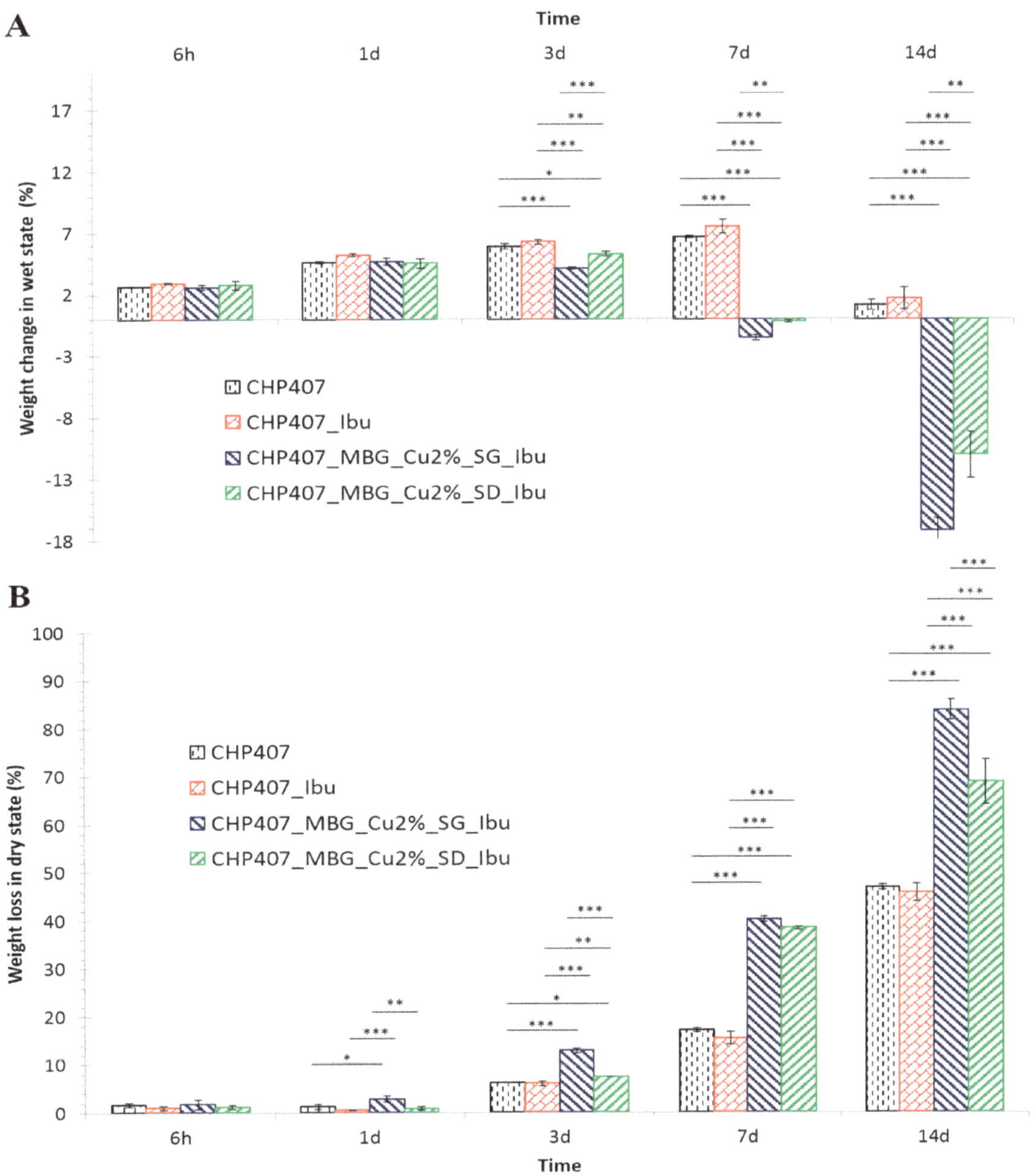

Figure 5. Swelling (**A**) and weight loss (**B**) of CHP407, CHP407_Ibu, CHP407_MBG_Cu2%_SG_Ibu and CHP407_MBG_Cu2%_SD_Ibu gels evaluated at 6 h, 1d, 3d, 7d and 14d.

SEC analysis was also performed on the residual polymer phase collected on day 14 (Figure 6).

A

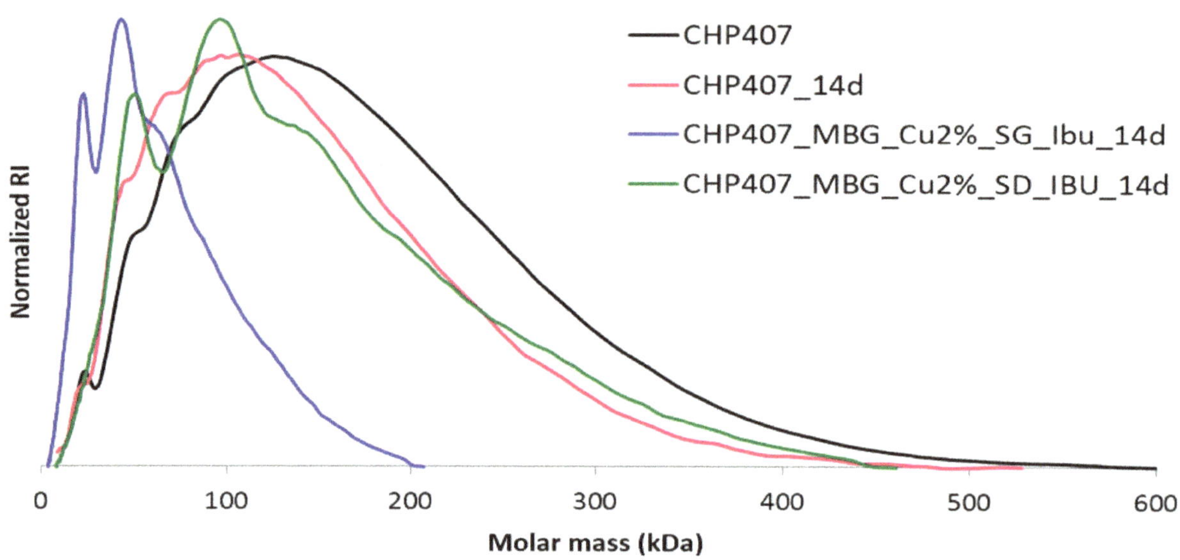

B

	M_n (Da)	D
CHP407	71670	1.7
CHP407_14d	64260	1.6
CHP407_MBG_Cu2%_SG_Ibu_14d	28746	1.6
CHP407_MBG_Cu2%_SD_Ibu_14d	28381	1.8

Figure 6. Molecular weight distribution (normalized refractive index (RI) vs. molar mass) (**A**) and estimated M_n and D values (**B**) of as synthesized CHP407 and residual CHP407 collected from CHP407, CHP407_MBG_Cu2%_SG_Ibu and CHP407_MBG_Cu2%_SD_Ibu gels incubated in aqueous medium for 14 days.

SEC revealed that the high destabilization of MBG containing gels in aqueous medium is ascribable to a progressive polymer chemical degradation, which was almost absent in pure CHP407 and CHP407_Ibu gels. In fact, CHP407 number average molecular weight decreased of about 60% and 10% in MBG-containing and pure hydrogel samples, respectively. In analogy with data concerning the bio-stability for poly(ether urethane)-based biomedical devices, such as pacemaker leads, this behavior can be ascribed to the occurrence of metal ion-mediated oxidation induced by the copper ions progressively released within the gels and the surrounding medium, which trigger the oxidative degradation of the polymer network [38,39].

3.3.3. Ion/Drug Release Test

Ibuprofen release profile from CHP407-based gels was assessed in physiological-like conditions, that is, Trizma® buffer at 37 °C (Figure 7).

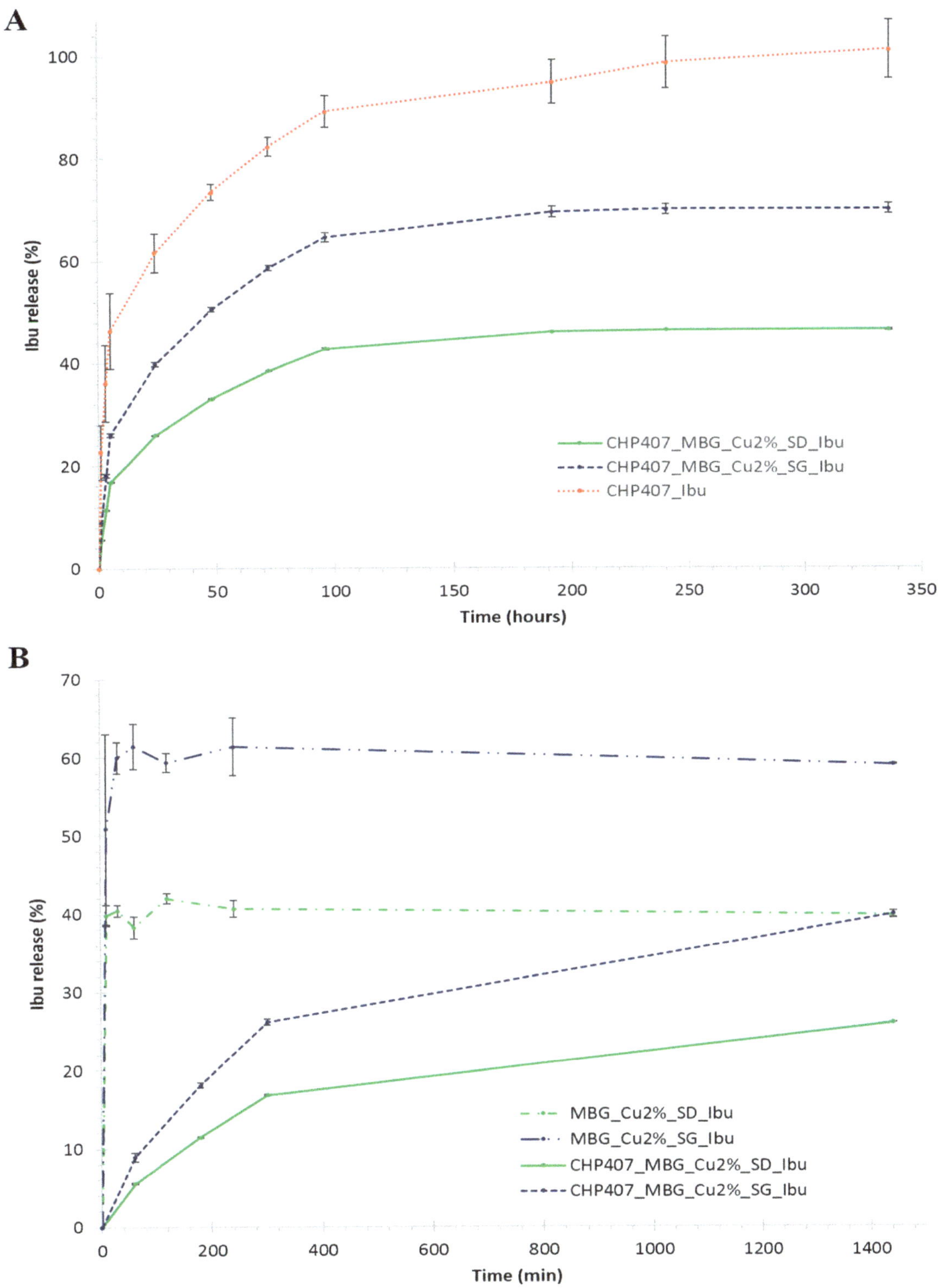

Figure 7. (**A**) Ibuprofen release (%) profile from CHP407_Ibu, CHP407_MBG_Cu2%_SG_Ibu and CHP407_MBG_Cu2%_SD_Ibu hydrogels. (**B**) Comparison among ibuprofen release profiles assessed from CHP407_MBG_Cu2%_SG_Ibu, CHP407_MBG_Cu2%_SD_Ibu, MBG_Cu2%_SD_Ibu and MBG_Cu2%_SD_Ibu.

Figure 7A compares ibuprofen release profiles from CHP407_Ibu, CHP407_MBG_Cu2%_SG_Ibu and CHP407_MBG_Cu2%_SD_Ibu up to 14 days observation time. A complete release of the drug was observed from the gels loaded with ibuprofen as such, with a release of 98.6 ± 5.0% at day

10. On the other hand, MBG-loaded gels showed a sustained and prolonged release of the drug, with a percentage release of 70.0 ± 1.0% and 46.4 ± 0.1% from CHP407_MBG_Cu2%_SG_Ibu and CHP407_MBG_Cu2%_SD_Ibu, respectively, after 14 days incubation. Moreover, starting from day 8 the release profile reached a plateau value for both particle-loaded gels, thus suggesting an incomplete ibuprofen release. However, this phenomenon cannot be avoided, being correlated to the progressive pore occlusion due to the dissolution of silica-based MBG framework and its re-precipitation as silica gel at the pores mouth, in accordance with observations reported by Mortera et al. [40], who, in addition, also reported a significant change of the delivery curves as a function of the release medium volume. To further investigate this aspect, the release profile of ibuprofen from MBG_Cu2%_SG_Ibu and MBG_Cu2%_SD_Ibu alone was studied in the same release conditions (in term of powder/medium volume ratio) adopted for hybrid hydrogel testing. As a matter of fact, both MBG_Cu2%_SG_Ibu and MBG_Cu2%_SD_Ibu showed a plateau ibuprofen release of 61.3 ± 3.7% and 40.6 ± 1.0% after 30 and 10 min incubation time, respectively. The significant difference in the maximum amount released can be attributed to the very high surface reactivity of spray-dried systems when soaked in aqueous media, leading to enhanced dissolution/re-precipitation phenomena and consequent hindered pore accessibility [16]. By comparing ibuprofen release kinetics from free MBGs and hydrogels containing MBG particles within the first 4 h, the role exerted by the polymeric matrix in modulating the release profile of ibuprofen was clearly highlighted (Figure 7B). In fact, a significant reduction ($0.0001 < p < 0.001$) in the initial burst release upon MBG incorporation within CHP407 gels was observed, with approx. 85% burst release reduction for both kinds of particles investigated. The release profile of copper ions from the developed hybrid formulations was also studied, showing a trend similar to that assessed for ibuprofen (Figure 8).

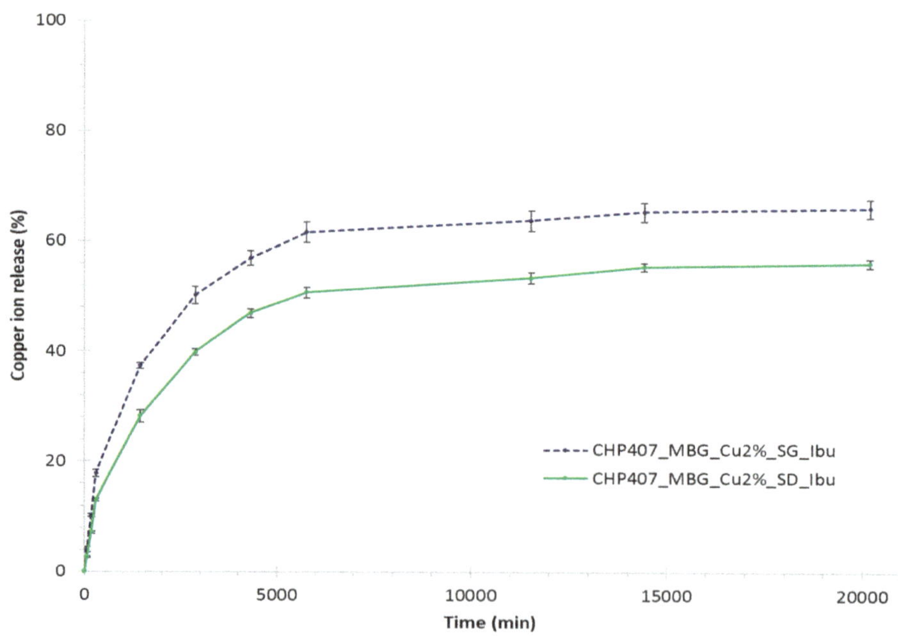

Figure 8. Copper ion release (%) profile from CHP407_MBG_Cu2%_SG_Ibu and CHP407_MBG_Cu2%_SD_Ibu gels.

After 14 days of incubation in aqueous medium, the 66.1 ± 1.6% and 56.1 ± 0.8% (corresponding to 291.5 ± 7.1 ppm and 192.3 ± 2.7 ppm, respectively) of the copper initially present in the MBG framework was released from CHP407_MBG_Cu2%_SG_Ibu and CHP407_MBG_Cu2%_SD_Ibu, respectively. These amounts fully agree with our previous results obtained for Cu-substituted MBGs without ibuprofen [16], highlighting that drug loading within MBG porous structure did not suppress or hinder the capability to release therapeutic ions through ion-exchange reactions. The incorporation of Cu-substituted MBGs within the polymeric phase successfully decreased the undesirable initial burst release of Cu^{2+} species typically observed for particles alone ($0.0001 < p < 0.001$). Indeed, after 1h incubation in similar releasing conditions, CHP407_MBG_Cu2%_SG_Ibu and CHP407_MBG_Cu2%_SD_Ibu released an amount of copper ions approximately 72 % and 61 % lower compared to the corresponding free MBG particles. Both ibuprofen and copper ions were released faster from CHP407_MBG_Cu2%_SG_Ibu compared to CHP407_MBG_Cu2%_SD_Ibu, in accordance with the higher surface area of MBG_Cu2%_SG_Ibu compared to MBG_Cu2%_SD_Ibu, which accounts for a faster molecule diffusion, either ions or drugs, through MBG porous network.

To clarify the ion/drug release mechanism, the equation of Korsmeyer-Peppas was employed to estimate the release exponent n within the timeframe 1–5 h (being Korsmeyer-Peppas equation valid up to 60% release). Ibuprofen delivery from CHP407_Ibu gels turned out to be a purely Fickian diffusion-driven release, with an n exponent of 0.45 ± 0.04. On the other hand, CHP407_MBG_Cu2%_SG_Ibu and CHP407_MBG_Cu2%_SD_Ibu gels released ibuprofen with an anomalous mechanism (n value of 0.66 ± 0.03 and 0.68 ± 0.01 for CHP407_MBG_Cu2%_SG_Ibu and CHP407_MBG_Cu2%_SD_Ibu, respectively), being the drug first diffused from the MBGs within the hydrogel and then through the hydrogel in the surrounding releasing medium. Interestingly, the release exponent clearly highlighted the coexistence of diffusion and ion exchange reactions when copper species were released, being n values higher than 0.89 (n value of 0.94 ± 0.08 and 0.90 ± 0.07 for CHP407_MBG_Cu2%_SG_Ibu and CHP407_MBG_Cu2%_SD_Ibu, respectively).

Taken together the obtained data proved the ability of the developed platform to co-deliver copper ions and ibuprofen with a sustained release profile. The final released concentration can be finely modulated to target the required therapeutic effect with no associated toxicity, by taking advantage of the several degrees of freedom offered by the hybrid system, such as the initial particle concentration within the gel solution (before gelation) and the amount of ion/drug loaded inside the MBG nanocarriers.

4. Conclusions

In this work, a first attempt toward the design of a hybrid sol-gel formulation able to simultaneously co-release copper ions (exerting pro-angiogenic and anti-bacterial effects) and an anti-inflammatory drug (ibuprofen) was successfully achieved. To this aim, Cu-substituted MBG (2% mol) particles were loaded with ibuprofen through an incipient wetness technique, resulting in a high loading capacity, and then embedded within PEU-based thermosensitive gels at the highest possible concentration (20 mg/mL), according to an optimized incorporation protocol. Full characterization of the resulting hybrid systems was performed to highlight the effects of particle encapsulation on gelation kinetics as well as on ions/drug release mechanism. The incorporation of MBG particles within the sol-gel systems did not negatively affect their capability to undergo a temperature-driven sol-to-gel transition within a few minutes. The progressive release of Cu^{2+} species was found to play a significant role on the stability of the gels in an aqueous environment and catalyzed the oxidation of the PEU chains. The co-release of copper ions and ibuprofen from hybrid formulations was sustained and prolonged over time for up to more than one week, with a strongly reduced initial burst effect compared to MBG particles alone (2%–4% vs. 7%–14% Cu^{2+} release and 6%–9% vs. 38%–61% ibuprofen release from hybrid MBG-polyurethane formulations and free MBG particles, respectively). However, the release profile of both copper species and ibuprofen was affected by the progressive occlusion of mesopores resulting from the dissolution and the re-precipitation of silica-based MBG framework in the form of a silica gel at the pore entrance [40–42].

Taken together the obtained data proved the ability of the proposed hybrid thermosensitive formulation to concentrate and maintain the MBG carriers at the pathological site and to guarantee in situ and prolonged co-release of ions and drugs, thus opening the way to the design of multifunctional platforms for advanced treatment of compromised tissue healing. The high versatility of the proposed approach lies in the possibility to modulate the relative amount of the organic and inorganic components, by changing the initial particle concentration within the hydrogel solution (before gelation), and/or the initial drug loading and the chemical composition of MBGs, in order to design systems able to co-release ions and pharmaceutics with concentrations and kinetics adapted to the targeted applications and not producing cytotoxic effects.

The versatility of the herein developed hybrid sol-gel systems could thus pave the way to the treatment of a great variety of pathological conditions of soft (e.g., non-healing wounds) and hard (e.g., delayed bone healing) tissues.

Author Contributions: Conceptualization, M.B., C.P., S.F. and R.L.; methodology, M.B., C.P. and R.L.; validation, M.B., C.P., S.F. and R.L.; formal analysis, M.B., C.P. and R.L.; investigation, M.B., C.P. and R.L.; resources, M.B., C.P. and R.L.; writing—original draft preparation, M.B., C.P., S.F. and R.L.; writing—review and editing, S.F., G.C. and C.V.-B.; visualization, M.B.; supervision, S.F., G.C. and C.V.-B.; funding acquisition, C.V.-B.

References

1. Kargozar, S.; Montazerian, M.; Hamzehlou, S.; Kim, H.W.; Baino, F. Mesoporous bioactive glasses: Promising platforms for antibacterial strategies. *Acta Biomater.* **2018**, *81*, 1–19. [CrossRef] [PubMed]
2. Vishnu Priya, M.; Sivshanmugam, A.; Boccaccini, A.R.; Goudouri, O.M.; Sun, W.; Hwang, N.; Deepthi, S.; Nair, S.V.; Jayakumar, R. Injectable osteogenic and angiogenic nanocomposite hydrogels for irregular bone defects. *Biomed. Mater.* **2016**, *11*, 035017. [CrossRef] [PubMed]
3. Lowe, S.B.; Tan, V.T.G.; Soeriyadi, A.H.; Davis, T.P.; Gooding, J.J. Synthesis and High-Throughput Processing of Polymeric Hydrogels for 3D Cell Culture. *Bioconjug. Chem.* **2014**, *25*, 1581–1601. [CrossRef] [PubMed]
4. Zhu, M.; Zhu, Y.; Zhang, L.; Shi, J. Preparation of chitosan / mesoporous silica nanoparticle composite hydrogels for sustained co-delivery of biomacromolecules and small chemical drugs. *Sci. Technol. Adv. Mater.* **2013**, *14*, 045005. [CrossRef] [PubMed]
5. Zhao, P.; Liu, H.; Deng, H.; Xiao, L.; Qin, C. Colloids and Surfaces B: Biointerfaces A study of chitosan hydrogel with embedded mesoporous silica nanoparticles loaded by ibuprofen as a dual stimuli-responsive drug release system for surface coating of titanium implants. *Colloids Surf. B Biointerfaces* **2014**, *123*, 657–663. [CrossRef] [PubMed]
6. Lunter, D.J. Evaluation of mesoporous silica particles as drug carriers in hydrogels. *Pharm. Dev. Technol.* **2017**, *23*, 826–831. [CrossRef] [PubMed]
7. Kim, B.S.; Chen, Y.; Srinoi, P.; Marquez, M.D.; Lee, T.R. Hydrogel-Encapsulated Mesoporous Silica-Coated Gold Nanoshells for Smart Drug Delivery. *Int. J. Mol. Sci.* **2019**, *20*, 3422. [CrossRef] [PubMed]
8. Lei, L.; Liu, Z.; Pingyun, Y.; Yuan, P.; Jin, R.; Wang, X.-d.; Jiang, T.; Chen, X. Injectable colloidal hydrogel with mesoporous silica nanoparticles for sustained co-release of microRNA-222 and aspirin to achieve innervated bone regeneration in rat mandibular defects. *J. Mater. Chem. B* **2019**, *7*, 2722–2735. [CrossRef]
9. Fiorilli, S.; Molino, G.; Pontremoli, C.; Iviglia, G.; Torre, E.; Cassinelli, C.; Morra, M.; Vitale-Brovarone, C. The incorporation of strontium to improve bone-regeneration ability of mesoporous bioactive glasses. *Materials* **2018**, *11*, 678. [CrossRef]
10. Zhou, Y.; Han, S.; Xiao, L.; Han, P.; Wang, S.; He, J.; Chang, J.; Wu, C.; Xiao, Y. Accelerated host angiogenesis and immune responses by ion release from mesoporous bioactive glass. *J. Mater. Chem. B* **2018**, *6*, 3274–3284. [CrossRef]
11. Wu, C.; Zhou, Y.; Xu, M.; Han, P.; Chen, L.; Chang, J.; Xiao, Y. Copper-containing mesoporous bioactive glass scaffolds with multifunctional properties of angiogenesis capacity, osteostimulation and antibacterial activity. *Biomaterials* **2013**, *34*, 422–433. [CrossRef] [PubMed]
12. Wang, X.; Cheng, F.; Liu, J.; Smått, J.H.; Gepperth, D.; Lastusaari, M.; Xu, C.; Hupa, L. Biocomposites of copper-containing mesoporous bioactive glass and nanofibrillated cellulose: Biocompatibility and angiogenic promotion in chronic wound healing application. *Acta Biomater.* **2016**, *46*, 286–298. [CrossRef] [PubMed]
13. Bari, A.; Bloise, N.; Fiorilli, S.; Novajra, G.; Vallet-Regí, M.; Bruni, G.; Torres-Pardo, A.; González-Calbet, J.M.; Visai, L.; Vitale-Brovarone, C. Copper-containing mesoporous bioactive glass nanoparticles as multifunctional agent for bone regeneration. *Acta Biomater.* **2017**, *55*, 493–504. [CrossRef] [PubMed]
14. Li, H.; Li, J.; Jiang, J.; Lv, F.; Chang, J.; Chen, S.; Wu, C. An osteogenesis / angiogenesis-stimulation artificial ligament for anterior cruciate ligament reconstruction. *Acta Biomater.* **2017**, *54*, 399–410. [PubMed]

15. Romero-sánchez, L.B.; Marí-beffa, M.; Carrillo, P.; Ángel, M.; Díaz-cuenca, A. Copper-containing mesoporous bioactive glass promotes angiogenesis in an in vivo zebrafish model. *Acta Biomater.* **2018**, *68*, 272–285. [CrossRef] [PubMed]
16. Pontremoli, C.; Boffito, M.; Fiorilli, S.; Laurano, R.; Torchio, A.; Bari, A.; Tonda-Turo, C.; Ciardelli, G.; Vitale-Brovarone, C. Hybrid injectable platforms for the in situ delivery of therapeutic ions from mesoporous glasses. *Chem. Eng. J.* **2018**, *340*, 103–113. [CrossRef]
17. Vergara-figueroa, J.; Alejandro-mart, S.; Pesenti, H. Obtaining Nanoparticles of Chilean Natural Zeolite and its Ion Exchange with Copper Salt (Cu^{2+}) for antibacterial applications. *Materials (Basel)* **2019**, *12*, 2202. [CrossRef]
18. Rosenberg, M.; Vija, H.; Kahru, A.; Keevil, C.W.; Ivask, A. Rapid in situ assessment of Cu-ion mediated effects and antibacterial efficacy of copper surfaces. *Sci. Rep.* **2018**, *8*, 8172. [CrossRef]
19. Barralet, J.; Gbureck, U.; Habibovic, P.; Vorndran, E.; Gerard, C.; Doillon, C.J. Angiogenesis in Calcium Phosphate Scaffolds by Inorganic Copper Ion Release. *Tissue Eng. Part A* **2009**, *15*, 1601–1609. [CrossRef]
20. Charnay, C.; Bégu, S.; Tourné-Péteilh, C.; Nicole, L.; Lerner, D.A.; Devoisselle, J.M. Inclusion of ibuprofen in mesoporous templated silica: Drug loading and release property. *Eur. J. Pharm. Biopharm.* **2004**, *57*, 533–540.
21. Boffito, M.; Gioffredi, E.; Chiono, V.; Calzone, S.; Ranzato, E.; Martinotti, S.; Ciardelli, G. Novel polyurethane-based thermosensitive hydrogels as drug release and tissue engineering platforms: Design and in vitro characterization. *Polym. Int.* **2016**, *65*, 756–769. [CrossRef]
22. Alsirawan, M.B.; Mohammad, M.A.; Alkasmi, B.; Alhareth, K.; El-Hammadi, M. Development and validation of a simple HPLC method for the determination of ibuprofen sticking onto punch faces. *Int. J. Pharm. Pharm. Sci.* **2013**, *5*, 227–231.
23. Boffito, M.; Brancot, A.G.; Lima, O.; Bronco, S.; Sartori, S.; Ciardelli, G.; Torino, P. Injectable thermosensitive gels for the localized and controlled delivery of biomolecules in tissue engineering/regenerative medicine. *Biomed. Sci. Eng.* **2019**, *3*. [CrossRef]
24. El-Fiqi, A.; Kim, T.-H.; Kim, M.; Eltohamy, M.; Won, J.-E.; Lee, E.-J.; Kim, H.-W. Capacity of mesoporous bioactive glass nanoparticles to deliver therapeutic molecules. *Nanoscale* **2012**, *4*, 7475–7488. [CrossRef] [PubMed]
25. Vallet-Regí, M. Ordered mesoporous materials in the context of drug delivery systems and bone tissue engineering. *Chem. Eur. J.* **2006**, *12*, 5934–5943. [CrossRef] [PubMed]
26. Mellaerts, R.; Jammaer, J.A.; Van Speybroeck, M.; Chen, H.; Van Humbeeck, J.; Augustijns, P.; Van den Mooter, G.; Martens, J.A. Physical state of poorly water soluble therapeutic\rmolecules loaded into SBA-15 ordered mesoporous silica carriers:\rA case study with itraconazole and ibuprofen. *Langmuir* **2008**, *24*, 8651–8659. [CrossRef] [PubMed]
27. Gonzalez, G.; Sagarzazu, A.; Zoltan, T. Infuence of Microstructure in Drug Release Behavior of Silica Nanocapsules. *J. Drug Deliv.* **2013**, *2013*, 803585. [CrossRef] [PubMed]
28. Hong, S.; Shen, S.; Tan, D.C.T.; Ng, W.K.; Liu, X.; Chia, L.S.O.; Irwan, A.W.; Tan, R.; Nowak, S.A.; Marsh, K.; et al. High drug load, stable, manufacturable and bioavailable fenofibrate formulations in mesoporous silica: A comparison of spray drying versus solvent impregnation methods. *Drug Deliv.* **2016**, *23*, 316–327. [CrossRef]
29. López-Noriega, A.; Arcos, D.; Izquierdo-Barba, I.; Sakamoto, Y.; Terasaki, O.; Vallet-Regí, M. Ordered mesoporous bioactive glasses for bone tissue regeneration. *Chem. Mater.* **2006**, *18*, 3137–3144. [CrossRef]
30. Brás, A.R.; Merino, E.G.; Neves, P.D.; Fonseca, I.M.; Dionísio, M.; Schönhals, A.; Correia, N.T. Amorphous ibuprofen confined in nanostructured silica materials: A dynamical approach. *J. Phys. Chem. C* **2011**, *115*, 4616–4623. [CrossRef]
31. Zhang, Y.; Zhi, Z.; Jiang, T.; Zhang, J.; Wang, Z.; Wang, S. Spherical mesoporous silica nanoparticles for loading and release of the poorly water-soluble drug telmisartan. *J. Control. Release* **2010**, *145*, 257–263. [CrossRef]
32. Fiorilli, S.; Onida, B.; Bonelli, B.; Garrone, E. In situ infrared study of SBA-15 functionalized with carboxylic groups incorporated by a Co-condensation route. *J. Phys. Chem. B* **2005**, *109*, 16725–16729. [CrossRef]
33. Cauda, V.; Fiorilli, S.; Onida, B.; Vernè, E.; Vitale Brovarone, C.; Viterbo, D.; Croce, G.; Milanesio, M.; Garrone, E. SBA-15 ordered mesoporous silica inside a bioactive glass-ceramic scaffold for local drug delivery. *J. Mater. Sci. Mater. Med.* **2008**, *19*, 3303–3310. [CrossRef]

34. Wang, F.; Hui, H.; Barnes, T.J.; Barnett, C.; Prestidge, C.A. Oxidized mesoporous silicon microparticles for improved oral delivery of poorly soluble drugs. *Mol. Pharm.* **2010**, *7*, 227–236. [CrossRef]
35. Shen, S.C.; Ng, W.K.; Hu, J.; Letchmanan, K.; Ng, J.; Tan, R.B.H. Solvent-free direct formulation of poorly-soluble drugs to amorphous solid dispersion via melt-absorption. *Adv. Powder Technol.* **2017**, *28*, 1316–1324. [CrossRef]
36. Sliwinska-Bartkowiak, M.; Dudziak, G.; Gras, R.; Sikorski, R.; Radhakrishnan, R.; Gubbins, K.E. Freezing behavior in porous glasses and MCM-41. *Colloids Surf. A Physicochem. Eng. Asp.* **2001**, *187–188*, 523–529. [CrossRef]
37. Radhakrishnan, R.; Gubbins, K.E.; Sliwinska-Bartkowiak, M. Effect of the fluid-wall interaction on freezing of confined fluids: Toward the development of a global phase diagram. *J. Chem. Phys.* **2000**, *112*, 11048–11057. [CrossRef]
38. Thoma, R.J.; Tan, F.R.; Phillips, R.E. Ionic Interactions of Polyurethanes. *J. Biomater. Appl.* **1988**, *3*, 180–206. [CrossRef]
39. Coury, A.J. Chemical and Biochemical Degradation of Polymers Intended to be Biostable. In *Biomaterials Science: An Introduction to Materials in Medicine*, 3rd ed.; Elsevier: Amsterdam, The Netherlands, 2013; ISBN 9780123746269.
40. Mortera, R.; Fiorilli, S.; Garrone, E.; Verné, E.; Onida, B. Pores occlusion in MCM-41 spheres immersed in SBF and the effect on ibuprofen delivery kinetics: A quantitative model. *Chem. Eng. J.* **2010**, *156*, 184–192. [CrossRef]
41. Li, P.; Nakanishi, K.; Kokubo, T.; de Groot, K. Induction and morphology of hydroxyapatite, precipitated from metastable simulated body fluids on sol-gel prepared silica. *Biomaterials* **1993**, *14*, 963–968. [CrossRef]
42. Li, P.; Kangasniemi, I.; de Groot, K.; Kokubo, T.; Yli-Urpo, A.U. Apatite crystallization from metastable calcium phosphate solution on sol-gel-prepared silica. *J. Non-Cryst. Solids* **1994**, *168*, 281–286. [CrossRef]

11

How Does the CO_2 in Supercritical State Affect the Properties of Drug-Polymer Systems, Dissolution Performance and Characteristics of Tablets Containing Bicalutamide?

Agata Antosik-Rogóż [1,*], Joanna Szafraniec-Szczęsny [1,2], Krzysztof Chmiel [3], Justyna Knapik-Kowalczuk [3], Mateusz Kurek [1], Karolina Gawlak [2], Vittorio P. Danesi [4], Marian Paluch [3] and Renata Jachowicz [1]

1 Department of Pharmaceutical Technology and Biopharmaceutics, Faculty of Pharmacy, Jagiellonian University Medical College, Medyczna 9, 30-688 Krakow, Poland; joanna.szafraniec@uj.edu.pl (J.S.-S.); mateusz.kurek@uj.edu.pl (M.K.); renata.jachowicz@uj.edu.pl (R.J.)
2 Department of Physical Chemistry and Electrochemistry, Faculty of Chemistry, Jagiellonian University, Gronostajowa 2, 30-387 Krakow, Poland; gawlak@chemia.uj.edu.pl
3 Institute of Physics, Faculty of Science and Technology, University of Silesia, SMCEBI, 75 Pułku Piechoty 1a, 41-500 Chorzow, Poland; krzysztof.chmiel@smcebi.edu.pl (K.C.); justyna.knapik-kowalczuk@smcebi.edu.pl (J.K.-K.); marian.paluch@smcebi.edu.pl (M.P.)
4 Department of Drugs Sciences, University of Pavia, viale Taramelli, 12-27100 Pavia, Italy; vittoriopaolo.danesi01@universitadipavia.it
* Correspondence: agata.antosik@uj.edu.pl

Abstract: The increasing demand for novel drug formulations has caused the introduction of the supercritical fluid technology, CO_2 in particular, into pharmaceutical technology as a method enabling the reduction of particle size and the formation of inclusion complexes and solid dispersions. In this paper, we describe the application of $scCO_2$ in the preparation of binary systems containing poorly soluble antiandrogenic drug bicalutamide and polymeric excipients, either Macrogol 6000 or Poloxamer®407. The changes in the particle size and morphology were followed using scanning electron microscopy and laser diffraction measurements. Differential scanning calorimetry was applied to assess thermal properties, while X-ray powder diffractometry was used to determine the changes in the crystal structure of the systems. The dissolution of bicalutamide was also considered. Binary solid dispersions were further compressed, and the attributes of tablets were assessed. Tablets were analyzed directly after manufacturing and storage in climate chambers. The obtained results indicate that the use of supercritical CO_2 led to the morphological changes of particles and the improvement of drug dissolution. The flowability of blends containing processed binary systems was poor; however, they were successfully compressed into tablets exhibiting enhanced drug release.

Keywords: Bicalutamide; Poloxamer® 407; Macrogol 6000; supercritical carbon dioxide; solid dispersions; dissolution rate; amorphization

1. Introduction

The growing number of active pharmaceutical ingredients (APIs) are characterized by poor water solubility. Currently, more than 70% of APIs under development are considered as poorly water soluble and almost 40% present in the pharmaceutical industry possesses aqueous solubility less than 100 μg/mL. Most of them belong to the second class of the Biopharmaceutical Classification System (BCS). These compounds are characterized by low solubility and high intestinal membrane permeability [1].

Given that the oral bioavailability of active pharmaceutical ingredients depends on their solubility and/or dissolution rate, many methods of solubility improvement have been developed [2]. They include chemical modifications, such as prodrugs [3,4] or salt formation [5], physical processes as micronization or polymorph transitions, as well as the preparation of drug-carrier systems, including solid dispersions (SD) [6,7] and complexes with cyclodextrins [8–11]. Solid dispersions are defined as drug-carrier systems in which a hydrophobic active pharmaceutical ingredient is either molecularly dispersed in a hydrophilic matrix or exists as micro-fine crystals [12]. The matrix can be made from low molecular weight compounds, or more frequently, hydrophilic polymers. They provide the dissolution rate improvement, particle size reduction, reduction of agglomeration, wettability improvement that are achieved by solid dispersion [13,14]. They possess different functional groups, molecular weight, melting temperatures (T_m), and glass transition temperatures (T_g). They can be crystalline (poly(vinyl alcohol)), semicrystalline (poly L-lactic acid), or amorphous (polyvinylpyrrolidone). Moreover, each polymer is characterized by different abilities to maintain molecular dispersion of active substances [15]. Drug-polymer solid dispersions are formed using evaporation methods, such as spray drying, and melting methods, including extrusion. These techniques often require high temperatures, which can influence the stability of the active substance, or high amounts of solvents, which may increase product toxicity and affect the environment [16]. These undesirable effects can be avoided by using supercritical fluid technology for solid dispersion preparation. The most commonly used gas is carbon dioxide, which is a non-toxic, non-flammable and widely available substance. In the supercritical state, i.e., above the critical temperature (31.4 °C) and pressure (74 bar), it is viscous and permeable like gaseous substances, while the density is comparable with liquids. It can act as a solvent and/or as a plasticizer for many substances. Also, it is easy to remove from the product after processing, so it is possible to obtain a solvent-free product without a dedicated solvent removal process [16–19].

Currently, tablets are the most popular dosage form. This is due to the ease of administration, neutral taste, appropriate stability and low cost of manufacturing [20–23]. Given that compression is an integral part of tableting, the effect of applied the compression force on the physical stability of the drug needs to be considered, especially in the case of the compounds undergoing mechanically induced activation [24,25]. One of such is bicalutamide, a non-steroidal antiandrogen, which belongs to class II of the Biopharmaceutics Classification System, exhibiting low aqueous solubility (below 5 μg/mL) and high lipophilicity (logP = 2.92) [26]. Th drug undergoes polymorph transition (from physically stable form I to metastable form II) or amorphization upon mechanical treatment as a consequence of a need for the relaxation of stress field applied during milling [27,28]. Drug amorphization was previously described upon milling and spray drying with polyviylpyrrolidone (PVP) [29,30]. Given that glassy bicalutamide recrystallizes easily upon grinding or scratching, the effect of increased pressure on physical stability needs to be investigated deeply. Although many papers describe the effect of temperature and humidity on the stability of amorphous drugs, the effect of pressure applied to solid dispersions during tableting was rarely described [31]. Also, only a few papers describe how the tableting and storage of solid dispersions affect the dissolution performance of bicalutamide.

The polymers chosen for this study were polyethylene glycol (Macrogol 6000, PEG6000,) and Poloxamer® 407 (PLX407). These excipients are commonly used for solid dispersion preparation due to their solubilizing effects, surface adsorption, and wetting enhancement. Macrogols are widely used as carriers due to their low melting point, fast solidification, and capability of forming solid drug solutions [32,33]. However, the presence of a crystalline form may result in unstable formulations and lower dissolution rates [32]. For some drug-active substances, the improvement in solubility enhancement by Poloxamer is more efficient than by Macrogols [34]. Poloxamers, also called pluronics, are amphiphilic block copolymers consisting of hydrophilic ethylene oxide blocks (EO) attached to a central polypropylene oxide unit (PO) of hydrophobic character. They are widely used as carriers, mostly due to a low melting point. Moreover, the differences in the solubility of the constituent blocks of poloxamer macromolecule lead to thermo-responsive self-assembly in an aqueous environment, which is the additional advantage for solubility enhancement [35].

In our studies, we evaluated the use of the supercritical carbon dioxide ($scCO_2$) method as a way to obtain solid dispersions with bicalutamide, which were further (after mixing with excipients) compressed into tablets. The effect of tableting and storage in both normal and accelerated conditions was evaluated together with drug dissolution performance.

2. Materials and Methods

2.1. Materials

Bicalutamide (BCL, 99.3% purity, Hangzhou Hyper Chemicals Limited, Hangzhou, China) was used as an active substance: molecular formula $C_{18}H_{14}F_4N_2O_4S$, molecular weight 430.4 g/mol, solubility in water 3.7 μg/mL, logP = 2.92, pKa = 12.6, melting point 196 °C. Macrogol 6000 (PEG6000, Clariant, Muttenz, Switzerland): molecular formula $H(OCH_2CH_2)_nOH$, average n = 100, nonionic substance, melting point 65 °C, and Poloxamer® 407 (PLX407, BASF, Ludwigshafen am Rhein, Germany), molecular formula $HO(C_2H_4O)_a(C_3H_6O)_b(C_2H_4O)_aH$ a = 101, b = 56; average molecular weight 9840–14,600 g/mol, melting point 55 °C, freely soluble polymers were used as carriers. Carbon dioxide (CO_2; 99.99% purity, Pszczyna, Linde Gaz, Poland) was used as a supercritical fluid. Sodium lauryl sulfate (SLS; 98.8% purity; BASF) was used to prepare dissolution medium. Distilled water was used to prepare all the solutions. Cellulose microcrystalline (JRS Pharma, Rosenberg, Germany), sodium starch glycolate (DFE Pharma, Goch, Germany) and magnesium stearate (Merck, Darmstadt, Germany) were used as excipients to formulate tablets. All excipients used to formulate tablets were of pharmaceutical grade.

2.2. Methods

2.2.1. Solid Dispersion Preparation Using Supercritical Carbon Dioxide ($scCO_2$)

Bicalutamide and carriers, i.e., Macrogol 6000 or Poloxamer® 407, were mixed in a 1:1 weight ratio and loaded into a high-pressure reactor BR-300 (Berghof Products + Instruments GmbH, Eningen unter Achalm, Germany) equipped with a magnetic stirrer MR Hei-Standard (Heidolph Instruments, Schwabach, Germany), a heating mantle and a CHY 700T thermometer (CHY Firemate Co., Tainan City, Taiwan). To obtain supercritical conditions, carbon dioxide was pumped and compressed into a high-pressure reactor by a syringe pump SFT-10 (Supercritical Fluid Technologies Inc., Newark, NJ, USA). The process was conducted at 50 °C and 150 bar with Macrogol 6000 as a carrier, and at 60 °C and 160 bar with Poloxamer®407. In both cases, the magnetic stirrer was set at 500 rpm. The process parameters were monitored during the whole operation. The total mass of powder introduced into the high-pressure reactor was equal to 2 g. After the process, solid dispersions were pulverized through 1.8 mm sieve.

2.2.2. Scanning Electron Microscopy (SEM)

The morphological characterization of the samples was conducted using a Phenom Pro desktop electron microscope (Phenom World, Thermo Fisher Scientific, Waltham, MA, USA). Powdered samples were placed on the conductive adhesive tape glued to the specimen mount and measured in a holder for non-conductive samples. The acceleration voltage was equal to 10 kV. The stream of argon was used to remove the powder loosely bounded to the tape before the measurement.

2.2.3. Laser Diffraction Measurements

A Malvern Mastersizer 3000 (Malvern, UK) equipped with a HydroEV unit was used to determine particle size distribution. The samples were analyzed by the wet method using cyclohexane (reflective index, RI = 1.426) as a dispersant. Fraunhofer diffraction theory was applied to find the relationship between the particle size and the light intensity distribution pattern. The reported data represents the medians (D50 values) calculated as averages from ten series of measurements of each sample and the distribution span.

2.2.4. Powder X-Ray Diffraction (PXRD)

The diffraction patterns of the samples, i.e., pure substances, solid dispersions, and tablets, were registered at ambient temperature using an X-ray Rigaku Mini Flex II diffractometer (Tokyo, Japan) with a 5°/min step. Samples were scanned from 3° to 45°. Monochromatic Cu Kα radiation (λ = 1.5418 Å) was used.

2.2.5. Differential Scanning Calorimetry (DSC)

The thermal properties of the solid dispersions, raw bicalutamide, and carriers were examined using a differential scanning calorimetry (DSC) 1 STARe System (Mettler-Toledo, Greifensee, Switzerland). The measuring device was equipped with an HSS8 ceramic sensor with 120 thermocouples and a liquid nitrogen cooling station. The instrument was calibrated for temperature and enthalpy using zinc and indium standards. The glass transition temperature, crystallization, and melting were determined as the midpoint of the glass transition step, the onset of the exothermic peak, and the peak of the endothermic event, respectively. The samples were measured in an aluminum crucible (40 µL). The sample mass used for DSC experiments varied between 7 to 10 mg. All measurements were carried out with and without annealing (T = 323 K; t = 10 min). The experiments were performed from 273 to 478 K, with a heating rate equal to 10 K/min.

2.2.6. Preparation of Tablet Blends

The composition of each three formulations containing raw BCL or solid dispersions are presented in Section 3.3. Bicalutamide or solid dispersions were manually mixed with excipients: cellulose microcrystalline as a filler for 3 min, sodium starch glycolate as a disintegrant for 3 min and magnesium stearate as a lubricant for 1 min, in the porcelain dish.

2.2.7. Tableting Process and Tablet Characterization

The compression of tablets blends was performed using a single punch tableting machine (Korsch EK0, Berlin, Germany) equipped with the round flat punches which are 8 mm in diameter; each tablet type contained 50 mg of the active substance. Punches were equipped with tensiometers connected to a computer by Esam Traveler 1 Data Acquisition System Master Unit, type 0508-S-ESA (ESA Messtechnik GmbH, München, Germany). To obtain tablets that possess satisfactory properties, the pressure force applied on a blend containing raw bicalutamide and solid dispersions was equal to 7 kN (140 MPa) and 2 kN (40 MPa), respectively.

The mass uniformity of tablets was measured based on the method described in European Pharmacopoeia (Ph. Eur.) 9.0. The hardness, thickness and diameter of 20 randomly selected tablets were measured using hardness tester apparatus (VanKel VK200, Agilent Technologies, Santa Clara, CA, USA) and expressed as a mean value with standard deviation. The friability test was performed using a Pharma Test apparatus (Pharma Test Apparatebau AG, Hainburg, Germany). The disintegration time of the tablets was measured in distilled water at 37 °C using an Electrolab ED-2 SAPO (Electrolab, Mumbai, India) disintegration apparatus at 30 strokes/min.

2.2.8. Dissolution Studies

The dissolution studies were carried out using the method recommended by the Food and Drug Administration (FDA) for BCL tablets, i.e., United States Pharmacopeia (USP) paddle apparatus (II type), and the parameters, i.e., 50 rpm, 1000 mL of 1% SLS solution, 37 ± 0.5 °C. The analysis was performed in a Vision Elite 8 apparatus (Hanson Research, Chatsworth, CA, USA) equipped with a Vision G2 AutoPlus Autosampler, and an AutoFill sample collector (Hanson Research, Chatsworth, CA, USA). Samples, i.e., raw BCL, physical mixture, and solid dispersions obtained by supercritical carbon dioxide methods, containing the equivalent of 50 mg of the active substance, as well as prepared tablets, were poured into the beakers. A volume of 5 mL of the samples was withdrawn from each dissolution vessel at predefined intervals, filtered, diluted, and assayed spectrophotometrically at $\lambda = 272$ nm (UV-1800 Shimadzu, Shimadzu Corporation, Kyoto, Japan). After the collection of each sample, the dissolution medium was replaced with the same volume of pure one. The tests were carried out in triplicate, and the results represent averages with their standard deviations.

2.2.9. Contact Angle Measurements

A DSA255 drop shape analyzer (Krüss, Hamburg, Germany) was used to measure the contact angles using a sessile drop technique. A droplet of distilled water of volume equal to 2 μL was deposited on the surface of prepared tablets.

2.2.10. Stability Studies

Tablets were packed into PVC/Al blisters and placed in climate chambers (Memmert GmbH + Co. KG, Schwabach, Germany) and stored in either 25 °C/60% relative humidity (long-term conditions) or 40 °C/75% relative humidity (accelerated conditions). After six-month storage, tablets were analyzed for the following parameters: mass, hardness, thickness, contact angle, and dissolution rate of bicalutamide. The solid dispersion was analyzed after its preparation. The tablets' properties were evaluated just after the preparation and after the stability studies.

3. Results and Discussion

3.1. Solid-State Characteristics of Solid Dispersions

Based on the SEM results (Figure 1), raw bicalutamide exhibited elongated crystals of smooth surfaces. They were hexagonal and 30–160 μm long (Figure 1A). The median of the particle size distribution determined using a laser diffraction measurements laid was 81.7 μm (Table 1). The analysis of microphotographs of carriers indicated that Macrogol 6000 exhibited irregular particles of smooth surface and length not exceeding 100 μm (Figure 1B). In the case of the particles of Poloxamer® 407, they were smooth and spherical, of a diameter varying between 50 μm and 250 μm (Figure 1C). The medians of the particle size were 113 μm and 180 μm for PEG6000 and PLX407, respectively (Table 1). However, the distribution span for PEG6000 was much higher than for the other compounds, which indicated a wide distribution. The analysis of the particle size distribution revealed the presence of dust particles in each sample visible as a distribution tail within the region below 10 μm (Figure 2). In the case of bicalutamide and PLX407 the distributions were narrow and symmetrical (despite said tails), while in the case of Macrogol, the particle size was distributed uneven, with a maximum shift towards big particles. The distribution curve is skewed to the left, which can explain the differences between the size calculated from the SEM picture and laser diffraction measurements. The particles visualized using an electron microscope represent the fraction described by the extended distribution shoulder visible on the left side of the plot (pictures showing greater particles at the same magnification were not representative enough and are not presented here), while the laser diffraction assessed all the particles present in the sample.

After the treatment of BCL-PEG6000 binary mixtures by a supercritical carbon dioxide at 130 bar and 50 °C in the high-pressure reactor, solid dispersions were pulverized and white, free-flowing powders were obtained. In the case of solid dispersion with Poloxamer® 407, prepared at higher process parameters, i.e., pressure 140 bar, temperature 60 °C. The obtained sample also was white; however, its structure was foamy. After pulverized, white, free flowing powder was obtained.

Solid dispersions morphology was analyzed using SEM. The obtained results showed that the sample containing Macrogol 6000 exhibited irregular particles of a smooth surface with well-visible incorporated particles of different contrast. They were identified as the crystals of the active substance (Figure 1D). The particles of the solid dispersion with Poloxamer® 407 were rough, with visible inclusions of BCL crystals (Figure 1E).

Table 1. Particles size distribution of raw bicalutamide and carriers, results obtained by the laser diffraction method.

Substance	D_{50} (μm)	Span
Bicalutamide	81.7	1.70
Macrogol 6000	113.0	3.18
Poloxamer® 407	180.0	2.02
BCL-PEG6000	1120	2.01
BCL-PLX407	356	2.90

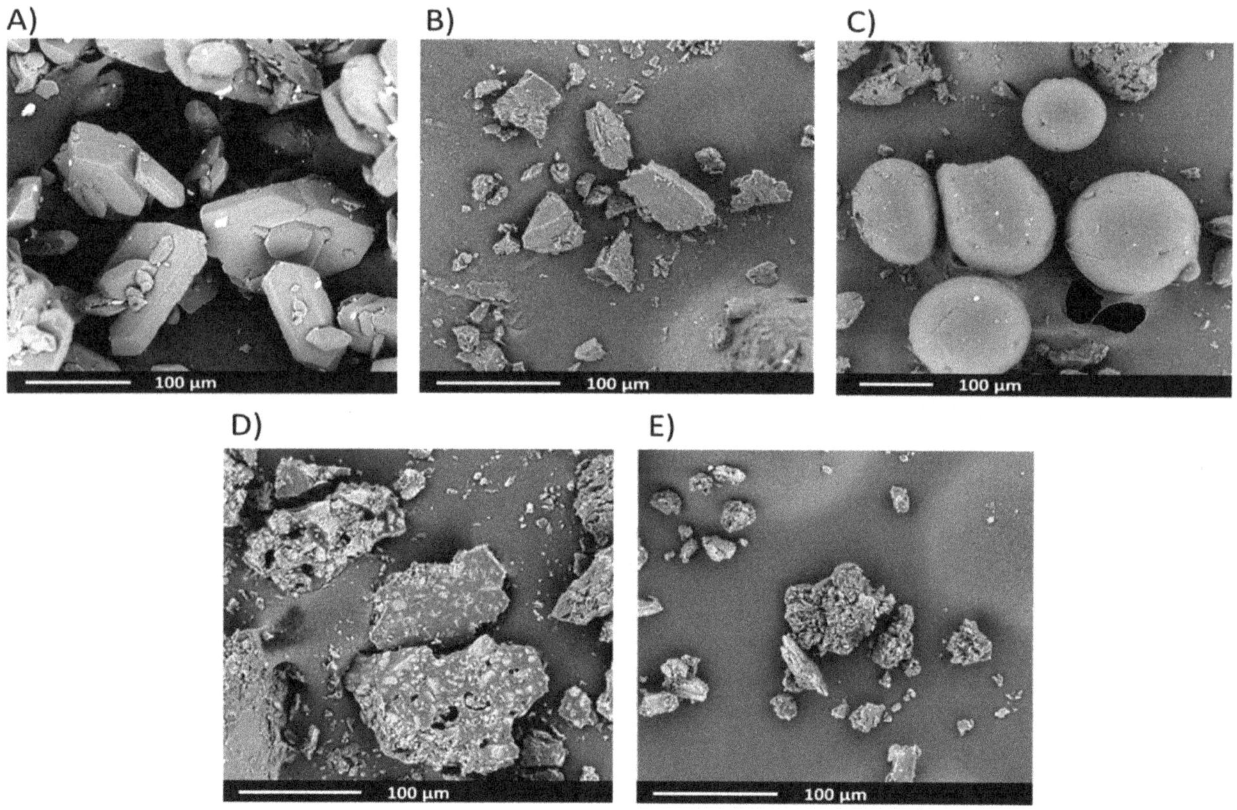

Figure 1. SEM image of raw bicalutamide (**A**), PEG6000 (**B**), PLX407 (**C**), BCL-PEG6000, (**D**) and BCL-PLX407 (**E**) solid dispersions.

The laser diffraction measurements revealed that solid dispersions exhibited a wide particle size distribution, in both cases skewed to the left, with two visible modes (Figure 2). The median of BCL-PEG6000 solid dispersion particles lay above 1 mm, which could be a result of the intense laser light diffraction on big particles and the presence of a well-resolved mode of the distribution curve. In the case of solid dispersion with Poloxamer® 407, the median of the particle size distribution was equal to 356 μm (Figure 2).

The thermal properties were obtained using differential scanning calorimetry (DSC). The presence of an endothermic peak with an onset at 196 °C corresponds to the melting temperature of form I polymorph of bicalutamide (Figure 3). After the treatment with supercritical CO_2, decreases in bicalutamide crystallinity in both obtained solid dispersions were noticed. This was confirmed by a decrease in the melting temperature of the active substance. For the solid dispersion prepared with Macrogol 6000, the melting of bicalutamide was recorded as an onset at 152.6 °C. The presence of the second endothermic peak with the onset at 60 °C corresponds to the melting point of the carrier. In the case of solid dispersions with Poloxamer® 407, the glass transition temperature was recorded at −6.2 °C. Bicalutamide crystallization occurred at 145.4 °C, while it melted at 167.4 °C. This indicated that the treatment with supercritical CO_2 led to drug amorphization. However, the system was characterized by very low physical stability in ambient conditions, expressed as a negative value of T_g. It resulted from low values of PLX407 T_g, −65 °C, combined with T_g of amorphous form of bicalutamide equal to 55 °C [36,37].

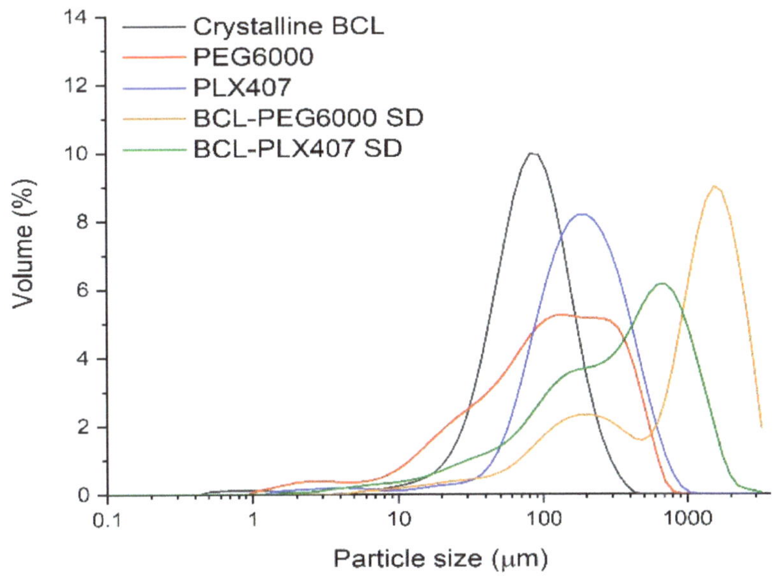

Figure 2. The particle size distribution of raw bicalutamide, polymers, and solid dispersions.

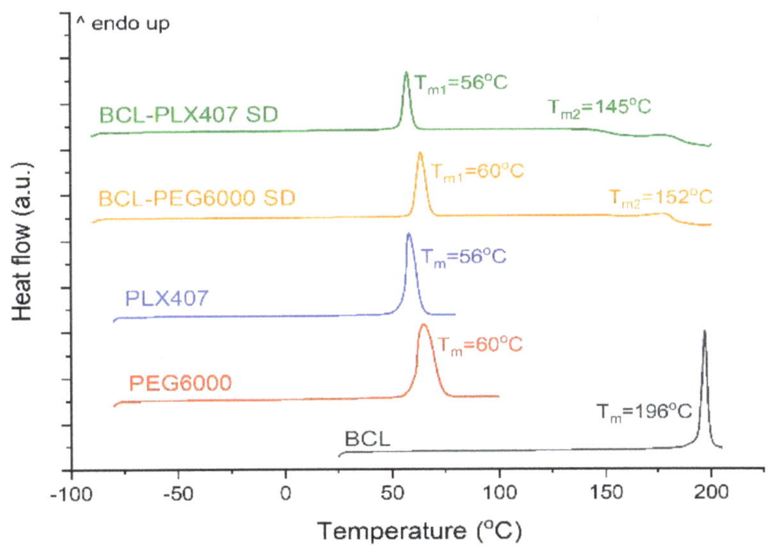

Figure 3. Scanning differential calorimetry of raw bicalutamide, polymers, and solid dispersions.

The molecular structure of each compound and solid dispersions was assessed using X-ray diffractometry. The diffraction pattern of raw bicalutamide is characteristic for crystalline form I polymorph, rich in distinctive Braggs peaks at 2θ equal to 6.2°, 9.5°, 12.3°, 14.3°–14.6°, 17.0°, 19.0°, 20.0°, and 24.0° (Figure 4). In the case of the used carriers, the diffraction patterns showed only two signals for each component, resulting from the semi-crystalline nature of the polymers. A decrease in the drug crystallinity was noticed in both types of solid dispersions. It was demonstrated by the decrease in the intensity and broadening of the peaks (Figure 4). Interestingly, the positions of the peaks shifted in comparison with the initial form of the drug. This indicated the recrystallization into the second polymorph of BCL, with the Braggs peaks positioned at 12.8°, 17.4°, 19.5°, 23.7–24.3°, and 25.4° [27].

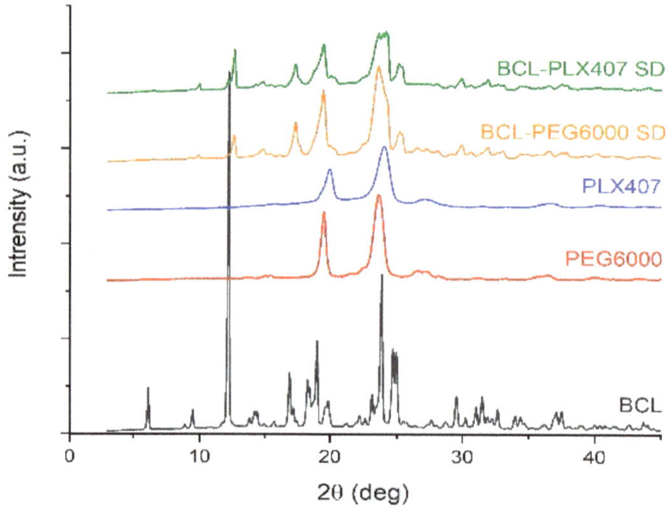

Figure 4. X-ray diffraction of raw bicalutamide and carriers, i.e., Macrogol 6000 and Poloxamer® 407, and solid dispersions.

3.2. Bicalutamide Dissolution

The preparation of solid dispersions using the supercritical carbon dioxide method with Macrogol 6000 and Poloxamer®407 led to a decrease in bicalutamide crystallinity, which resulted in dissolution improvement. The dissolution profiles of bicalutamide were very similar in both types of solid dispersions (Figure 5). After 1 h, 74.80 ± 1.66% of the drug dissolved from BCL-PEG6000 solid dispersion, and 77.43 ± 6.01% from the BCL-PLX407 one. The amount of bicalutamide dissolved from solid dispersions was approximately nine times greater than that determined for crystalline bicalutamide (form I polymorph), as 8.85 ± 1.02% of pure drug dissolved. No significant differences in the drug dissolution characteristics were noticed after the physical mixing of the active substance with any of the two polymers (approximately 12% of drug dissolved from each mixture). This confirms that the hydrophilic character of the carriers was not a crucial factor driving drug dissolution, and the dissolution improvement was related to the changes that occurred after the treatment with supercritical CO_2. During the process, the drug substance was dissolved in the polymer in supercritical CO_2, and the magnetic stirrer ensured uniform mixing of the ingredients. In the process of carbon dioxide removal, the sample solidified as a result of the rapid decrease in pressure. It provided homogenous distribution of the drug substance in the carrier.

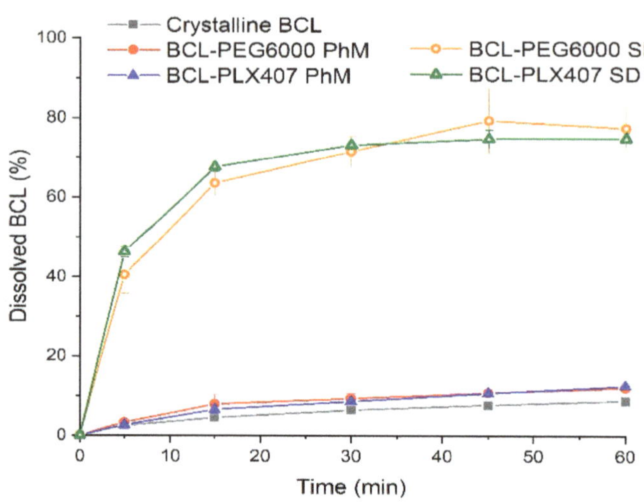

Figure 5. Dissolution of bicalutamide from solid dispersions with Macrogol 6000 and Poloxamer®407 in comparison with physical mixtures and crystalline bicalutamide (form I polymorph).

3.3. Characteristics of Tablets Containing BCL-PEG6000, BCL-PLX407 Solid Dispersions and Raw BCL

The three types of tablets were prepared using the direct compression method. The BCL-PEG6000 and BCL-PLX407 solid dispersions and raw bicalutamide were mixed with cellulose microcrystalline, sodium starch glycolate, and magnesium stearate to formulate tablets (Table 2). The obtained results revealed that hardness, thickness and friability were satisfactory.

Table 2. The composition of tablets containing BCL-PEG6000 and BCL-PLX407 solid dispersions and raw bicalutamide.

Substance	Tablets					
	Raw BCL		Solid Dispersion			
			BCL-PEG6000		BCL-PLX407	
	Content of Compounds in One Tablet					
	mg	%	mg	%	mg	%
BCL	50.00	41.67	-	-	-	-
BCL-Polymer (SD)	-	-	100.00	58.82	100.00	58.82
Cellulose Microcrystalline	64.00	53.33	64.00	37.65	64.00	37.65
Sodium starch glycolate	4.80	4.00	4.80	2.82	4.80	2.82
Magnesium stearate	1.20	1.00	1.20	0.71	1.20	0.71

The analysis of hardness showed that the tablets containing solid dispersions were characterized by higher hardness than those with raw bicalutamide (Table 3). This resulted from the binding properties of the used carriers, which also affected the disintegration time. Tablets containing solid dispersions disintegrated for longer than tablets with raw bicalutamide. Moreover, the tablets with BCL-PLX407 solid dispersion exhibited a six-fold longer disintegration time than those with BCL-PEG6000 solid dispersion, 24 min 22 s and 4 min 23 s, respectively. The difference was caused by the properties of poloxamer, which behaves like a binding substance [38]. During the compression process, particles tend to aggregate and increase the number of direct contact points between them, which extends tablet disintegration. Despite the surface activity and solubilizing activity of the polymer, a great content of poloxamer in the sample can retard tablet disintegration due to the gelling properties of the polymer [38–40].

Table 3. The properties of tablets containing solid dispersions (SD) and crystalline bicalutamide.

System \ Parameter	Mass (mg)	Thickness (mm)	Hardness (kp)	Friability (%)	Disintegration Time (min:s)	Contact Angle (°)
SD BCL-PEG6000	169.3 ± 7.0	3.60 ± 0.04	2.87 ± 0.63	0.0	4:23	50.8
SD BCL-PLX407	168.1 ± 5.8	3.43 ± 0.04	2.28 ± 0.64	0.4	24:22	55.8
Raw BCL	121.5 ± 3.6	2.08 ± 0.04	1.97 ± 0.25	0.6	00:31	85.4

The use of hydrophilic polymers in solid dispersion resulted in an increase in the wettability of the surface in comparison with the tablets containing raw bicalutamide. The tablets containing solid dispersions were more hydrophilic. They exhibited lower values of contact angles than the tablets with crystalline BCL:50.8° and 55.8° for the tablets containing PEG6000 and PLX407, respectively.

The X-ray diffraction analysis indicated that the active substance was amorphous. The presence of a broad halo instead of the Braggs peaks characteristic for crystalline drug substances, visible in Figure 4, indicated that bicalutamide was amorphous in all tested tablets (Figure 6). We assumed that this resulted from the propensity of bicalutamide to undergo activation upon mechanical treatment [10,12,27]. This means that the material gains some amount of energy which needs to be released. The relaxation of the stress field, applied during compression, occurs in several ways, including amorphization, as in the case of investigated tablets.

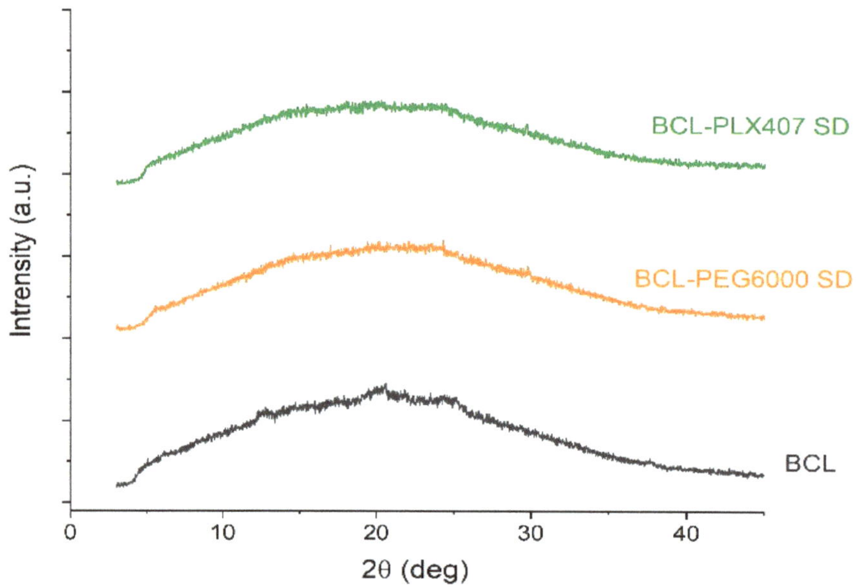

Figure 6. Diffraction patterns of tablets containing raw bicalutamide and solid dispersions.

As shown in Figure 7, bicalutamide release from the tablets indicated that the use of solid dispersions in tablets significantly enhanced drug release. This resulted from the improved wettability and amorphization of bicalutamide upon compression. After 1 h, 80.16 ± 8.56% and 56.61 ± 4.84% of the drug released from the tablets with PEG6000 and PLX407 solid dispersions, respectively. From tablets containing raw bicalutamide, 17.99 ± 1.70% dissolved, which was two times greater in comparison with the drug alone. Although the dissolution of bicalutamide from both solid dispersions was comparable at each time point, the differences in profiles were noticeable between solid dispersions (Figure 5) and corresponding tablets. After 30 min, 28% more bicalutamide was dissolved from tablets containing BCL-PEG6000 solid dispersion in comparison with the BCL-PLX407 tablets.

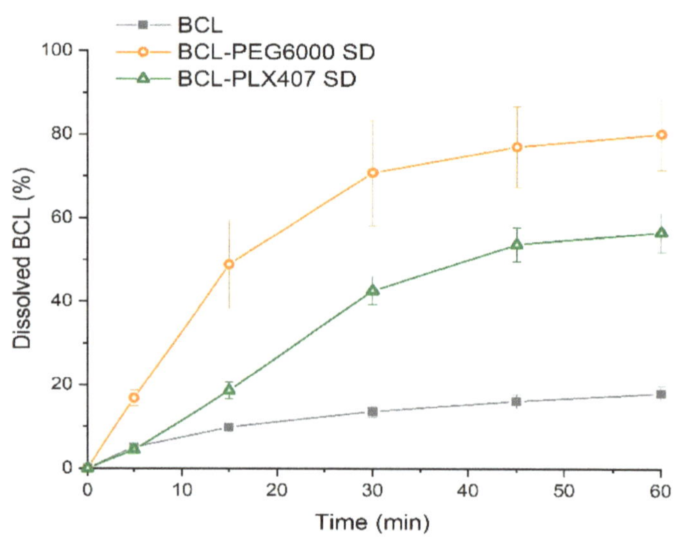

Figure 7. Dissolution profile of tablets containing solid dispersions and raw bicalutamide.

The prepared tablets were evaluated for stability upon storage. The results of the studies after six months revealed that the storage in both the long-term and accelerated conditions affected the properties of the tablets (Table 4) in comparison with tablets analyzed immediately after preparation (please refer to Table 3).

Table 4. Properties of tablets after six months of storage.

Parameter / System	Mass (mg)	Hardness (kp)	Thickness (mm)	Disintegration Time (min:s)	Contact Angle (°)
		25 °C, 60% RH			
SD BCL-PEG	168.3 ± 3.5	2.47 ± 0.15	3.66 ± 0.01	04:57	48.9
SD BCL-PLX	174.5 ± 5.1	2.63 ± 0.51	3.53 ± 0.05	27:10	58.9
		40 °C, 75% RH			
SD BCL-PEG	177.0 ± 4.4	1.80 ± 0.36	3.73 ± 0.08	04:59	59.8
SD BCL-PLX	175.9 ± 5.5	1.25 ± 0.07	3.76 ± 0.06	14:39	53.8

In both types of tablets, drug release decreased after storage, regardless of the storage conditions (Figure 8A,B). However, less noticeable changes occurred for tablets stored at 25 °C and 60% RH. The amount of dissolved bicalutamide was 70.42% and 50.82% in the case of tablets containing solid dispersion with PEG6000 and PLX407, respectively. On the contrary, 32.01% of bicalutamide was released from BCL-PEG6000 tablets stored in accelerated conditions, which was a 2.5-fold decrease, in comparison with the freshly prepared tablets.

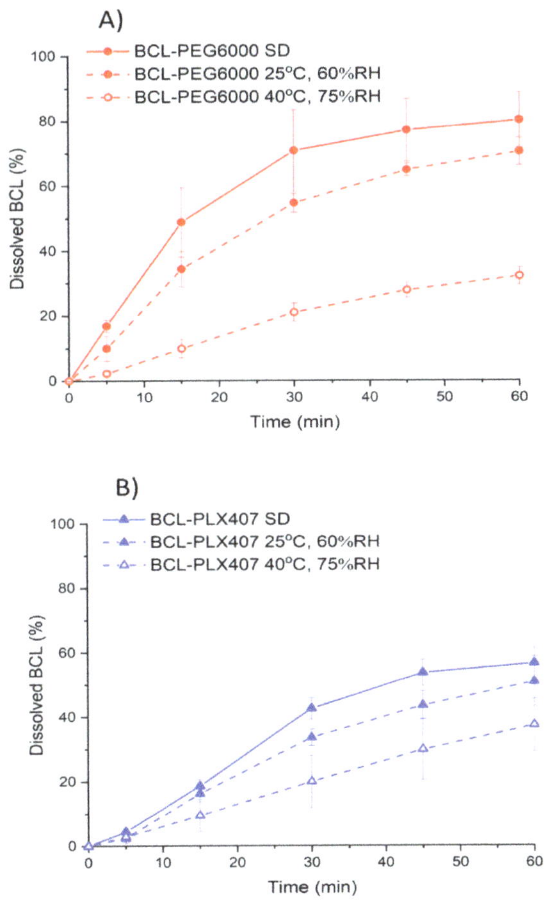

Figure 8. Release profiles of bicalutamide from tablets containing solid dispersion with either PEG6000 (**A**) or PLX4087 (**B**) after stability studies, in comparison with tablets analyzed after preparation.

Moreover, after the six-month stability studies, no phase transition of the drug substance occurred (Figure 9). The diffraction patterns did not change in comparison with those measured for tablets directly after compression (Figure 6). The bicalutamide remained amorphous, as confirmed by the halo visible in the diffractograms (Figure 9). This indicated that water absorbed from the air in the climate chambers did not cause drug recrystallization.

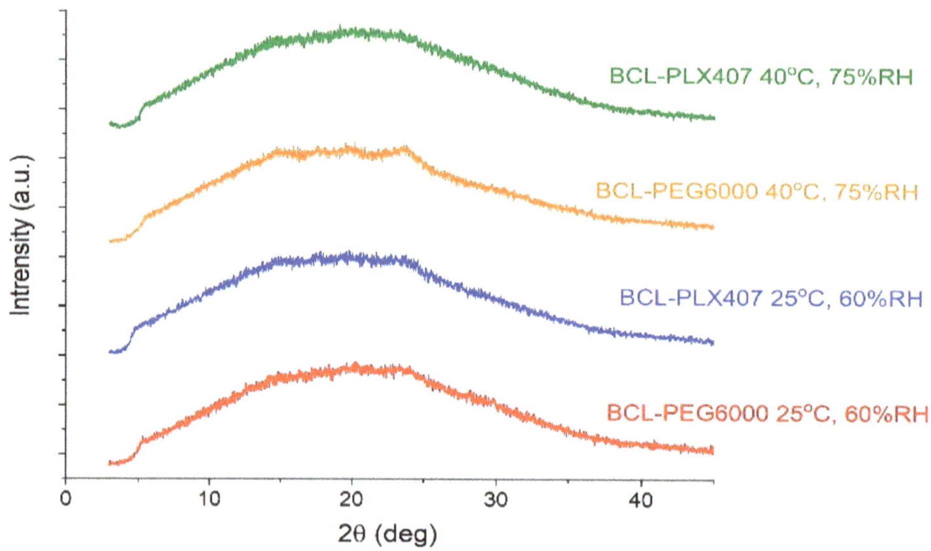

Figure 9. Diffraction patterns of bicalutamide in tablets with solid dispersions after stability studies.

4. Conclusions

This study has examined the effect of supercritical carbon dioxide treatment on the properties of binary systems containing bicalutamide and Macrogol 6000 or Poloxamer® 407. The dissolution and attributes of tablets were evaluated. The $scCO_2$ influenced not only the size and shape of the particles of the processed substances, but also the dissolution characteristics of bicalutamide from solid dispersions. Supercritical conditions induced a decrease in the crystallinity of the active substance. The obtained solid dispersions were successfully formulated in tablets. The tableting process induced the amorphization of the drug substance. This phenomenon confirmed the sensitivity of bicalutamide on mechanical activation. After 1h, the amount of bicalutamide dissolved from tablets with PEG6000 remained unchanged. In the case of tablets containing Poloxamer®407, the amount of released substance decreased by 20%. However, the compression affected the dissolution profiles of the drug substance in comparison with solid dispersion. The stability studies indicated that storage conditions affected the tablets' properties. The amount of the released drug decreased regardless of the storage conditions. However, in the stability studies after six months, the diffraction patterns did not change, which indicated that the physical state of the active substance was unchanged.

Author Contributions: A.A.-R.—writing original draft, investigation; J.S.-S.—writing, review and editing, investigation; K.C.—investigation; J.K.-K.—investigation; M.K.—investigation; K.G.—investigation; V.P.D.—investigation; M.P.—conceptualization, project administration; R.J.—conceptualization, review, supervision. All authors have read and agreed to the published version of the manuscript.

References

1. Thiry, J.; Kok, M.; Collard, L.; Frere, A.; Krier, F.; Fillet, M.; Evrard, B. Bioavailability enhancement of itraconazole-based solid dispersions produced by hot melt extrusion in the framework of the Three Rs rule. *Eur. J. Pharm. Sci.* **2017**, *99*, 1–8. [CrossRef]
2. Fujii, M.; Okada, H.; Shibata, Y.; Teramachi, H.; Kondoh, M.; Watanabe, Y. Preparation, characterization, and tableting of a solid dispersion of indomethacin with crospovidone. *Int. J. Pharm.* **2005**, *293*, 145–153. [CrossRef]
3. Abet, V.; Filance, F.; Recio, J.; Alvarez-Builla, J.; Burgos, C. Prodrug approach: An overview of recent cases. *Eur. J. Med. Chem.* **2017**, *127*, 810–827. [CrossRef]
4. Huttunen, K.M.; Raunio, H.; Rautio, J. Prodrugs—From Serendipity to Rational Design. *Pharm. Rev.* **2011**, *63*, 750–771. [CrossRef]
5. Serajuddin Abu, T.M. Salt formation to improve drug solubility. *Adv. Drug Del. Rev.* **2007**, *59*, 603–616. [CrossRef] [PubMed]

6. Benes, M.; Pekarek, T.; Beranek, J.; Havlicek, J.; Krejcik, L.; Simek, M.; Tkadlecova, M.; Dolezal, P. Methods for the preparation of amorphous solid dispersions—A comparative study. *J. Drug Del. Sci. Tech.* **2017**, *38*, 125–134. [CrossRef]
7. Newman, A.; Knipp, G.; Zografi, G. Assessing the Performance of Amorphous Solid Dispersions. *J. Pharm. Sci.* **2012**, *101*, 1355–1377. [CrossRef]
8. He, Y.; Ho, C. Amorphous Solid Dispersions: Utilization and Challenges in Drug Discovery and Development. *J. Pharm. Sci.* **2015**, *104*, 3237–3258. [CrossRef] [PubMed]
9. Huang, Y.; Dai, W.-G. Fundamental aspects of solid dispersions technology for poorly soluble drugs. *Acta Pharm. Sinica B* **2014**, *4*, 18–28. [CrossRef]
10. Jermain, S.V.; Brough, C.; Williams, R.O. Amorphous solid dispersions and nanocrystal technologies for poorly water-soluble drug delivery. *Int. J. Pharm.* **2018**, *535*, 379–392. [CrossRef]
11. Vo, C.; Park, C.; Lee, B.-J. Current trends and future perspectives of solid dispersions containing poorly water soluble drugs. *Eur. J. Pharm. Biopharm.* **2013**, *85*, 799–813. [CrossRef] [PubMed]
12. Craig, D. The mechanisms of drug release from solid dispersions in water-soluble polymers. *Int. J. Pharm.* **2002**, *231*, 131–144. [CrossRef]
13. Eloy, J.O.; Marchetti, J.M. Solid dispersions containing ursolic acid in Poloxamer 407 and PEG 6000: A comparative study of Fusion and solvent methods. *Powder Tech.* **2014**, *253*, 98–116. [CrossRef]
14. Altamimi, M.A.; Neau, S.H. Investigation of the in vitro performance difference of drug-Soluplus® and drug-PEG 6000 dispersions when using spray drying or lyophilization. *Saudi Pharm. J.* **2017**, *25*, 419–439. [CrossRef] [PubMed]
15. Weuts, I.; Van Dycke, F.; Voorspoels, J.; De Cort, S.; Stokbroekx, S.; Leemans, R.; Brewster, M.E.; Xu, D.; Segmuller, B.; Turner, Y.T.; et al. Physicochemical Properties of the Amorphous Drug, Cast Films, and Spray Dried Powders to Predict Formulation Probability of Success for Solid Dispersions Etravirine. *J. Pharm. Sci.* **2011**, *100*, 260–274. [CrossRef] [PubMed]
16. Milovanovic, S.; Djuris, J.; Dapcevic, A.; Madarevic, D.; Ibric, S.; Zizovic, I. Soluplus®, Eudragit®, HPMC-AS foams and solid dispersions for enhancement of Carvedilol dissolution rate prepared by supercriticial CO_2 process. *Polym. Test.* **2019**, *76*, 54–64. [CrossRef]
17. Nuchuchua, O.; Nejadnik, M.R.; Goulooze, S.C.; Ljescovic, N.J.; Every, H.A.; Jiskoot, W. Characterization of drug delivery particles produced by supercritical carbon dioxide technologies. *J. Supercrit Fluids* **2017**, *128*, 244–262. [CrossRef]
18. Abuzar, S.M.; Hyun, S.-M.; Kim, J.-H.; Park, H.J.; Kim, M.-S.; Park, J.-S.; Hwang, S.-J. Enhancing the solubility and bioavailability of poorly water-soluble drugs using supercritical antisolvent (SAS) process. *Int. J. Pharm.* **2018**, *532*, 1–13. [CrossRef]
19. Badens, E.; Masmoudi, Y.; Mouahid, A.; Crampon, C. Current situation and perspectives in drug formulation by using supercritical fluid technology. *J. Supercrit Fluids* **2018**, *134*, 274–283. [CrossRef]
20. Vasconcelos, T.; Sarmento, B.; Costa, P. Solid dispersion as strategy to improve oral bioavailability of poor water soluble drugs. *Drug Disc. Today* **2007**, *12*, 1068–1074. [CrossRef]
21. Wei, Q.; Keck, C.; Muller, R. Preparation and tableting of long-term stable amorphous rutin using porous silica. *Eur. J. Pharm. Biopharm.* **2017**, *113*, 97–107. [CrossRef] [PubMed]
22. Krasnyuk, I.I.; Koval'skii, I.V.; Nikulina, O.I.; Belyatskaya, A.V.; Krasnyuk, I.I.; Kharitonov, Y.Y.; Grikh, V.V.; Obidchenko, Y.A.; Vorob'ev, A.N. Preparation and investigation of tabletted medicinal formulations of a solid dispersion of rutin. *Pharm. Chem. J.* **2015**, *49*, 481–485. [CrossRef]
23. Abebe, A.; Akseli, I.; Sprockel, O.; Kottala, N.; Cuitino, A.M. Review of bilayer tablet technology. *Int. J. Pharm.* **2014**, *461*, 549–558. [CrossRef] [PubMed]
24. Wlodarski, K.; Tajber, L.; Sawicki, W. Physicochemical properties of direct compression tablets with spray dried and ball milled solid dispersions of tadalafil in PVP-VA. *Eur. J. Pharm. Biopharm.* **2016**, *109*, 14–23. [CrossRef] [PubMed]
25. Patel, S.; Kou, X.; Hou, H.; Huang, Y.; Strong, S.C.; Zhang, G.G.Z.; Sun, C.C. Mechanical Properties and Tableting Behavior of Amorphous Solid Dispersions. *J. Pharm. Sci.* **2017**, *106*, 217–223. [CrossRef]
26. Antosik, A.; Witkowski, S.; Woyna-Orlewicz, K.; Talik, P.; Szafraniec, J.; Wawrzuta, B.; Jachowicz, R. Application of supercritical carbon dioxide to enhance dissolution rate of bicalutamide. *Acta Pol. Pharm.* **2017**, *74*, 1231–1238.

27. Németh, Z.; Sztatisz, J.; Demeter, Á. Polymorph transitions of bicalutamide: A remarkable example of mechanical activation. *J. Pharm. Sci.* **2008**, *97*, 3222–3232. [CrossRef]
28. Vega, D.R.; Polla, G.; Martinez, A.; Mendioroz, E.; Reinoso, M. Conformational polymorphism in bicalutamide. *Int. J. Pharm.* **2007**, *328*, 112–118. [CrossRef]
29. Szafraniec, J.; Antosik, A.; Knapik-Kowalczuk, J.; Kurek, M.; Syrek, K.; Chmiel, K.; Paluch, M.; Jachowicz, R. Planetary ball milling and supercritical fluid technology as a way to enhance dissolution of bicalutamide. *Int. J. Pharm.* **2017**, *533*, 470–479. [CrossRef]
30. Szafraniec, J.; Antosik, A.; Knapik-Kowalczuk, J.; Gawlak, K.; Kurek, M.; Szlęk, J.; Jamróz, W.; Paluch, M.; Jachowicz, R. Molecular Disorder of Bicalutamide-Amorphous Solid Dispersions Obtained by Solvent Methods. *Pharmaceutics* **2018**, *10*, 194. [CrossRef]
31. Szafraniec-Szczęsny, J.; Antosik-Rogóż, A.; Knapik-Kowalczuk, J.; Kurek, M.; Szefer, E.; Gawlak, K.; Chmiel, K.; Peralta, S.; Niwiński, K.; Pielichowski, K.; et al. Compression-Induced Phase Transition of Bicalutamide. *Pharmaceutics* **2020**, *12*, 438. [CrossRef] [PubMed]
32. Bley, H.; Fussnegger, B.; Bodmeier, R. Characterization and stability of solid dispersions based on PEG/polimer blends. *Int. J. Pharm.* **2010**, *390*, 165–173. [CrossRef] [PubMed]
33. Betageri, G.V.; Makarla, K.R. Enhancement of dissolution of glyburide by solid dispersion and lyophilization techcniques. *Int. J. Pharm.* **1995**, *126*, 155–160. [CrossRef]
34. Chutimaworapan, S.; Ritthidej, G.C.; Yonemochi, E.; Oguchi, T.; Yamamoto, K. Effect of Water-Soluble Carriers on Dissolution Characteristics of Nifedipine Solid Dispersions. *Drug Dev. Ind. Pharm.* **2000**, *26*, 1141–1150. [CrossRef]
35. Sancheti, P.P.; Vyas, V.M.; Shah, M.; Karekar, P. Development and characterization of bicalutamide poloxamer F68 solid dispersion system. *Pharmazie* **2008**, *8*, 571–575.
36. Szafraniec, J.; Antosik, A.; Knapik-Kowalczuk, J.; Chmiel, K.; Kurek, M.; Gawlak, K.; Odrobińska, J.; Paluch, M.; Jachowicz, R. The Self-Assembly Phenomenon of Poloxamers and Its Effect on the Dissolution of a Poorly Soluble Drug from Solid Dispersions Obtained by Solvent Methods. *Parmaceutics* **2019**, *11*, 130. [CrossRef]
37. Szczurek, J.; Rams-Baron, M.; Knapik-Kowalczuk, J.; Antosik, A.; Szafraniec, J.; Jamróz, W.; Dulski, M.; Jachowicz, R.; Paluch, M. Molecular Dynamics, Recrystallization Behavior, and Water Solubility of the Amorphous Anticancer Agent Bicalutamide and Its Polyvinylpyrrolidone Mixtures. *Mol. Pharm.* **2017**, *14*, 1071–1081. [CrossRef]
38. Kaul, G.; Huang, J.; Chatlapalli, R.; Ghosh, K.; Nagi, A. Quality-by-Design Case Study: Investigation of the Role of Poloxamer in Immediate-Release Tablets by Experimental Design and Multivariate Data Analysis. *AAPS Pharm. Sci. Tech.* **2011**, *12*, 1064–1076. [CrossRef]
39. D'souza, A.A.; Shegokar, R. Polyethylene glycol (PEG): A versatile polymer for pharmaceutical applications. *Expert Opin. Drug Del.* **2016**, *13*, 1257–1275. [CrossRef]
40. Szafraniec, J.; Antosik, A.; Knapik-Kowalczuk, J.; Chmiel, K.; Kurek, M.; Gawlak, K.; Paluch, M.; Jachowicz, R. Enhanced Dissolution of Solid Dispersions Containing Bicalutamide Subjected to Mechanical Stress. *Int. J. Pharm.* **2018**, *542*, 18–26. [CrossRef] [PubMed]

Permissions

All chapters in this book were first published by MDPI; hereby published with permission under the Creative Commons Attribution License or equivalent. Every chapter published in this book has been scrutinized by our experts. Their significance has been extensively debated. The topics covered herein carry significant findings which will fuel the growth of the discipline. They may even be implemented as practical applications or may be referred to as a beginning point for another development.

The contributors of this book come from diverse backgrounds, making this book a truly international effort. This book will bring forth new frontiers with its revolutionizing research information and detailed analysis of the nascent developments around the world.

We would like to thank all the contributing authors for lending their expertise to make the book truly unique. They have played a crucial role in the development of this book. Without their invaluable contributions this book wouldn't have been possible. They have made vital efforts to compile up to date information on the varied aspects of this subject to make this book a valuable addition to the collection of many professionals and students.

This book was conceptualized with the vision of imparting up-to-date information and advanced data in this field. To ensure the same, a matchless editorial board was set up. Every individual on the board went through rigorous rounds of assessment to prove their worth. After which they invested a large part of their time researching and compiling the most relevant data for our readers.

The editorial board has been involved in producing this book since its inception. They have spent rigorous hours researching and exploring the diverse topics which have resulted in the successful publishing of this book. They have passed on their knowledge of decades through this book. To expedite this challenging task, the publisher supported the team at every step. A small team of assistant editors was also appointed to further simplify the editing procedure and attain best results for the readers.

Apart from the editorial board, the designing team has also invested a significant amount of their time in understanding the subject and creating the most relevant covers. They scrutinized every image to scout for the most suitable representation of the subject and create an appropriate cover for the book.

The publishing team has been an ardent support to the editorial, designing and production team. Their endless efforts to recruit the best for this project, has resulted in the accomplishment of this book. They are a veteran in the field of academics and their pool of knowledge is as vast as their experience in printing. Their expertise and guidance has proved useful at every step. Their uncompromising quality standards have made this book an exceptional effort. Their encouragement from time to time has been an inspiration for everyone.

The publisher and the editorial board hope that this book will prove to be a valuable piece of knowledge for researchers, students, practitioners and scholars across the globe.

List of Contributors

Michelina Catauro, Elisabetta Tranquillo and Federico Barrino
Department of Engineering, University of Campania "Luigi Vanvitelli", via Roma 29, I-81031 Aversa, Italy

Ignazio Blanco
Department of Civil Engineering and Architecture and UdR-Catania Consorzio INSTM, University of Catania, Viale Andrea Doria 6, 95125 Catania, Italy

Francesco Dal Poggetto
Ecoricerche srl, via Principi Normanni 36, 81043 Capua Caserta, Italy

Daniele Naviglio
Department of Chemical Sciences, University of Naples Federico II, via Cintia, 80126 Naples, Italy

Jethro Medina
Department of Physics and Astronomy, Rowan University, Glassboro, NJ 08028, USA

Dave Jao and Ye Xue
Department of Physics and Astronomy, Rowan University, Glassboro, NJ 08028, USA
Department of Biomedical Engineering, Rowan University, Glassboro, NJ 08028, USA

Xiao Hu
Department of Physics and Astronomy, Rowan University, Glassboro, NJ 08028, USA
Department of Biomedical Engineering, Rowan University, Glassboro, NJ 08028, USA
Department of Biomedical and Translational Sciences, Rowan University, Glassboro, NJ 08028, USA

Katarzyna Wasilewska and Katarzyna Winnicka
Department of Pharmaceutical Technology, Medical University of Bialystok, Mickiewicza 2c, 15-222 Bialystok, Poland

Maria Laura Coluccio, Valentina Onesto, Stefania De Vitis, Luca Tirinato, Gerardo Perozziello, Patrizio Candeloro and Natalia Malara
Department of Experimental and Clinical Medicine, University Magna Graecia, 88100 Catanzaro, Italy

Giovanni Marinaro
Institute of Process Engineering, Technische Universität Dresden, 01069 Dresden, Germany
Institute of Fluid Dynamics, Helmholtz-Zentrum Dresden-Rossendorf (HZDR), 01328 Dresden, Germany

Mauro Dell'Apa and Francesco Gentile
Department of Electrical Engineering and Information Technology, University Federico II, 80125 Naples, Italy

Alessandra Imbrogno
Emerging Materials & Devices, Tyndall National Institute, Cork T12 R5CP, Ireland

Enzo Di Fabrizio
Department of Applied Science and Technology, Polytechnic University of Turin, 10129 Torino, Italy

Zhanna K. Nazarkina, Boris P. Chelobanov and Irina V. Romanova
Institute of Chemical Biology and Fundamental Medicine, Siberian Branch, Russian Academy of Sciences, Novosibirsk 630090, Russia

Vera S. Chernonosova and Pavel P. Laktionov
Institute of Chemical Biology and Fundamental Medicine, Siberian Branch, Russian Academy of Sciences, Novosibirsk 630090, Russia
Meshalkin National Medical Research Center, Ministry of Health of the Russian Federation, Novosibirsk 630055, Russia

Andrey A. Karpenko
Meshalkin National Medical Research Center, Ministry of Health of the Russian Federation, Novosibirsk 630055, Russia

Rafael R. Castillo, Daniel Lozano and María Vallet-Regí
Departamento de Química en Ciencias Farmacéuticas, Facultad de Farmacia, Universidad Complutense de Madrid, Plaza Ramón y Cajal s/n, 28040 Madrid, Spain
Centro de Investigación Biomédica en Red—CIBER, 28029 Madrid, Spain
Instituto de Investigación Sanitaria Hospital 12 de Octubre—imas12, 28041 Madrid, Spain

Xiangyu Zheng, Hongli Li, Yi He, Mingwei Yuan, Renyu Yang, Nianfeng Jiang, Minglong Yuan and Cui Yang
National and Local Joint Engineering Research Center for Green Preparation Technology of Biobased Materials, Yunnan Minzu University, Kunming 650500, China

Meili Shen
National and Local Joint Engineering Laboratory for Synthesis Technology of High Performance Polymer, Jilin University, Changchun 130012, China

Lisa Haddick, Karin Möller, Hanna Engelke and Thomas Bein
Department of Chemistry and Center for Nano Science, University of Munich (LMU), Butenandtstrasse 5-13, 81377 Munich, Germany

Wei Zhang, Sören Reinhard and Ernst Wagner
Pharmaceutical Biotechnology and Center for Nano Science, University of Munich (LMU), Butenandtstrasse 5-13, 81377 Munich, Germany

Adam Chyzy, Monika Tomczykowa and Marta E. Plonska-Brzezinska
Department of Organic Chemistry, Faculty of Pharmacy with the Division of Laboratory Medicine, Medical University of Bialystok, Mickiewicza 2A, 15-222 Bialystok, Poland

Monica Boffito, Rossella Laurano and Gianluca Ciardelli
Department of Mechanical and Aerospace Engineering, Politecnico di Torino, Corso Duca degli Abruzzi 24, 10129 Torino, Italy

Carlotta Pontremoli, Sonia Fiorilli and Chiara Vitale-Brovarone
Department of Applied Science and Technology, Politecnico di Torino, Corso Duca degli Abruzzi 24, 10129 Torino, Italy

Agata Antosik-Rogóż, Mateusz Kurek and Renata Jachowicz
Department of Pharmaceutical Technology and Biopharmaceutics, Faculty of Pharmacy, Jagiellonian University Medical College, Medyczna 9, 30-688 Krakow, Poland

Joanna Szafraniec-Szczęsny
Department of Pharmaceutical Technology and Biopharmaceutics, Faculty of Pharmacy, Jagiellonian University Medical College, Medyczna 9, 30-688 Krakow, Poland
Department of Physical Chemistry and Electrochemistry, Faculty of Chemistry, Jagiellonian University, Gronostajowa 2, 30-387 Krakow, Poland

Karolina Gawlak
Department of Physical Chemistry and Electrochemistry, Faculty of Chemistry, Jagiellonian University, Gronostajowa 2, 30-387 Krakow, Poland

Krzysztof Chmiel, Justyna Knapik-Kowalczuk and Marian Paluch
Institute of Physics, Faculty of Science and Technology, University of Silesia, SMCEBI, 75 Pułku Piechoty 1a, 41-500 Chorzow, Poland

Vittorio P. Danesi
Department of Drugs Sciences, University of Pavia, viale Taramelli, 12-27100 Pavia, Italy

Index

www.ingramcontent.com/pod-product-compliance
Lightning Source LLC
LaVergne TN
LVHW082147200926
848484LV00008B/2116

* 9 7 9 8 8 8 7 4 0 0 7 0 9 *